cultural aging

cultural aging

Life Course, Lifestyle, and Senior Worlds

Stephen Katz

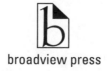

broadview press

Library and Archives Canada Cataloguing in Publication

Katz, Stephen

Cultural aging : life course, lifestyle, and senior worlds / Stephen Katz.
Includes bibliographical references and index.

ISBN 1-55111-577-8

1. Aging. 2. Gerontology. 3. Older people. I. Title.
HQ1061.K38 2005   305.26   C2004-906600-5

Broadview Press Ltd. is an independent, international publishing house, incorporated in 1985. Broadview believes in shared ownership, both with its employees and with the general public; since the year 2000 Broadview shares have traded publicly on the Toronto Venture Exchange under the symbol BDP.

We welcome comments and suggestions regarding any aspect of our publications—please feel free to contact us at the addresses below or at broadview@broadviewpress.com.

North America:

PO Box 1243, Peterborough,
Ontario, Canada K9J 7H5

P.O. Box 1015
3576 California Road, Orchard Park, NY, USA 14127

Tel: (705) 743-8990; Fax: (705) 743-8353
E-mail: customerservice@broadviewpress.com

UK, Ireland, and continental Europe:

NBN Plymbridge
Estover Road
Plymouth PL6 7PY UK

Tel: 44 (0) 1752 202301
Fax: 44 (0) 1752 202331
Fax Order Line: 44 (0) 1752 202333
Customer Service:
cservs@nbnplymbridge.com
Orders:
orders@nbnplymbridge.com

Australia and New Zealand:

UNIREPS,
University of New South Wales
Sydney, NSW, 2052
Australia

Tel: 61 2 9664 0999
Fax: 61 2 9664 5420
E-mail:
info.press@unsw.edu.au

Broadview Press Ltd. gratefully acknowledges the financial support of the Government of Canada through the Book Publishing Industry Development Program for our publishing activities.

www.broadviewpress.com

Edited by Betsy Struthers
Book design and composition by George Kirkpatrick

PRINTED IN CANADA

To Mickey and Shirley, my beloved parents,

makers of the arts of life.

Contents

Acknowledgements   9
Introduction   11

Part One: Aging, Life Course, and the Cultural Politics of Expertise   21

Chapter 1: Imagining the Life Span: From Premodern Miracles to
           Postmodern Fantasies   23
Chapter 2: Charcot's Older Women: Bodies of Knowledge at the
           Interface of Aging Studies and Women's Studies   37
Chapter 3: The Government of Detail: The Case of Social Policy on
           Aging, *Stephen Katz and Bryan Green*   53
Chapter 4: Reflections on the Gerontological Handbook   70
Chapter 5: Critical Gerontological Theory: Intellectual Fieldwork and
           the Nomadic Life of Ideas   85
Chapter 6: Creativity Across the Life Course? Titian, Michelangelo,
           and Older Artist Narratives, *Stephen Katz and
           Erin Campbell*   101

Part Two: Lifestyle and the Fashioning of Senior Worlds   119

Chapter 7: Busy Bodies: Activity, Aging, and the Management of
           Everyday Life   121
Chapter 8: Exemplars of Retirement: Identity and Agency Between
           Lifestyle and Social Movement, *Stephen Katz and
           Debbie Laliberte-Rudman*   140

Chapter 9:   Forever Functional: Sexual Fitness and the Aging Male
             Body, *Barbara L. Marshall and Stephen Katz*   161
Chapter 10: Growing Older Without Aging? Postmodern Time and
             Senior Markets   188
Chapter 11: Spaces of Age, Snowbirds, and the Gerontology of Mobility:
             The *Elderscapes* of Charlotte County, Florida   202

Afterword: Aging Together   233

             References   235
             Index   263

Acknowledgements

There are many people to thank whose support and guidance over the years have made these essays possible. My colleagues at Trent University, especially Jim Conley, Barbara Marshall, Deborah Parnis, Jim Struthers, and Andrew Wernick, provided constant encouragement. Trent's Committee on Research generously awarded funds from the Social Sciences and Humanities Research Council of Canada at key moments, including a Trent University Research Fellowship in 2001-02 for a partial teaching release to work on this book. Anne Brackenbury from Broadview Press breathed life into this book, and its publication owes a great deal to her enthusiasm and creative elaboration of my original proposal. The historical material for several of these essays was collected at the Wellcome Library for the History and Understanding of Medicine in London, and I thank the librarians and staff there who were so helpful and knowledgeable.

To my friends abroad, who read earlier versions of these papers, provided insightful commentary, or offered me the opportunities to discuss my work at conferences and invited presentations, I am immensely grateful. These include Anne Basting, Simon Biggs, Lawrence Cohen, Thomas R. Cole, David J. Ekerdt, (the late) Ellen Gee, Mike Featherstone, Margaret Morganroth Gullette, Jyrki Jyrkämä, Teresa Mangum, Victor W. Marshall, Pirjo Nikander, Chris Phillipson, Ruth Ray, Susan Squier, and Kathleen Woodward. Jaber F. Gubrium and W. Andrew Achenbaum have been career mentors for me and model critical thinkers. Susan Murphy, Peri Ballantyne, Ann Robertson, and other members and staff at the Institute for Human Development, Life Course, and Aging at the University of Toronto always made me feel welcome and treated my contributions as valuable. Many of the ideas in these essays got their first airing in my classes on aging at Trent, and I thank my students for their patience, curiosity, and stimulating responses. Debbie Laliberte-Rudman and Pia Kontos, as Ph.D. students at the University of Toronto, stretched my theoretical research as we worked together on their graduate programs of study.

which I and others became concerned (Katz, 1992). A recent incarnation of this trend is the Global Aging Initiative (GAI) sponsored by the influential Center for Strategic and International Studies (CSIS) in the United States (see www.csis.org/gai). The GAI researchers work with a Commission on Global Aging whose advisory board includes representatives from some of the world's largest multinational corporations and policy research institutes. According to the GAI, global aging not only poses a "mounting fiscal burden" that threatens global economic prosperity, but also weakens the forces of geopolitical security due to the divergent demographics between developed and developing countries.

However, clustered around this new era of aging and its collective or global ageism are "new aging" cultures—that is, new enclaves of lifestyle and retirement which foster new identities and ways *to be* older in body, mind, and spirit. Within these cultures the life course is no longer a singular, industrialized experience based on prescribed developmental social roles terminating in old age, but a more indeterminate process with several beginning, overlapping, and end points and contingent life transitions. Indeed, life course transitions can be distributed across several possible life courses within one's lifetime. Whereas aging has been a process registered in linear biological, chronological, psychological, and social terms, today these are joined by the lateral and spatial movements of cultural aging as culture itself has come to play a dominant and powerful role in late capitalist societies.

The majority of the essays in this book have appeared earlier as published book chapters and journal articles. However, their collection here into one text represents my current thinking, and their combination creates a much stronger commentary on the knowing and experiencing of aging today than any one of the essays alone could accomplish. The essays look at cultural aging in two domains, organized into two parts of the book. Part One, "Aging, Life Course, and the Cultural Politics of Expertise," consists of six essays that probe the historical, textual, political, and cultural practices of gerontological knowledge and associated fields of expertise that have constituted aging as a problem of truth. Although each essay tackles a different set of issues, often in different historical periods, they engage the common practical stories of how we came to know ourselves as aging.

"Imagining the Life Span: From Premodern Miracles to Postmodern Fantasies" explores the images of longevity found in popular medical treatises from the Renaissance to the early nineteenth century, with a focus on how miraculous accounts of centenarians' lives created the basis for a philosophical, scientific approach to aging during the Enlightenment.

"Charcot's Older Women: Bodies of Knowledge at the Interface of Aging Studies and Women's Studies" is a critique of Jean-Martin Charcot's *Clinical Lectures on the Diseases of Old Age* (1881), recognized as a pioneering, nineteenth-century scientific text on old age. Less acknowledged in gerontology, however, are the elderly women of Paris's Salpêtrière Hospital who were Charcot's research subjects. By looking at the feminist research on Charcot, hysteria, and the history of the Salpêtrière, the essay questions how revisiting Charcot and "his" women can strengthen the connection between aging studies and women's studies.

"The Government of Detail: The Case of Social Policy on Aging," co-authored with Bryan S. Green, my colleague at York University, examines the linguistic shaping of social policy reports on aging and the textual designs through which political rationalities become articulated and conveyed to the public. Here we apply Foucault's work on "governmentality" to the American *Developments in Aging* (1987) to critique the use of detail as a compelling technique in social policy discourse and as a moral practice that situates senior citizens as subordinate and dependent.

"Reflections on the Gerontological Handbook" considers, from a genealogical standpoint, how and why the handbook genre has become so authoritative in aging studies and what cultural biases are hidden within its scientific rhetorics and professional formats.

In the next essay on "Critical Gerontological Theory: Intellectual Fieldwork and the Nomadic Life of Ideas," I distill the discursive and intellectual dynamics that lie behind the recent subfield of critical gerontology and propose that the subfield's criticality derives from the gerontological tradition of fracturing, transfiguring, borrowing, and recombining theoretical ideas from outside of aging studies. The discussion also takes up the work of Bourdieu and Deleuze and Guattari to suggest that critical thinking in gerontology is a "nomadic" enterprise, best understood through an exercise in intellectual "fieldwork."

The final essay in Part One, "Creativity Across the Life Course? Titian, Michelangelo, and Older Artist Narratives," was co-authored with Erin Campbell, who teaches and researches Renaissance and Early Modern art history at the University of Victoria. We address several historical questions about late-life style and artistic biography within the field of cultural production. How do older artist narratives construct a gerontological discourse about art and creativity? Is there an older, mature, or late-life artistic style, and, if so, what does it actually demonstrate and how is it recognized? Are late works always great works? Our conclusions suggest art history and aging studies have a great deal to contribute to each other.

In all these writings I am struck by the power of ideas: how they both shape and overflow their sanctioned boundaries; establish and defy theoretical stasis; wander unpredictably between metaphor, myth, and fact; and default on their assigned places in scientific progress to become other things and join other forces. Thus, the critique of such ideas is not simply aimed at their role as the constructing, subjectifying means by which our political ideologies are fed to us. Critique here is also an act related to what Foucault called a critical *curiosity* that,

> ... evokes the care one takes of what exists and what might exist; a readiness to find what surrounds us as strange and odd; a readiness to throw off familiar ways of thought and to look at the same things in a different way; a passion for seizing what is happening now and what is disappearing; a lack of respect for the traditional hierarchies of what is important and fundamental. (1997, p. 325)

Critical curiosity is the attitude that is further exemplified in Part Two of the book, "Lifestyle and the Fashioning of Senior Worlds," whose five essays examine the contradictory issues of imagery, identity, experience, body, and place that accompany the contingencies of cultural aging. Here two issues in particular arise. First, there is the contradictory relation between negative and positive aging. The new aging cultures have replaced aging stereotypes of decline, disease, and dementia with empowering values of independence, activity, well-being, and mobility. From such values have flowed more positive and realistic images around growing older so that the ageism of the doom-and-gloom demographic scenarios is offset by the anti-ageism of new aging cultures. However, this anti-ageism is not without problems of its own of course, which is why a primary recurring theme of the essays is the complementarity that exists between the negative and positive in that nexus of forces where government, population, gerontology, consumerism, retirement, and later life intersect. One way to understand this intersection is to borrow from sociologist Arlie Hochschild's (1994) examination of the commercial spirit of feminism in women's advice literature. According to Max Weber, the historical commercial "spirit of capitalism" drew on the revolutionary well-springs of Protestantism; likewise, says Hochschild, a commercial "spirit" of domestic life in the late twentieth century is drawing on the revolutionary well-springs of feminism. Thus, according to Hochschild's focal analogy, "feminism is to the commercial spirit of intimate life as Protestantism is to the spirit of capitalism" (p. 12). And perhaps what is occurring in our case is similar: the positive, political energies of the grey movement are dispersed and redeployed in the service of a commercial spirit of a seniors' market culture.

Second, there is the issue of the conflation between anti-ageism and *anti-aging*, where we find a fascinating admixture of scientific, cosmetic, and pharmacological "defense against time" advice discourses and "age-defying" practices based on lifestyle and "attitude." The proliferation of techniques around exercise, cosmetic surgery, diets, and beauty products has also created an anxiety-riven culture where, as Kathleen Woodward wryly notes, "at precisely the historical moment that the elderly are appearing on the historical stage in record numbers, many are vanishing into the crowd, no longer visibly marked as old" (1991, p. 161). Although such anti-aging techniques create an illusion of consumer democracy by projecting a world in which everyone can have age-defiant beautiful bodies, it is the elite celebrities of Hollywood to whom homage is paid for their anti-aging heroism—until, that is, such celebrities become "too old" to be seen in films. As the title of the essay "Growing Older Without Aging?" suggests, we can only grow older "successfully" according to the new cultural standards, if we carefully separate out, mask, or eliminate the signs of aging while doing so.

However, the other side of the paradox of arrested aging is the fantasy of interminable youth. But would it not sound either comical or grotesque to be forever pregnant, forever infantile, forever mentally challenged, forever menopausal, forever pubescent, or forever dying? Would we really wish the biological, geological, or cosmological orders of existence neither to age, nor change in time, nor regenerate themselves through cycles of birth and death? Could we imagine buildings and fine furniture not becoming more beautiful and valuable by weathering, or fine wines and cheeses not improving through curing, fermenting, and ripening? Could civilizations mature outside of the temporal dynamics and millennia of development, which made them "great"? So why has "forever" become attached to being "young" when such an idea makes so little sense everywhere else. One response is that the vacuity of popular anti-aging culture is allowed to prepossess every social register related to aging because of the contradictory cultural forces that shape our expectations of living well and aging well in a society that has become uncertain

of its life course identities and ethics. It is not simply the senior marketers, the makers of Viagra, the Sun City developers, or the anti-wrinkle
industry—all of whom receive considerable criticism in the following
essays—that saturate our public consciousness with quixotic images of
aging. It is also their investment in the wider social and economic project
in postmodern timelessness, where speed, impermanence, and immortality take priority over biography, history, and aging. This project, when
conjoined to the neoliberal dream of the end of state-supported dependency, becomes one in which "seniors" become lifestyle specialists as
active, acquiring, risk-managing, consumer citizens.

These two issues are raised in the first essay in Part Two, "Busy Bodies:
Activity, Aging, and the Management of Everyday Life." This essay discusses the role of "activity" as part of a larger disciplinary discourse in
the management of everyday life for older people in the context of a
neoliberal "active society." By examining the theoretical and practical
aspects of activity in the gerontological field and how activity has become
a keyword in radical and popular vocabularies for narratives of the self,
the essay concludes with a summary of interviews with retirees who
understand the contradictory correlation in their lives between "activity"
and "freedom."

"Exemplars of Retirement: Identity and Agency Between Lifestyle and
Social Movement," was co-written with Debbie Laliberte-Rudman, while
she was completing her original and exciting Ph.D. dissertation at the
University of Toronto on new-aging images of retirement. We joined
forces to explore the relation between agency and identity in later life by
examining two cases: first, the individualized images of the "retired worker" and "opportunity-seeking consumer" as exemplars of retiree identities as represented in a Canadian newspaper; and, second, the image of
the Third Age learner in the historical development of the British
Universities of the Third Age (U3A).

"Forever Functional: Sexual Fitness and the Aging Male Body," was
written with and inspired by Barbara L. Marshall, my colleague at Trent
University. It traces the ideas and practices in gerontology and sexology
that transformed the problem of male sexual *fitness* from a nineteenth-
century patriarchal politics of life, centred on regeneration, population,
and nation, to a twentieth-century idealization of successful aging
premised on heterosexual functionality across the life course. The
research also details the influence of the so-called Viagra revolution on
the technologization of male sexuality and the fostering of a new crisis-
ridden midlife ageism.

"Growing Older Without Aging?: Postmodern Time and Senior Markets" is an essay directly focussed on the commercial "fashioning" aspect of senior worlds. It discusses why critical studies of aging link the diversity and paradoxes of later life to the advent of a "postmodern life course" and how marketing strategies target "ageless" consumers in order to create a cultural blurring of traditional age boundaries. By looking at the rhetoric and images of aging in consumer culture generally, and marketing literature in particular, this essay illustrates the lucrative interaction between positive aging, anti-ageism, and anti-aging.

The final essay in Part Two is called, "Spaces of Age, Snowbirds, and The Gerontology of Mobility: The *Elderscapes* of Charlotte County, Florida." Based on a fieldwork project I conducted in Florida in 1998-99, this research is about the cultural aging of spaces or *elderscapes* in an area unique for the size of its retired and aging population. Places of retirement and aging have become increasingly important to gerontological issues of mobility, residence, community, and autonomy. Hence, the main part of this essay is about Canadian "snowbird" migrational culture in Charlotte County, Florida, and theorizes its relevance to spatial gerontology and the sociology of aging. Conclusions propose a fresh approach to understanding retirement "flow" as well as retirement "time" that might contribute to a *gerontology of mobility* for the twenty-first century.

As is evident from this Introduction and throughout the essays, I affiliate my position with the cultural and gerontological critics who point to the emergence of cultural aging and its problematical "positive," "successful," and "active" mandates as a new form of ageism and an element of current bio-demographic politics and its enforced ethics of self-care and individual responsibility. Hence, the overlapping themes of political control and cultural constructivism are prominent in the essays. However, the essays also seek out the possibilities of resistance as part of the aging process. Cultural aging, despite its configuration in regimes of life course and technologies of expertise, is also an opportunity to go beyond the disciplining bounds of consumer practices and neoliberal, market practices and to defy both negative and positive ageism. The contradictory identities of cultural aging can also subvert its spaces, temporalities, and subjectivities, by cultivating an alternative politics of representation and living in time, rather than against it. For example, the essay on "Exemplars of Retirement" suggests that the promise of the new aging and the resolution of debates about agency and identity lie beyond the bounds of the privileged site of individual subjectivity in more collective forms of negotiated identity. The example of the lifelong learner is thus revisited to illustrate how agency becomes a potent social force not necessarily because of its resistance to "structure" or dominant discourse, but because it is experienced and located through collective engagement. Similarly, the essay on "Spaces of Age" contends that the retiree groups in southern Florida who occupy experimental, intercultural social spaces also use their considerable biographical assets to counter their marginalization by the dominant culture.

Ultimately, aging is a great equalizer precisely because it submits all forms of life and matter to common principles of truth and provides us with the communal opportunities to share our lives through time, narrative, memory, generation, and heritage. These are the realities that bolster genuine anti-ageism and counteract the illusory appeal of being "forever young." In his essay on "The End of Temporality," Frederic Jameson asserts that the end of temporality is a "situation" of postmodernity,

> … characterized as a dramatic and alarming shrinkage of existential time and the reduction to a present that hardly qualifies as such any longer, given the virtual effacement of that past and future that can alone define a present in the first place. We can grasp this development more dramatically by thinking our way back to an age in which it was still possible to conceive of an individual (or existential) life as a biographical destiny. (2003, p. 708)

We certainly cannot return to such a time as the one described by Thomas R. Cole in the late medieval society where "only the bells of the monastery or parish would have broken the natural rhythms of daily life" and "all time belonged to God" (1992b, p. 14). Nor can we simply reinvent past notions of personal destiny or spiritual eternity and enfold them into our battles with consumer timelessness. We can, however, critically refuse the "effacement" of the past and the future in the "shrinkage" of the present, and work to reconnect these with new and wide-ranging timelines as we learn to extend the radical actions of those who went before us to those who will follow. The essays in this book undoubtedly raise more issues and questions than they can possibly address, but their overall purpose is to invite readers, whether they browse selected essays or read them in order, to exercise their own critical curiosity about cultural aging today.

PART ONE: AGING, LIFE COURSE, AND THE CULTURAL POLITICS OF EXPERTISE

one

Imagining the Life Span: From Premodern Miracles to Postmodern Fantasies

As I write this chapter, Dr. Deepak Chopra's *Ageless Body, Timeless Mind: The Quantum Alternative to Growing Old* (1993) is the hottest selling commodity in advice literature (*Globe and Mail*, Toronto, 17 August 1993). Blending bits of historical wisdom on keeping old age at bay with postmodern self-discipline on keeping the body supposedly ageless, this book, like so many published today on living the long life, appeals to our cultural preoccupation with challenging the limits of the human life span. The human life span, whatever duration it assumes, is a peculiar kind of fact because it represents a possibility that is rarely achieved. Unlike life expectancy, which is a statistical figure based on the average person's length of life, the life span is "the extreme limit of human longevity," that is, the longevity of the longest living individuals (Gruman, 1966, p. 7). Hence, it embodies the boundaries of human existence, and, in our culture, the scientific community sets these boundaries at 110 years. However, if one considers the life span to be more than an indisputable biological fact and examines it as a discursive or imagined production, symbolic of a culture's beliefs about living and aging, then one can also glimpse something of the larger social and ideological orders from which such beliefs derive their significance. In other words, the life span provides an intellectual key to how general discourses of existence are organized, whether such discourses are conceived in biological, philosophical, political, theological, or consumerist terms.

In this chapter, I am interested in the human life span as it has been historically imagined in medical hygiene literature and culturally constituted in postmodern culture. Historical literature is a valuable source of insight for understanding not only the discursive dimensions of the past, but also the postmodern life course today, when the idealization of long life has become such a lucrative component of consumer culture. In their exhaustive research studies, notable gerontological historians, such as W. Andrew Achenbaum, Thomas Cole, Carole Haber, and David Troyansky, have transformed the dusty passages of historical treatises into a vibrant and critical dimension of contemporary gerontological scholarship.[1] Their work has focussed on aging and old age in their time as relational, socially constructed phenomena that mediate the cultural production of knowledges, images, and bodies. This chapter contributes to this growing body of research by also considering how images of timelessness in the human life span reflect cultural priorities around bodily life. Since the Renaissance, the possibility of timeless living has been pursued with scientific rigour and popular fascination. In the nineteenth century, medical, demographic, and insurance industry investigations proved the life span to be fixed, thus dismissing as fanciful premodern images of excessive longevity. In postmodern culture, as the conclusion will suggest, the prospect of an endless life has been revived through consumer images of perpetual youth and a blurring of traditional lifecourse boundaries (Featherstone and Hepworth, 1991). Zygmunt Bauman says of the "postmodern strategy of survival," that, compared to "traditional ways of dabbling with timelessness ... instead of trying (in vain) to colonize the future, it dissolves it in the present. It does not allow the finality of time to worry the living—by slicing time (all of it, exhaustively, without residue) into short-lived, evanescent episodes. It rehearses mortality, so to speak, by practising it day by day" (1992a, p. 29).

Facts and Imagination in the Premodern Life Span

Popular literature on the history of the body and old age is often laced with romantic and positivist tendencies that diminish the historical complexity and contingency of the past. Thus, premodern historical writings on the life span are cast as pre-scientific and pre-gerontological, mired in the superstition, magic, and ignorance which the celebrated laboratory breakthroughs of modern science eventually overcame. However, if we consider "facts" in a different way, one less judged from the presentist viewpoints of twentieth-century science, then, as Lorraine Daston comments, there is a strong relationship between "facts," "evidence," *and* "miracles" (1991). She further claims that, during the Enlightenment, preternatural phenomena, such as monstrous births or prodigies, lost their status as religious signs and became increasingly naturalized. Furthermore, she says of these phenomena: "Long marginal to scholastic natural philosophy, and now stripped of their religious significance, they had become the first scientific facts. The very traits that had previously unfitted them for use in natural philosophy, and which had then disqualified them from use in theology, made this new role possible" (1991, p. 109).

In other words, the science of the Enlightenment challenged the traditional division of the natural and preternatural, assuming that the latter should be investigated as extensions of the former. Rather than separating the marvels, anomalies, and oddities from scientific inquiry, scientists from Francis Bacon to Charles Darwin would insist that by studying them more directly one could truly learn about nature. Similarly, premodern writers on aging imagined that the lives of centenarians and cases of excessive longevity, however marvellous, were facts that illustrated the rationality of human existence and the contours of the human life span. This partially explains the "bizarre" coupling in the same texts of scientific observations with fantastical beliefs in the longevity of life, as noted by Troyansky (1989, p. 113).

How then, during and after the Renaissance, did writers on medicine and hygiene interpret individual cases of excessive longevity as acceptable facts? In turn, how did these facts reflect the historical construction of a humanist, rational outlook on human nature? By excessive longevity I am referring to persons who supposedly lived between 100 and 200 years. The works of Luigi Cornaro (supposedly 1464-1566) and Francis Bacon (1561-1626) are cited in the historical literature as exemplary cases of late Renaissance reformulations of the human life span.[2] Cornaro, a sixteenth-century Venetian nobleman, first published his treatise, *How to Live One Hundred Years and Avoid Disease* (one of its many translated titles), in Padua in 1558. He went on to write revised editions as he supposedly progressed past the centenarian mark, and remained healthy until his death in 1566 at the presumed age of 102 years, although other reports claim that he only lived to be 96 years (Minois, 1989, p. 271). It is more likely that Cornaro falsified his date of birth in order to claim to be a centenarian (Lind, 1988, p. 5). However, his actual age is not as relevant as his imagined one, which became a fact and a foundational aspect of the literature in the following centuries. Cornaro became ill between the ages of 35 and 40. Physicians told him that unless he lived "a sober and orderly" life, he would soon die (Cornaro, 1935, p. 33). He simplified and reduced his diet, exercised and slept regularly, and made sure to enjoy his gardens and artistic activities. At the age of 83 he wrote,

> ... the life which I live at this age, is not a dead, dumpish, and sowre life; but cheerful, lively and pleasant .... Yet I am sure, that my end is farre from me: for I know (setting casualities aside) I shall not die but by a pure resolution: because that by the regularitie of my life I have shut out death all other wayes. (1935, p. 50)

Cornaro's text was widely translated, distributed, and quoted throughout Europe (Gruman, 1966, p. 71; Troyansky, 1989, pp. 79, 111) and the United States (Cole, 1992b, p. 147). In England it went through 50 editions (Gruman, 1966, p. 71). His treatise was not unique in that its focus on the means for prolonging life typified a general preoccupation of Renaissance humanist writers. However, his popularity in medical literature was a consequence of his combining a fabulously detailed confessional on self-discipline with a practical demonstration of Galen's principles of moderation and balance of the body's humours.[3] Indeed, Cornaro can be considered one of the earliest proponents of an Enlightenment approach to aging because he focussed on the miraculous lives of centenarians, his own life in this case, as *evidence* for a scientific approach to old age. While Freeman may exaggerate that "Luigi Cornaro, exemplary of his age, wrote a little book and changed his world" (1965, p. 16), Cornaro did inaugurate a literary tradition that inspired writers up until the early twentieth century to create similarly optimistic longevity models of their own.

Francis Bacon's treatise, *The Historie of Life and Death* (1977 [1638]),[4] is one of the most recognized attempts at bringing a scientific emphasis to the human life span and life expectancy. Bacon, while opposing the traditional theory of the humours (Minois, 1989, p. 274), stressed the related Galenic idea that dryness is a primary characteristic of aging.[5]

> Age is a great but slow dryer; for all naturall bodies not rotting or putrefying, are dryed by Age, being the measure of time, and the effect of the in-brcd spirit of bodies, sucking out bodies moysture there by decaying, and of the outward ayre, multiplying above the

inward spirits, and moysture of the body, and so destroying them.
(Bacon 1977 [1638], pp. 27-28)

As for life expectancy Bacon explains that people lived longer in biblical
times and, since the flood of Noah, life spans have contracted to an outside limit of 100 years (1977 [1638], p. 74). Bacon recommends the use of
life-prolonging medicines such as betel nut, poppy-juice, tobacco, and
other stimulants that thicken the blood and strengthen the spirit.
"Venery" or sex is also useful for stirring up the spirits and causing "heat."
Finally, advantageous emotional states are joy, sorrow, grief, and compas-
sion, since fear, anger, and envy shorten life. Perhaps Bacon offers very
little beyond traditional and commonsensical ideas about health and old
age; however, the importance of his work is that it repositioned longevity
as evidence of the systematicity of human nature. Furthermore, Bacon's
prestige as a scientist added legitimacy to the growing literature on prolonging the life span (Gruman, 1966, p. 81; Boyle and Morriss, 1987, p. 99).

In the spirit of Cornaro and Bacon, writers from the seventeenth to the
early nineteenth centuries continued to explore the mysteries of longevity. Their narratives on the human life span combined neo-Galenic practicalities and Enlightenment optimism with a widening focus on evidence.
For example, Dr. John Smith, in his *The Portrait of Old Age* (1752 [1666]) follows tradition and makes reference to the Galenic processes of coldness
and dryness that characterize life in old age, along with fear, which is "the
most notorious trouble of the mind" (p. 135). However, this text attempts
to integrate traditional notions of aging with those of medicine, itself
recently inspired by William Harvey's discovery of the circulation of
blood. In fact Smith provides an allegorical interpretation of the twelfth
chapter of Ecclesiastes in terms of its foretelling the circulation of blood
(Livesley, 1975, p. 15). In so doing, he states that while "the lives of the
Patriarchs before the flood were extended to almost a thousand years,"
after the flood "God abbreviates the course of man's life, and seems precisely to set it at one hundred and twenty years" (Smith, 1752 [1666], p. 5).
And, even at this precise old age, Smith asks "Is there not something in
man ... altogether independent of the body? and perfectly free from the
frailties of age?" (p. 25). In other words, is there not a natural state of grace
beyond corporeality where "man" may flourish in old age?

For Smith as for Bacon, the assertion that the human life span was at
least 100 years was an important element in their theoretical models.
Further evidence was to come by way of a series of miraculous cases, the
most popular of which was the Englishman Thomas Parr. Parr died at the

reputed age of 152 in 1635. Apparently he married twice—first at the age of 80 and again at the age of 120 (Gould and Pyle, 1898, p. 373). His autopsy was performed and given scientific credibility by William Harvey (Haber, 1983, p. 54), who claimed of Parr that his death was the result of an overly rich life in his latter days at Court in London. Parr's case, like Cornaro's, was important enough to warrant mention in medical books for almost three centuries. There were many other popular reports as well. Dr. James Keill of Northampton, England reported in 1706 that John Boyles, a button maker, was believed to have died at the age of 130 years (Haber, 1983, p. 59). James Easton, in *Human Longevity* (1799), collected the names of 1,712 centenarians who lived from A.D. 66 to 1799, offering little in the way of substantiation. These were the kinds of marvellous facts that bolstered the Enlightenment's optimistic claim that the capabilities of the human body revealed the munificence of the natural order and the mysteries of the life force.[6]

The early nineteenth century produced two important texts: *The Code of Health and Longevity* (1807) by Sir John Sinclair and *An Essay on the Disorders of Old Age* (1817) by Sir Anthony Carlisle. The investigations of Sinclair and Carlisle follow the same discursive track laid out in the texts on old age in the previous century; they contain the familiar list of remarkable cases of human longevity, focussing on Thomas Parr, along with detailed proposals for dietary, exercise, and behavioural regimes that would ensure long life. However, a marked difference is their insistence on more medical intervention in the study of aging. Sinclair complains of a lack of postmortem evidence "to ground any positive opinion regarding the effects of old age, and the causes of death of old men" (Sinclair, 1807, p. 62). He admits that some of his information has been researched from hospital and workhouse reports (p. 39). Surgeon and anatomist Carlisle, writing his treatise for the Royal College of Surgeons in London, also advocates a more important role for medicine:

> The age of Sixty may, in general, be fixed upon as the commence-ment of senility. About that period it commonly happens, that some signs of bodily infirmity begin to appear, and the skilful [*sic*] med-ical observer may then be frequently able to detect the first serious aberrations from health. (Carlisle, 1817, p. 13)

The texts of Carlisle and Sinclair signal a growing trend in the nine-teenth century to construct old age as a clinical problem, one for which the centuries' old tales of Parr and others would play a dwindling role as evidence.[7]

Longevity as Modern Scientific Inquiry

By the mid-nineteenth century, the study of old age and the aging process had become increasingly distinct from traditional ideas about the life span. Modern medicine had reconstructed the body in terms of pathological anatomy, displacing degenerative processes to micro-levels of tissues and cells and gradually separating old age as a special part of the life course, one marked by systematic signs of senescence (Cole, 1992b, ch.9; Haber, 1983, 1986; Kirk, 1992). Von Kondratowitz reports in his study of the medicalization of old age that as the nineteenth century progressed there were fewer references in mortality statistics to death "due to old age" and more references to death due to specific illnesses in old age (1991, p. 154). The concept of death from old age as the obstacle to be overcome was essential to Enlightenment longevity arguments. Death as a consequence of specific diseases in and of old age signals very different kinds of epistemological inquiries, therapeutic systems, and concepts of the aged subject.

Thus, while longevity literature was still popular in the nineteenth and early twentieth centuries, there were important differences in approach. For example, Thomas Bailey's *Records of Longevity* (1857) introduces a skepticism about the marvellous "facts" of the past. His work consists of a fabulous list of over 300 pages which rank in alphabetical order cases of persons in England and Wales who lived to be between 100 and 185 years, with obituary-like descriptions of each case. However, departing from the earlier literature, Bailey admits that, "It is true, that many of these alleged facts are deficient in that strict verification which would enable a man to speak positively as to the truth of the statements ...." (1857, p. 4). The Austrian doctor Arnold Lorand's *Old Age Deferred* (1912) represents another departure. While he too quotes the cases of Thomas Parr (p. 60) and Henry Jenkins (p. 61), who apparently lived to be 169, Lorand's concern is with heredity and environment, ideas relatively foreign to the Enlightenment's principle of the life span as a symbolic marker of the laws of nature. Elie Metchnikoff, who coined the term *gerontology*, writes in his *The Prolongation of Life: Optimistic Studies* (1907), that "Centenarians are really not rare" (p. 86). He concludes that, "human beings may reach the age of 150, but such cases are certainly extremely rare, and are not known from the records of the last two centuries" (p. 88). Again, the secret to longevity is heredity, a modern scientific issue. Just as the glands were Lorand's key to long life, for Metchnikoff it was the intestines.

The most salient expression of the modern perspective on longevity is William J. Thoms's book, *Human Longevity: Its Facts and Its Fictions* (1873).[8] Thoms was the deputy librarian for the House of Lords. His investigation questions the sensationalizing of and lack of evidence for excessive cases of longevity:

> The duration of human life has hitherto been treated almost exclusively by Naturalists and Physiologists—men eminently qualified by their professional attainments to do full justice to the subject, so far as relates to the scientific conclusions to be deduced from the facts before them. They have, however, taken as facts what are really, in the majority of cases, mere assertions, and, by arguing from false premises, have arrived at very erroneous and unjustifiable conclusions. (1873, p. vii)

Thoms settles accounts with the past by delineating the common sources of evidence—baptismal certificates, tombstone inscriptions, and personal recollections—and describes the inaccuracies that can taint them. He says, "it is surely no unreasonable law to lay down that certificates of baptism, unsupported by corroborative testimony, cannot be received as evidence of longevity" (p. 37). Sometimes more than one child can have the same name, or the father and son can have the same name. An inquirer needs to check more thoroughly evidence such as dates of public or armed forces registrations, employment records, place and time of marriage, and numbers of children (p. 40).

In the remainder of the book, Thoms takes on a variety of cases of extreme longevity to prove his points about misleading evidence. In the end, he disproves most of the famous cases, including those of Thomas Parr and Henry Jenkins. The evidence, or the new concept of evidence, simply does not support the apocryphal stories of their lives. Of Parr's story Thoms concludes, "In the absence of a single scrap of information in support of any one of the minute particulars recorded of the 'old, old man', it seems impossible to arrive at any other conclusion than the particulars in question have no other foundation than idle gossip" (p. 92). After refuting Jenkins's case, Thoms advises that, "I hope the time is not far distant when the reputed age of Henry Jenkins will no longer interfere with scientific inquiry into the average duration of Human Life" (p. 84).

Thoms's work was not met everywhere with sympathy, especially since Jenkins had been honoured with a monument in Yorkshire and Parr had been interred in Westminster Abbey (Gruman, 1966, p. 74). Nevertheless, his investigations destroyed the idea that an individual could conserve vital powers and extend life beyond the normal range of statistical and medical probabilities. In so doing, Thoms contributed to a medical fixing of the human life span that would be supported in other bureaucratic domains such as life insurance,[9] pension, and retirement structures. Previous assumptions had been that a person could live to about 200 years given the right physical, moral, and environmental conditions. One can hardly question that a life span of 80 or 90 years, implied by Thoms, is obviously more realistic than one of 200 years. However, Thoms's work had a more important impact: it signalled the shift in concept from the human life span as a philosophical-medical fact, with miraculous possibilities, to a clinical-biological certainty. As such, the modern concept of the life span conferred to the aged body a fixed period of time. This fixing corresponded to the growing cultural and governmental differentiation of old age in the late nineteenth and early twentieth centuries.

The modern period produced a dual concept of the life span. On the one hand, excessive longevity was still possible according to popular hygiene literature, which became gradually separate from the medical framework.[10] On the other hand, the life span was a scientific, demographic fact that operated within prescribed statistical limits. This fact was primarily established by the Belgian statistician Adolphe Quételet in *A Treatise On Man and the Development of His Faculties* 1968 ([1842]). Quételet's statistical calculations on the norms, curves, and variations of the "average man" numerically verified that the "biblical count of three-score and ten closely reflected the maximum length of human existence" (Haber, 1983, p. 42).[11]

Conclusions: Postmodern Timelessness

This chapter has supported the view that the medical and hygiene writers on longevity from the late Renaissance to the early nineteenth century imagined the life span to be substantiated by the knowable and miraculous laws of nature. Non-presentist evaluations of the popularity of excessive longevity cases, such as that of Thomas Parr, show them to reflect the optimistic rationalism of the Enlightenment and its neo-Galenic medical regimes. From the mid-nineteenth century onwards changing administrative and medical perspectives on old age radically altered the image of the life span by reclassifying the aged body in terms of temporal finitude. The vitality of living was no longer dependent upon personal discipline, moderation, and diet, but upon laws of development within the body's cells and tissues. Where the Enlightenment's medicine, science, and philosophies constructed old age as a special but integral part of life, modernity's forms of calculation, division, and hierarchy separated it as a distinct, developmental stage. The scope of this chapter prevents me from elaborating this final point, but other authors have rigorously and insightfully done so.[12] Instead we return to the question of the postmodern present, where the life span has been infused with rich cultural imagery based on the commodification, rather than the scientificity, of timelessness.

Western culture is still curious about reports of longevity. Texts, such as David Davies's *The Centenarians of the Andes* (1975) and G.Z. Pitskhelauri's *The Prolongevity of Soviet Georgia* (1982), and numerous documentaries on apparently exceptionally long-living peoples from remote habitats, reanimate the traditional interest in exceeding commonplace life span limits. In addition, with increasing demographic evidence that life expectancy is drawing closer to life span potential, Westerners ideally anticipate long, active, healthy lives. However, the features of postmodern aging also derive from cultural industries that distribute pleasure and leisure across an unrestricted range of objects, identities, styles, and expectations. In so doing, such industries recast the life span in fantastical ways, in particular, in the masking of age and the fantasy of timelessness.

With different emphases Bauman (1992b), Cole (1992b, pp. 227-51), Conrad (1992), Featherstone and Hepworth (1991), Moody (1988a, 1993), and Woodward (1991) note that the postmodern life course is characterized by a number of overlapping, often disparate conditions associated with the blurring of traditional chronological boundaries and the integration of formerly segregated periods of life. Fixed definitions of childhood, middle age, and old age are eroding under pressure from two cultural directions that have accompanied the profound shifts in the political economy of labour, retirement, and social inequality. First, since the 1960s gerontological writers, in their critique of negative ageist stereotypes and practices, have produced more accurate and positive images that bespeak the vitality, creativity, empowerment, and resourcefulness attainable in old age. In some instances the positivity of the discourse has repressed important issues in old age.[13] Secondly, elderhood has been reconstructed as a marketable lifestyle that connects the commodified values of youth with body-care techniques for masking the appearance of age.[14] This development is aligned to the stratifying tactics of late capitalism whereby lifestyle hierarchies intersect with the complex of differences based on class, ethnicity, nationality, and gender (see Featherstone and Hepworth, 1986). For older persons it means that the significance of age, positive and negative, dissolves in the fast-paced economy of images dominated by exercise, diet, cosmetic management. and leisure activities. The chances of experiencing the aging of the body in a meaningfully temporal, open, and unalienated way are slim. Thus, the postmodern life course engenders a simulated life span, one that promises to enhance living by stretching middle age into a timelessness hitherto associated only with the likes of Luigi Cornaro and Thomas Parr.

Harry Moody flags the film *Cocoon* as a "postmodern fable" (1993, p. xxxiii). In it, as in postmodern culture itself, "freedom is actually a massive form of denial and an escape from history" (p. xxxviii). However, I also envision that the postmodern fantasy of living outside of time will provide the impetus for older individuals to resist Western society's dominant obligations. Ethnographic research has already documented this process in local situations. For example, Haim Hazan, in his case study of a London Day Centre for older persons (1986), records that a beauty class was poorly attended (p. 320), as were fitness classes, "because members preferred to be engaged in activities where competition and testing out of achievements were not required" (p. 317). From the cultural history of the past, as well as the present, we might also hope to learn that even the most universal of images, such as the life span, opens a discursive window onto that which passes for the timeless truths about living, aging, and dying.

Notes

This essay began its life span as a conference paper presented at the lively *Images of Aging* conference held at Trent University, 21-24 May 1992, where I first became introduced to many of the issues on cultural aging pursued in this book. Conference presenters were invited to revise and expand their papers for a book edited by organizers Mike Featherstone and

Andrew Wernick, entitled *Images of Aging: Cultural Representations of Later Life* (London: Routledge, 1995, pp. 61-75). I was very pleased that my essay was included and I thank the publishers for permission to reprint it here.

1. As the references and citations in this essay demonstrate, I am indebted to the many excellent secondary sources available on the history of old age. Some of the leading publications in this area are the following. Medieval history: Burrow (1986), Goodich (1989), Sears (1986), and Sheehan (1990). History of death and dying: Ariès (1981) and Elias (1985). American history: Achenbaum (1978, 1983), Chudacoff (1989), Fischer (1978), Graebner (1980), Gratton (1986), Haber (1983), Quadagno (1982), and Van Tassel and Stearns (1986). European history: Kohli (1986b), Laslett (1989), Minois (1989), Pelling and Smith (1991), Stearns (1982), and Troyansky (1989). Literary and cultural history: Achenbaum (1995), Freeman (1979), Cole (1992b), and Covey (1991). History of women and aging: Premo (1990) and Jalland and Hooper (1986).

2. Livesley contends that the detailed attention paid to the aging process by Cornaro and Bacon was due, in part, to their hypochondria (1975, p. 12). Freeman also mentions that Bacon "was a bit of a hypochondriac who stuffed himself with varieties of evil tasting drugs" (1965, p. 17).

3. Cornaro's manual frames the body in the traditional Galenic mold, as dependent "on the harmonie of humours and elements" (Cornaro, 1935, p. 41). However, Cole (1992b, p. 96) and Gruman (1966, p. 68) point out that Cornaro also challenged the reign of Galenic hygiene because of his individual optimism and desire for long life. I tend to disagree with Turner's rather rigid assessment that Cornaro conceived of his dietary regime "within an exclusively religious framework as a defence against the temptations of the flesh" (1991, pp. 161-62). While Cornaro's text is narrated with theological reference points, his concern is less with spiritual afterlife than with the earthly pleasures of good health.

4. Bacon's work, originally in Latin, was *Historia Vitae et Mortis*, the third part of a longer text called *Instauratio Magna*, published in 1623. The full title of the English translation of 1638 is *The Historie of Life and Death, With Observations Naturall and Experimentall for the Prolonging of Life* (Lind, 1988, p. 4).

5. Unfortunately, Bacon died in 1626 at the age of 65, after getting ill on a freezing winter day while stuffing a chicken with snow in order to prove that cold can preserve flesh. Faithful to his convictions, he chose to recover in a damp, rather than dry bed, which led to his death from bronchitis. So much for the scientific method.

6. Examples of eighteenth-century medical texts which express these sentiments are George Cheyne, *An Essay on Health and Long Life* (1725); John Floyer, *Medicina*

Gerocomica: Or the Galenic Art of Preserving Old Men's Habits (1724); Benjamin Rush, *Medical Inquiries and Observations* (1797); and Christopher Hufeland, *The Art of Prolonging Life* (1797).

7. A characteristic of the life span in all historical periods is that it is a male construction. Then, as now, it seems that women's lives were marginal to the medical understanding of the human life course, except in discussions of reproduction. As Carlisle admits, "I pass over the diseases of women, because it would be improper to introduce them in a work, which is addressed to general readers" (1817, p. 89).

8. I am thankful to Carole Haber (1983: 42-43) and Gerald Gruman (1966: 74) for signalling the historical importance of Thoms's work.

9. Lorraine Daston mentions that while life insurance has a long history, it had little to do with people's age or mortality tables until the nineteenth century (1988, p. 168). See also Haber (1983, pp. 42-46) for discussion of the social scientific limiting of the life span and the degradation of old age. For theoretical discussions that link insurance technologies to the governing of risk see the relevant chapters in *The Foucault Effect: Studies in Governmentality* (Burchell *et al.*, 1991).

10. Cole (1992b) describes how health reform, religion, medicine, and quackery in the United States intersected in ways that kept alive the discourse of prolongevity.

11. Quételet's influence in aging studies is acknowledged in gerontology. See Birren and Clayton (1975), Boyle and Morriss (1987, p. 190), Haber (1983, pp. 41-42), and Kirk (1992, p. 489). One of the more interesting treatments of Quételet is Bookstein and Achenbaum (1993). They argue that Quételet's "social physics," once introduced into gerontology, produced unfortunate consequences because, "both the controversy over Quételet and the existence of alternative models of statistical reasoning seem to have been ignored or overlooked by the founders of modern gerontology" (p. 25). While Quételet's work had already been criticized in the field of biometrics, gerontologists in the pursuit of methodological rigour and professional credibility embraced his erroneous calculation techniques.

12. In addition to the historians cited above, see Held (1986), Kohli (1986a), Mayer and Schoepflin (1989), and Modell (1989).

13. See Cole (1986), Harper and Thane (1989), and Moody (1988a). Moody rightly complains that "Late life is hailed as a time to keep busy, to remain involved with others, engaged in activities. But vigorous activity and sustained meaning are not the same thing. In fact, frenzy of activity can simply mask an emptiness of shared meaning" (1988a, p. 238). Cole more philosophically says:

> The currently fashionable positive mythology of old age shows no more tolerance or respect for the intractable vicissitudes of aging than the old

negative mythology. While health and self-control were seen previously as virtues reserved for the young and middle-aged, they are now demanded of the old as well. Unable to infuse decay, dependency, and death with moral and spiritual significance, our culture dreams of abolishing biological aging. (1986, p. 129)

14. A representative text is Jeff Ostroff's *Successful Marketing to the 50+ Consumer* (1989). Of course there is no end to media examples that target the 50-, 60-, and 70-somethings. A striking term in this discourse is "down-aging," which means, "making it fashionable to be 50, look 40 and act 30" ("The New Middle Age," *The Globe and Mail Report on Business*, Toronto, May 1993: 47). For a critical account of "Gold in Gray," see Minkler (1991).

two

Charcot's Older Women: Bodies of Knowledge at the Interface of Aging Studies and Women's Studies

On the one hand, it seems that gerontology has been a haven for women scholars and practitioners and for the interests of older women. Even a cursory glance at the development of the field in North America reveals the important contributions made by women in the United States such as Ruth Cavan, Carroll Estes, Meredith Minkler, Bernice Neugarten, Matilda White Riley, and Ethel Shanas.[1] In Canada, women such as Neena Chappell, Anne Martin-Matthews, Susan McDaniel, Sheila Neysmith, and Blossom Wigdor, among many others, have inspired much of Canadian gerontology's major theoretical interventions and academic achievements. As well gender issues have surfaced significantly within gerontology, especially in studies of care giving, retirement, intergenerational relations, and health services. Much recent work on women and aging, including collections of essays and special issues of journals, attest to the strength of this development.[2] And on a popular level, the fact that celebrated feminists such as Betty Friedan, Germaine Greer, and Gloria Steinem have turned their attention to aging and written personal accounts of the subject also reveals that the link between age and gender is a crucial one. In fact, as Julie McMullin reminds us, aging studies in general has made it quite obvious that one simply does not study old people, but older women and older men (1995, p. 37).

On the other hand, both women's studies and aging studies have accused each of ignoring the other. In 1993 Beth Hess, in her afterword to the special issue of the *Journal of Aging Studies* on socialist feminism, observed that it was easier to bring women into gerontological professional associations, such as the Gerontological Society, than it was, and is, to "bring new perspectives into the research agenda and dominant paradigms of academic gerontology, even though the majority of elderly in modern societies are female, and even though as a relatively new and low-status field, gerontology was more welcoming to women than other fields" (1993, p. 195). Further, it has been pointed out that gerontological considerations of gender, however widespread, often suffer from the "gender-as-variable" or the "add-and-stir" dilemma, that is, that gender is not developed as a politically sophisticated and theoretically innovative impetus for rethinking the diversity of older women's lives, but rather is "added" in an empirical fashion to an already constituted gerontological vision of social relations. As an example we might consider the distinction advanced by Sheila Neysmith between "caring for" and "caring about." According to Neysmith, "caring for" is based on enumerating the "specification of tasks associated with the activities of daily living," while "caring about" involves the often invisible "emotional and mental labour" behind such tasks, the understanding of which would require historical critiques of gender as a social construction and caring practices as social problems (1995, p. 115).

In their introduction to the collection *Connecting Gender and Ageing: A Sociological Approach* (1995) editors Sara Arber and Jay Ginn offer another reason why gender is reduced to a variable. The quantitative and policy-driven imperatives of mainstream gerontology, they conclude, are at methodological variance with the qualitative and theory-driven mandates of feminist scholarship. In the end, according to Julie McMullin, gender-as-variable approaches result either in "gender ageing theory," where gender is added to sociological approaches to aging, or "feminist ageing theory," where age relations are added to feminist theory—and neither approach is adequate to the task of integrating gender and age (1995, p. 31).

While women's studies have reproached gender-blind and theory-poor work in gerontology, they have also come under parallel criticism from gerontologists and researchers in associated aging studies. Beginning perhaps with Myrna Lewis and Robert Butler's 1972 charged essay "Why Is Women's Lib Ignoring Old Women" and Donna Beeson's

1975 "Women in Studies of Aging," a series of articles and books has followed that has targeted feminisms and feminists for not taking the extra
step and bridging anti-sexism with anti-ageism, women abuse with elder
abuse, and women's liberation with elder liberation in both heterosexual
and lesbian dimensions.[3] Some of the reasons for such neglect have been
attributed to the young age of most feminist scholars and, as Shulamit
Reinharz rightly observes, because "feminists, just as everybody else, have
been socialized in our aging-phobic and geronto-phobic culture" (1986, p.
507). More profoundly, as Kathleen Woodward suggests, the insistence
that "anatomy is not destiny" has led feminists to disregard how, in old
age, anatomy is—unavoidably—destiny, and that "we cannot detach the
body in decline from the meanings we attach to old age" (1991, p. 19).

Given their entangled connections, where then might women's studies
and aging studies join together to enliven scholarly exploration and theoretical critique to transform the various inequities foisted upon human
difference in our society? One important area is empowerment, Meredith
Minkler suggests (1996). Another is making explicit the link between sexism and ageism so that, in the words of Reinharz, "the major contribution
that the issue of aging can make to feminism is the mandate to re-examine all feminist theory in light of this dimension. And the major contribution that feminism can make for those concerned with aging is to provide
a model and some of the personnel of a successful social movement"
(1986, p. 512). Jon Hendricks (1993) and Sheila Neysmith (1995) both urge
that aging studies re-examine its foundational premises by taking into
consideration feminist revampings of biased scientific objectivity and the
emotional conditions of qualitative research. Attention to the rhetoric of
age studies is also critical. Innovations in language and critical scrutiny of
metaphors can shake up and feminize gerontological conventions. Sarah
F. Pearlman's coining of "Late Mid-Life Astonishment" as a new developmental transition for women between the ages of 50 and 60 is just such a
case in point (1993).

To contribute to this project of connecting women's studies and aging
studies, I want here to turn to the rise of gerontological knowledge itself,
especially to the epistemological centrality of bodies, both gendered and
aged, to the formation of gerontological knowledge.[4] How have bodies of
knowledge and knowledge of bodies co-constituted each other? While
my book *Disciplining Old Age* runs off after this question in the direction of
Foucault's work, gender is not its main focus. This chapter, then, is about
missing bodies—specifically, the missing bodies of older women in the
history of gerontological literature inspired by the great nineteenth-cen-

tury French clinician, Jean-Martin Charcot, doyen of Paris's Salpêtrière Hospital for women. My specific focus is Charcot's *Clinical Lectures on the Diseases of Old Age*, originally published in France in 1867, with a second edition in 1874. In 1881 two English translations appeared: the first by William Tuke for the New Sydenham Society in London and the second an American edition promoted by physician Alfred Loomis who added his own essays and lectures (the American edition is the source material for this essay). In *Disciplining Old Age* I, like other cultural gerontologists, position Charcot's text as the point of departure for a critique of the founders of gerontology and geriatrics such as Elie Metchnikoff who coined the term *gerontology*, Ignatz Nascher who invented geriatrics, and G. Stanley Hall who brought old age into the purview of psychology. I find myself now struck less by the book's reputation as a founding scientific text that sparked the medicalization of old age than by the basis of its subject material: the women stuck in Paris's immense Salpêtrière Hospital. While most histories on gerontology, aging, and old age accent the canonical power of Charcot's text, few of them comment on the bodies and identities of these women who formed gerontology's first institutionalized population of aged subjects. As far as I know, the feminist literature has also avoided them. Thus, Charcot's text not only stands at the contested interface between the practices of scientific culture, technologies of difference, and the corporeal worlds of older women, but also discloses the absence of the critical traffic that should be passing between aging studies and women's studies. As well it signals the barrier between the sociology of the body and the history of medicine. So, here I explore the ways in which Charcot's work, the disciplinary imperatives of the human sciences, and the sexual politics of the Salpêtrière Hospital—all so crucial to feminist and cultural histories of hysteria—came together in the late nineteenth century to inaugurate a distinct knowledge about old age and a problematization of its subjects.

Charcot and The Salpêtrière

The name Salpêtrière comes from "saltpeter," the Paris hospital having originally been part of a sixteenth-century arsenal. By the mid-1600s it had become a public hospital for destitute women and prostitutes; later it also became a women's prison. According to Christopher Goetz, in the seventeenth and eighteenth centuries the Salpêtrière was the largest asylum in Europe, holding between 5,000 and 8,000 persons at a time when the entire population of Paris was only 500,000. "Part asylum, part prison, part old people's home," in the words of Mark Micale, "this remarkable hybrid institution housed for over two centuries every imaginable form of social and medical "misfit" from the lowliest sectors of Parisian life" (1985, p. 707). Its reputation as a terrible and terrifying place of confinement on the edge of the city, what Yannick Ripa refers to as the "capital of female suffering" in mid nineteenth-century Paris (1990, p. 9), did not prevent it from becoming a popular and frequently visited site where its unfortunate inmates were subjected to the humiliation of public display and exhibition.

The first medical facility appeared at the Salpêtrière in the early 1780s, over 130 years after its founding. Philippe Pinel (1795-1826), the celebrated liberal reformer of the early nineteenth century, transformed the hospital through such changes as improved nutrition, the removal of chains, and the demolition of the old basement cells. In turn, these opened the Salpêtrière to a new generation of medical researchers for by 1850 it "offered an untapped and incomparable variety of patient material" (Goetz, 1987, p. xxiii). It was into this space of untapped and incomparable patient material, the majority of it female and much of it elderly, that Jean-Martin Charcot stepped, first as an intern between 1848-52 and later, after passing his exams in 1862, as an attending physician, professor, and chief medical officer. Charcot stayed at the Salpêtrière until his death in 1893, remaking the hospital into a world-renowned site of medical authority and a cultural centre for the innovation of photographic techniques, the perfection of the art of public lectures, and the demonstration of fascinating new therapies based on hypnosis and electric shock.

With its 5,000 patients, the late nineteenth-century Salpêtrière provided Charcot with the opportunity to enlarge through his own authority the stature of the medical profession in Parisian culture. Inside the hospital he reclassified patients, amassed data, oversaw new scientific facilities, and added a publications press to handle the outpouring of published material. By 1886 the Salpêtrière had over 100 buildings on 51 hectares of land. Often compared to Napoleon, Charcot was indeed the emperor of a countersite or *heterotopia* in the sense that Foucault gave to the term: the Salpêtrière was "a kind of effectively enacted utopia in which the real sites, all the other real sites that can be found within the culture, are simultaneously represented, contested, and inverted" (Foucault, 1986, p. 24). According to Jan Goldstein (1987), outside the hospital Charcot entertained Paris's medical, literary, and political elites at the Tuesday soirées at his sumptuous residence which was outfitted with, among other things,

Asian antiques and Gobelins tapestries. In the year after his death in 1893, a street in Paris bore his name as did a number of diseases, disorders, and medical techniques which he discovered.

The force that articulated the inside and the outside of this world of the Salpêtrière was the Charcot lectures. First held in regular wards and later in a new amphitheatre, these were well-publicized, precisely prepared and memorized, and delivered with dramatic panache. An American physician visiting the Salpêtrière reported, for example, that Charcot's lectures "left on the mind of the student a series of mental pictures of patients and of lessons which no amount of private study could possibly produce" (quoted in Goetz, 1987, p. xxx). Charcot's orchestration of medical theatrics involved props, diagrams, photographs, pharmaceutical gadgetry, and, most importantly, the patients, or better, the patients' bodies: the silenced, material resources manipulated by Charcot to ground his theories and astonish his audiences. Because it was the Salpêtrière, these bodies were female, a crucial fact that I will elaborate in a moment. The point to be emphasized here, however, is that Charcot, his lectures, and the bodies of his female patients intersected at angles that made disciplined medical knowledge the showpiece of Parisian modernity and scientific progress. At the center of this intersection was Charcot's recreation of hysteria as a predominant pathology. The important, rich, feminist and critical histories of hysteria have argued persuasively that much of the success of the Charcotian enterprise depended on its construction of hysteria as a proliferative, positivist, and performative science.[5] Building on this work, I raise a further question: why have scholars paid such little attention to the senilizing of women's bodies in light of their sophisticated analysis of hysteria?

According to Jan Goldstein (1987), hysteria was a way of proliferating and widening a zone of nervous diseases intermediate between sanity and insanity, the normal and the pathological, and the physical and the psychological. Under Charcot's reign the physicians and psychiatrists at the Salpêtrière, especially those eager to be acknowledged by him, happened to discover more women suffering from hysteria and classified more kinds of observations and problems as hysterical than did their counterparts at other institutions. Photographs documenting case histories of hysterical women were collected in three volumes of the *Iconographie photographie de la Salpêtrière* (1876-77, 1878, 1879-80; see Didi-Huberman, 1982). In fact the establishment of photography studios at the hospital was inspired by the disciplinary will to represent, circulate, and codify this new horizon of female suffering. Between 1882 and 1893 Charcot, according to Daphne de

Marneffe (1991), devoted over one-third of his lectures to the subject of hysteria, some of which Freud heard when he studied at the Salpêtrière between October 1885 and February 1886 and whose influence would remain with him back in Vienna. Thus, hysteria was a proliferative discursive machine whose parts—texts, bodies, photographs, lectures, case studies, careers, and rhetorics—produced a knowledge of femininity that eclipsed all the alternatives. This leads to a second point, which is that the science of hysteria was an intensely positivist one.

Charcot's medical beliefs in the evidential powers of observation, the scrupulous keeping of records, the pathologizing mapping of patients' bodies, and, above all, the disavowal of religious or premodern perspectives—all point to his faith in positivism. As he says in the introduction to his lectures on old age: "The new physiology absolutely refuses to look upon life as a mysterious and supernatural influence which acts as its caprice dictates, freeing itself from its law.... It purposes to bring all the vital manifestations of a complex organism to workings of certain apparatuses, and the action of the latter to the properties of certain tissues of certain well-defined elements. It does not seek to find out the essence or the why of things" (Charcot, 1881, p. 12). In terms of hysteria, Charcot's positivism was a challenge to previously held religious or mystical ideas about demonic possession, witchcraft, and miracle cures. Positivism was also at the core of his methodology, based as it was on a mechanics of seeing and describing patients rather than of listening or responding to them. In his obituary to Charcot, Freud aptly describes him as "a *visuel*, a man who sees" (quoted in Marneffe, 1991, p. 93).

Critics have also pointed out that Charcot's positivist attempts to territorialize hysteria with such exactitude disclose the arbitrary, biased, and constructed nature of his theories and conclusions. Sander Gilman, for example, has explored the connection between Charcot's work on hysteria and contemporary racist and anti-Semitic discourses on heredity and degeneration (1988).[6] Daphne de Marneffe has argued convincingly that,

> Charcot's and his colleagues' firm belief in their own objectivity itself constituted a threat to that very objectivity: first, by making them unable to question their own role in constructing the picture of the disease; and second, through their inability to see their own participation in recreating the pathogenic conditions of their patients' lives—neglect, lack of empathy, and exploitation. (1991, p. 106)

Marneffe's focus on the lives of the patients brings us to the third and final point about Charcot's hysteria, which is that beneath its intellectual capital as a lofty human science, however discredited it was later to become, lay the realities of the outcast women of the Salpêtrière and their enactments of hysteria.

In 1870, the Salpêtrière restructured its wards so that women diagnosed with epilepsy and hysteria were put together. Charcot was in charge of both. Several commentators maintain that many of the women who exhibited uncontrollable movements and fits during Charcot's lectures on hysteria, were in fact acting, even simulating and imitating the seizures of their epileptic ward-mates. Further, the medical authorities actually encouraged such stigmatizing chicanery with the result that a group of favourite hysterics became celebrated through the theatrics of Charcot's lectures. As Elaine Showalter has put it, the *grande hysterié* convulsive seizure was the showstopping "specialty of the house at the Salpêtrière" (1985, p. 150). Charcot was himself aware of this problem, but claimed that such dramatic manifestations were part of the disease.[7] Women diagnosed as hysterical may or may not have performed hysteria, but hysteria was a type of performance nevertheless: spectacular bodies did fantastical things, often under hypnotic conditions, in front of amused audiences under the watchful directorship of Charcot or one of his associates.

Thus, Charcot's hysteria, with its technical and institutional apparatuses and casts of patients, was a proliferative, positivist, and performative science. It invented an ontological depth to femininity with a stunning display of surfaces. An expansive literature from women's studies, cultural history, and psychiatry attests to hysteria's importance as a symbol of the raw sexualization of everyday life in Western society.[8] With these insights in mind, I turn to explore Charcot's work on old age.

Charcot's *Clinical Lectures on the Diseases of Old Age*

Charcot's *Clinical Lectures on the Diseases of Old Age* consists of 21 lectures; in the 1881 American edition Alfred Loomis adds ten more of his own. In his introduction Charcot outlines clearly his intentions as a medical researcher and the institutional connection between the Salpêtrière and its elderly female population. Besides the "lunatics, idiots, and epileptics," he writes, the "remainder of the population of this asylum consists of about twenty-five hundred females, who, with some few exceptions, belong to the least-favored portion of society." He divides these women into two categories, the first of which is explicitly comprised of older women:

> The first is composed of women who are, in general, over seventy years of age—for the administrative statutes have so decided it—but who, in all respects, enjoy an habitual good health, although misery or desertion has put them under the protection of public aid. Here, gentlemen, is where we shall find the materials which will serve us in making a clinical history of the affections of the senile period of life.
>
> The second category comprises women of every age—smitten, for the most part, with chronic, and, by repute, incurable diseases, which have reduced them to a condition of permanent infirmity. (1881, p. 17)

It is this first class of women—elderly, destitute, confined, but generally healthy—who, for Charcot, provided the cases and bodies for the advancement of geriatric research. The constitution of these women as clinical subjects also offered the opportunity for longitudinal study since, as Charcot notes, "we are here permitted to follow the patients through a long period of their existence, instead of being present only at a single episode of their history" (p. 18).

Although Charcot elaborates his project to identify the pathologies of old age, given the limits of nineteenth-century positivist medical science we are left wondering how this project was realized in relation to the daily lives of the Salpêtrière's 2,500 women. In certain cases Charcot does show how an individual case study contributes to the advancement of gerontological knowledge. An example is his discussion of a woman who is 103 years old and "in excellent health." Taking her temperature demonstrates that the body's temperature in old age is not lower than in the young, as previously believed; more importantly, Charcot insists that "rigorous observation shows us that, in certain respects, the organs of the aged perform their tasks with quite as much energy as those of adults" (p. 24).

In other lectures Charcot's diagnoses raise pertinent questions about the relationships between class, poverty, and health in these women. For instance, in his lecture on rheumatism, Charcot observes that the disease is "one of the most common infirmities of females, at least those of the poorer classes," afflicting eight out of one hundred women at the Salpêtrière" (p. 38). Later he adds that about three-fourths of the women attacked with nodular rheumatism "ascribe it to the prolonged influence of damp cold" (p. 151). He raises important medical issues of family and generational relations in a related case, commenting: "there is now in the Salpêtrière a woman that has nodular rheumatism, whose *daughter and grand-daughter* are already suffering pains in the smaller joints. Here are three generations successively attacked with the same disease" (p. 149; original emphasis). This interesting statement suggests the fascinating possibility that perhaps there were generations of women associated with the Salpêtrière. In another passage on rheumatism Charcot concludes that "uterine functions" such as menopause and pregnancy influence the disease (p. 153). How he actually learned this is a perplexity.

In spite of the occasional specific case, the lived world of Charcot's elderly women appears very distant in his lectures, precisely in part because of his scientific and sexist biases, which also plague his work on hysteria. Notwithstanding the preponderance of women in the Salpêtrière, statistical standards and norms, for example, are often posed in male terms. In the introduction Charcot lists the attributes of the "external appearance of an old man" (such as dry and loose skin, grey hair, a toothless mouth, and stooped posture) as signs of "a general atrophy of the individual" (pp. 20-21). More egregiously, in discussing fevers and febrility in old age, Charcot compares the aged to children and adults, but here the pathological aged figure is female and the normal adult figure is male; here we also see that the category of the adult and the category of the aged are understood to be mutually exclusive (pp. 32-33). Masculine pronouns pepper the text. For instance, although he has been citing evidence from cases of female patients, Charcot concludes that "the patient suffers spontaneous pains, quite vague in character, which pass off as he walks" (p. 145). Here we find a clear instance of how medical studies have generally identified the male body as the human body, even when the bodies on which such knowledge was built were female. In this instance too we see how, at the same time, the pathology of bodily aging is associated with the female body. As feminist critics have argued, nineteenth- and early twentieth-century representations of women's bodies and experiences often portrayed them as incoherent, biologically fouled misadventures. So we see, in a microcosm, the confusing overlap of the pathologies associated with aging with the politics of gender and youth. The old man is, as it were, feminized, and old age for both men and women is divorced from adulthood, thus implicitly infantilizing the older person.

The bodies of women, then, were at the site of the birth of geriatrics. But it is difficult to recover both their behaviour and the texture of their lives not only because of Charcot's scientific and sexist biases but also because, outside of his introductory remarks, he was not obliged by his nineteenth-century audience to talk about them.[9] This obligation belongs to us, however, and presents us with an exciting opportunity to see how the problematization of women and of old age emerged in tandem. Looking critically at what has been and can be made of this opportunity forms the last part of this chapter.

Charcot's Older Women, Aging Studies, and Women's Studies

Gerontologists and historians of old age rightfully acknowledge Charcot's *Clinical Lectures on the Diseases of Old Age* as a landmark text. Widely circulated, highly regarded, and often quoted, this work became a model text exemplifying how clinical research on the senile pathology of old age should be done. According to Joseph Freeman, it provided the "measuring stick" for geriatrics (1979, p. 46; see also Freeman, 1967). Indeed for many years Charcot's *Lectures* "remained," in the words of Trevor Howell, "the only serious textbook of Geriatrics" (1988, p. 62). Interestingly enough, W. Andrew Achenbaum has pointed out that one of the reasons why it was "the most influential work of the period" (1995, p. 37) is that the timing of the translations gave it "an importance as a model for future research in the United States far beyond its actual merits" because it corresponded to the advances being made in American medicine at the time (1978, p. 43).[10]

When it comes to discussing the women behind the science, work in aging studies has been far less discerning, however. The fact that Charcot's research was carried out in a poorhouse for women is usually raised but then left unelaborated. Cultural historian Thomas Cole points out that "Charcot's *Clinical Lectures* rarely gave much thought to the class or gender of the population on which they were based" and that "Charcot viewed these women as exemplars of physiological old age" (1992b, p. 201) but does not explore the question further. Jean-Pierre Bois includes only a short discussion of the Salpêtrière in his history of old age in France. Even Simone de Beauvoir, who asserts that "the Salpêtrière may be looked upon as the nucleus of the first geriatric establishment" (1972, p. 26), fails to go the extra step and speak about its women.

A more prominent exception to the trend is the work of Peter Stearns who, in his research on aging in France, insists that the old women of the Salpêtrière, rather than the old men of the Bicêtre, attracted more geriatric research because of the pervasive negative cultural attitudes toward older women. As he concludes in "Old Women: Some Historical Observations," "The available empirical evidence was combined with the judgement on menopause to cast post-menopausal women generally into limbo, with aesthetic contempt added to the whole unsavory brew" (1980, p. 45). Furthermore, as he writes in *Old Age in European Society*, the women, "being poor, often female and, above all, always old," were "open to any manipulative feelings a researcher might have in any event" (1977, p. 85). For Stearns, the distorted vision of female sexuality in part created the discursive background to the development of geriatric medicine. Stearns also astutely concludes as early as 1980 that one of the reasons why "older women have received relatively little attention from historians" is that "attention has been riveted on problems preoccupying other age groups, particularly those groups coinciding with the ages of a student audience and of the new generation of women's historians" (1980, p. 44).

Marjorie Feinson, in her essay "Where Are the Women in the History of Aging?" published five years later, cites Stearns's statement to buoy her contention that, despite the "proliferation of feminist scholarship, the historical experiences of aging women have not been examined systematically by either historians of aging, family historians, or feminist historians" (1985, p. 436). She proposes to remedy the situation by recovering from the past "shards of evidence," an apt archaeological metaphor that signals the scattered, unarticulated state of women's studies of aging at the time.[11] For Feinson these shards included evidence from witch-hunting and demographic history.

Feinson's dilemma is similar to the one I have been proposing with regard to Charcot's older women. On the one hand, we are witnessing a creative explosion of aging studies, women's studies, the sociology of the body and of medicine, and the cultural critique of modernity and its somber institutions; on the other hand, such important research seems to be missing some of the key material sites where women, aging, and the production of knowledge were co-disciplined. Thus, Charcot and the older women of the Salpêtrière represent an important puzzle whose shards or pieces await rejoining. One piece is the wider recognition of Charcot as a founding geriatrician and his lectures as disciplinary practices. As Brian Livesley has observed, "Charcot has not been identified previously as a Geriatrician and this aspect of his medical practice and expertise has been overlooked because of the great importance attached to his reputation as a Neurologist" (1975, p. 26). Another piece treats critical hysteria studies and the acuity of their research on women's bodies and professional discourses as a model for the historical study of aging and women. Was geriatrics, like hysteria, a proliferative, positivist, and performative science? Were theatrics and silenced patients as integral to Charcot's lectures on old age as they were to the lectures on hysteria? What relationship held between the sexual politics of old age and hysteria at the Salpêtrière? A third piece of the puzzle might be the representation of women in the gerontological texts that followed *Clinical Lectures on the Diseases of Old Age* whose authors commend Charcot and take up his positivist zeal to discover the secrets of the aged body.

Finally, there is a crucial piece of the puzzle lodged in the dilemma of silence on Charcot's older women, a dilemma that invites future research. Here I am thinking of interdisciplinary research on women and bodies such as, for example, the recent excellent collection *Deviant Bodies: Critical Perspectives on Difference in Science and Popular Culture*, edited by Jennifer Terry and Jacqueline Urla (1995). *Deviant Bodies* does not include discussions of aging bodies (or more specifically of Charcot or the Salpêtrière), but nonetheless it does provoke thought about them. The "generic human body" in the West embodies the binarisms of Western culture in its "more oppressive forms," the editors state, a binarism that I would argue includes that of young and old (Urla and Terry, 1995, p. 4). Hopefully we can look forward to this kind of critical work, which will shed light on Charcot's older women and draw the connections between aging studies and women's studies a step closer together.

Conclusions: Charcot Today

In their short professional histories, gerontology and geriatrics have attempted to shore up their disciplinary status by canonizing a set of nineteenth-century and early twentieth-century scientific texts. The male authors of these texts, most of them medical researchers, attempted to define the bodily, psychological, and demographic characteristics of aging and old age. In so doing, they tended to misrepresent women or neglect them altogether. Charcot's *Clinical Lectures on the Diseases of Old Age* is an important case in point. In spite of his ultimately narrow and negative portrayals of the aging process, even his critics regard his text as a pioneering articulation of clinical research and professional ingenuity.

Importantly, his *Lectures* were based on a relatively unknown but very large group of elderly women confined to the Salpêtrière Hospital who provided the subjects, cases, and bodies for his research.

Charcot is well-known within feminist cultural studies and psychoanalytic theory for his work with the hysterical bodies of women, bodies that we have come to assume were all young and, through Freud, were expressing in their theatricalized display a repressed sexuality, a desire that also has a long tradition of being associated with young, not older women. Given that Charcot based his research on the "senile period of life" of women, it is ironic that gerontological knowledge as it has developed throughout the first three-quarters of the twentieth century in particular has worked to silence, regulate, and negate women's bodies. At the same time, however, Charcot's Salpêtrière was, as I have suggested, a heterotopia. It is crucial to remember that not only was Charcot studying old age but he was studying it by virtue of the bodies of older women, most of whom were over 70 and enjoyed, as he put it, "an habitual good health." Concealed in the *Clinical Lectures*, in other words, is the model of late life as characterized by a preponderance of health, one embodied in women. Thus Charcot's Salpêtrière also animated and articulated the capacities, self-images, and energies of women in subject-constituting ways, ways which, I hope, we will learn more about in future research on the older women of this celebrated site.

Notes

The idea for this essay had been on my mind ever since reading Charcot's work for my book *Disciplining Old Age*. My actually writing it was in response to a phone call from Kathleen Woodward, Director at the time of the Center for Twentieth Century Studies at the University of Wisconsin-Milwaukee, asking me to submit a paper for a conference on *Women and Aging: Bodies, Cultures, Generations*, 17-21 April 1996, sponsored by the Center. It turned out to be a groundbreaking conference, and the feedback I received on the paper was helpful in rewriting it for publication in the *Journal of Women and Aging* 9(4), 1997, pp. 73-87. I am also grateful to the members of the Institute of Gerontology at the University of Michigan, in particular to W. Andrew Achenbaum, for their comments. Kathleen later wrote me from Paris saying that she was putting together a book based on the conference materials and wanted my paper. After enlarging and revising it according to her excellent editorial work,

"Charcot's Older Women" appeared in *Figuring Age: Women, Bodies, Generations*, edited by Kathleen Woodward (Bloomington, IN: Indiana University Press, 1999, pp. 112-27). It is reprinted here with permission of the publisher. The essay has also been translated into French: "Les vieilles dames de Charcot: Les corps de connaissance à l'interface des études sur l'âge et des études féministes," in *Vieillir jeunes, actifs et disponibles? Cahiers du genre* 31, 2001, pp. 105-28.

1. Neugarten, in fact, states: "I do not recall a single instance in which the fact that I was a woman worked to my disadvantage, or to my advantage, in my education or in my research career. I had encouragement all the way" (1988, p. 98).

2. See, for example, Leonard and Nichols (1994), Baines *et al.* (1991), and the following special issues of journals geared to interests of women: *The Gerontologist* 19.3 (1979), *Educational Gerontology* 17.2 (1991), and the *Journal of Aging Studies* 7.2 (1993) and 18.1 (2004). See also the *Journal of Women and Aging*.

3. Examples are Macdonald and Rich (1984), Copper and Rice (1988), Rosenthal (1990), Davis *et al.* (1993), and Pearsall (1997). As Corinne T. Field notes in her illuminating dissertation research (1997), early American feminists such as Elizabeth Cady Stanton (1815-1902), while well-recognized for their struggles for women's rights, are overlooked for their contributions to new ideals around female aging and the life course. Field's question is a valuable one: have the feminist chroniclers of the women's movement sidelined the women's movement's innovations in age studies?

4. See Laws (1995a) and Öberg (1996).

5. See, for example, Beizer (1994), Smith-Rosenberg (1985), and the many essays by Mark Micale on hysteria, both male and female, as well as his book *Approaching Hysteria* (1995).

6. On Charcot's hereditarian ideas, see Dowgibbin (1991) and Pick (1989) for a fuller account of the nineteenth- and early twentieth-century European preoccupation with questions of heredity and degeneration.

7. See McCarren's "'The Symptomatic Act' Circa 1900" (1995) in which she underscores the performative politics of Charcotian medicine by revisiting hysteria from the perspective of modern dance and staging. See also Owen (1971). Sigmund Freud, in a letter to his future wife on 24 November 1885, describing Charcot's lectures as engrossing and exhausting, also emphasizes the importance of performance in them: my "brain is sated as after an evening in the theatre" (quoted in Major, 1974, p. 388).

8. In "Hysteria Male/Hysteria Female" (1991), Mark Micale outlines the development of Charcot's work on male hysteria. Although Charcot's model of hysteria was based on his observation of women, he published case histories of over 60

male hysterics and treated many others. In 1882, at his request, the Salpêtrière opened a new *Service des hommes*, a 20-person infirmary for males suffering from nervous disorders. According to Micale, for Charcot, women "fall ill due to their vulnerable emotional natures and an inability to control their feelings. In contrast, men get sick from working, drinking, fighting, and fornicating too much. However, in members of both sexes, it should be noted, hysteria typically resulted from an excess of prescribed gender behaviours" (1991, p. 208).

9. Loomis's lectures seem to use mostly male examples though they also intermix women and men as if they constituted one—neuter—patient of old age. Loomis's lectures close the book, ending with one on "senile hypertrophy of the prostate gland," an obvious male condition. Loomis, a New York City physician and professor of pathology, delivered his lectures at New York's Bellevue Hospital.

10. Other scholars point to Charcot's influential role in medicalizing old age. See Cole (1992b), Haber (1983), and Kirk (1992).

11. Historical studies on women and old age include Jalland and Hooper (1986), Premo (1990), and Gratton and Haber (1993).

three

The Government of Detail: The Case of Social Policy on Aging

Stephen Katz and Bryan Green

The influence of Michel Foucault's work in the field of social policy studies has grown considerably in the past two decades, and this chapter examines its value to the study of aging and policy discourse. Social policy studies have been inspired mainly by Foucault's genealogical delineations of disciplinary power in *Discipline and Punish* (1979) and *The History of Sexuality Volume 1: An Introduction* (1980a). The former text, in revamping the criminological history of the prison system, recast modernity as a "disciplinary society" shaped by new forms of power following the decline of European sovereign regimes. The latter text depicted the frightening mastery with which nineteenth-century psychiatric expertise established a hierarchy of sexualized bodies and segmented the population into "normal" and "deviant" groups. In both studies the connection between the individual body and the social body, or population, was vital to the formation of modern politics. In particular Foucault radically historicized the notion of population. Extracting it from traditional demographic conceptions, he traced its discursive and political origins to the power/knowledge networks that grew out of the Enlightenment's social projects around health and wealth. Population thus emerged as a matrix of national, public control on several registers between the late seventeenth and the early twentieth centuries: Administrative authorities identified public risks and problematized spaces in urban environments; policing agencies standardized public behaviour and institutionalized problem groups (dependent, poor, "unproductive," delinquent, etc.); and professional power monitored and measured the health, growth, reproduction, and movements of the population. Indeed, Foucault believed that the modern state could not have attained its power without intervening in the life of the population, or what he called the "bio-politics of the population" (1980a, p. 139). The boldness of Foucault's work on disciplinary power and its implications for a simultaneous critique of traditional Marxist and humanist traditions inspired a broad and critical literature that illustrates the dense historical correlations between the rise of mercantile capitalism, European philosophies of individual rights and freedoms, and the disciplinary ruling of the population. Within these contexts the development of social policy documents and apparatuses seems a fitting piece to Foucault's picture of a "carceral" society, where "the power to punish is not essentially different from that of curing or educating" (1979, p. 303).

During the late 1970s Foucault also elaborated his ideas on liberal regimes of power, yet these have received less attention, until recently, in sociological and social policy studies than his work on discipline, power, sexuality, and bio-politics. One reason is that his critique of liberal politics appeared only in a handful of scattered essays and interviews, rather than in texts as popular as *Discipline and Punish* (1979) and *The History of Sexuality* (1980a), although these certainly touch on the paradoxical convergence of disciplinarity with liberal humanism. A second reason could be that, in comparison to longstanding Marxist and non-Marxist critical traditions in social policy studies, Foucault's gloss on liberal society has been criticized for being incomplete and unoriginal. Indeed, his focus on the rationalities of ruling and the autonomy of political reason (discussed below) would not be out of place in the writings of Max Weber or Frankfurt critical theorists such as Max Horkheimer or Theodor Adorno, among others. Thirdly, by neglecting to specify the positivity and productivity of liberal state power, as he did with disciplinary and other forms of power, Foucault never established a consistent position within ongoing policy and political science debates about the state itself.

Nevertheless, Foucault's work on liberal power and its constituent technologies, rationalities, and limits, encapsulated by his term *govern-*

mentality, has come to the fore of political theory as it has been expanded upon by adherents such as Nikolas Rose, Mitchell Dean, Colin Gordon, Pat O'Malley, and others. Some governmentality writers augment Foucault's ideas by adding elements from other discourses. For example, Rose (1999, pp. 49-51) and Miller and Rose (1990) adapt Bruno Latour's idea of "action at a distance" (Latour, 1986, 1987) to designate how political authority is extended over distances and territories via non-state agencies (e.g., philanthropists or urban planners). Others have revisited parts of Foucault's work, such as his comments on "pastoral power" (Foucault, 1983, pp. 213-15) and his definition of "government" as "the conduct of conduct" (pp. 220-21), to further their ideas about the politics of citizenry, selfhood, and welfare. Several recent collections as well as numerous papers in the British journal *Economy and Society* attest to the widening intellectual scope of governmentality (Barry, Osborne, and Rose, 1996; Dean, 1999; Rose, 1999).

This chapter explores the concept of governmentality in relation to social policy discourse and practice, illustrated by American policies on aging. In particular we wish to extend beyond our previous works (Green, 1993; Katz, 1996, 2000b) to examine how textual detail, linguistic style, professional vocabularies, and narrative coherence become representational techniques in the governance of later life, especially since such techniques are often neglected in governmentality studies. Before proceeding with our case study, it would be worthwhile to summarize what Foucault meant by governmentality and the relevant commentary that has materialized around it.

Foucault's paper, "Governmentality" (1991), is based on a lecture given in 1978, translated in 1979, and then largely overshadowed by his other work on sexuality.[1] In brief we can identify five basic themes that made the paper innovative and controversial: (1) the art of government, (2) the continuity of government, (3) the government of life, (4) the government of knowledge, and (5) the autonomy of governmental reason.

1. *The art of government.* Foucault says that in the seventeenth century treatises appear on "the art of government." These reveal a new problematic of government, prior to the establishment of professional discourses on "political science" or "policy studies," that moved beyond the Machiavellian prescriptions on how to achieve and maintain political sovereignty. Foucault remarks: "Having the ability to retain one's principality is not at all the same thing as possessing the art of governing" (1991, p. 90). Treatises by Adam Smith or John Locke made it clear that a new

problematic of government would have to address critical questions on how to rule, who should be ruled, the purposes of government, and the kinds of political rationalities to be used by government to protect and enhance the princehood and principality. The political break constituted by the "art of government" culminated in its liberal critique of sovereign power and the limits of government.

2. *The continuity of government.* Historically, a variety of governing bodies such as churches, regional councils, and aristocratic families ruled over subject populations according to the traditions of local authorities. The "art of government," however, focusses on what kind of technologies would enable the state to coordinate all the other forms of government into a complementary web of ruling apparatuses. For Foucault, government is dispersable; it can orchestrate many kinds of authority by folding them into the "state." Foucault says, therefore, that "government ties the state to society ... in the art of government the task is to establish a continuity, in both an upwards and a downwards direction" (1991, p. 91). Thus, the art of government stipulates that state power should circulate in a continuous fashion in order to bring all forms of traditional authority under its jurisdiction.

3. *The government of life.* Whereas in the Machiavellian problematic, sovereignty was exercised over territory and its subjects, the object of government is "things"—wealth and poverty, resources, climate, health, accidents, mobility, famines, death, migration and settlement, and most importantly, *life.* People also become things, as do their relations and interactions with each other. Hence, government sets in motion strategic, non-violent practices that bring to order the vagaries and contingencies of life through their objectification. Terms such as "political anatomy" and "political arithmetick," coined by British seventeenth-century economist and statistician William Petty (1690), became metaphors of the art of government. And, like the shift from the politics of death to a politics of life schematized by Foucault in *The History of Sexuality* (1980a) the shift from sovereign to governmental states transforms the population into a life-force of its own, determined by laws of health, morality, productivity, and reproductivity, and in need of supervision by the state.

4. *The government of knowledge.* The art of government became operationalized within the political realities of seventeenth- and eighteenth-century mercantilist states through a series of technical knowledges based on "sta-

tistics" (1991, pp. 6-7) and "police." Because the mercantilist economists needed to calculate how to create populational resources, control shipping over vast territories, rule colonial territories and peoples from distant imperial centres, predict the effects of trade, and tally the profits of war, they created statistical knowledges of ruling appropriate to the state. As Foucault says,

> Whereas statistics had previously worked within the administrative frame and thus in terms of the functioning of sovereignty, it now gradually reveals that population has its own regularities, its own rate of deaths and diseases, its cycles of scarcity, etc.; statistics shows also that the domain of population involves a range of intrinsic, aggregate effects, phenomena that are irreducible to those of the family, such as epidemics, endemic levels of mortality, ascending spirals of labour and wealth; lastly it shows that, through its shifts, customs, activities, etc., population has specific economic effects: statistics, by making it possible to quantify these specific phenomena of population, also shows that this specificity is irreducible to the dimension of the family. (1991, p. 99)

At the same time the eighteenth-century governmental science of police elucidated how the state should intervene into people's lives for the "public good." Police science as it developed in Germany has also been a topic of research for medical historians, such as George Rosen, whose characterization of it is apposite: "What national power required, as the rulers and their advisors saw it, was first of all a large population; second, that population should be provided for in a material sense; and thirdly, that it should be under the control of government so that it could be turned to whatever use public policy required" (1974, p. 123). Furthermore, police intervention paternalistically dealt with the provision of clean water, disease prevention, urban sanitation, housing, and hospitals. Hence, the enduring legacy of the policing model was not necessarily its establishment of healthy urban environments, but its problematization of poverty, unproductivity, deviance, and marginality. Foucault placed the police model at the core of Enlightenment populationist rationality: "When people spoke about police at this moment [from the end of the sixteenth to end of the eighteenth centuries], they spoke about the specific techniques by which a government in the framework of the state was able to govern people as individuals significantly useful for the world" (1988, p. 154). For the police model to operate its practitioners had to invent detailed knowledges of the social environment as a diagram of problems.

5. The autonomy of governmental reason. Statistics and police were just two of the early technical knowledges reinforced by the art of government in its bid to surmount the limitations of sovereign rule and widen the separation between types of state and types of government. As Foucault remarks, "It is the tactics of government which make possible the continual definition and redefinition of what is within the competence of the state and what is not, the public versus the private, and so on ...." (1991, p. 103). Needless to say, the divergences between capitalist, democratic, socialist, and authoritarian states are of lesser importance than the technologies and arts of government which they hold in common. Governmental reason has its own autonomy, therefore, and can be translated into an assemblage of political practices by a wide range of state and non-state authorities.

In addition to these five basic themes of Foucault's governmentality—the art, continuity, and autonomy of government, along with the government of life and knowledge—other writers have taken Foucault's perspective on the governmentalization of power to critique neoliberal regimes, insurance and risk-management programs, criminology, the professions, and the utilization of data technology and market rationalities in state enterprises (Chambon, Irving, and Epstein, 1999; Du Gay, 1996; Garland, 1997). The governmentality literature further emphasizes how personal conduct, freedom, choice, and responsibility are refigured as political resources and enfolded into the fabric of "the social" (Petersen and Bunton, 1997; Cruikshank, 1999). Questions have also been raised about the role of anti-welfarist agendas in compromising longstanding liberal ideas about individual freedoms and rights, mutating their meanings within new economic and political strategies. In this sense Mitchell Dean's interpretation is insightful: governmentality "defines a novel thought-space across the domains of ethics and politics, of what might be called 'practices of the self' and 'practices of government,' that weaves them together without a reduction of one to the other" (1994, p. 174).

Governmentality studies, both those of Foucault and others, also have been criticized along a number of fronts. Marxist theorists, such as Boris Frankel (1997), include governmentality writers among a long line of elite, pluralist, liberal, realpolitik thinkers whom he considers to be more apologetic than critical of their specific political cultures. While Frankel discounts the Anglo-Foucaultian school as a post-Marxist manifestation of the decline of the Left (especially in the United Kingdom and Australia), he does raise three important criticisms. First, some of the categories in the governmentality literature, such as "neoliberalism" or "the social," are used far too broadly and often in a universalistic and totalizing manner. Second, it is important to recognize that certain fiscal, national, and corporate forces and interests lie behind governmental technologies. These require scrutiny even where such forces and technologies may be relatively independent of each other. Third, the kind of diagnostic critique of the "present" made by governmentality thinkers does not necessarily lead to any particular form of action or inclination towards alternative forms of government. Countering this criticism, O'Malley, Shearing, and Weir (1997) argue that in Foucault's work, struggle, resistance, reversal, contingency, and contradiction are all elements of government. Yet, these authors also acknowledge that both critique and struggle seem to be increasingly absent from the governmentality literature. Likewise, Barry Hindess (1997) asks if "political rationalities" are always "governmental rationalities," and, if so, how can one particular rationality, such as liberalism, tie people to the state both as population-subjects and as free individuals?[22]

These criticisms point to the difficulties of theorizing the complex interactions between spheres of government, state, population, and economy, especially in a time when forms of rule have widened to include therapeutic, self-management, and lifestyle dimensions. They also mark out the ambiguous role of public social services today as neoliberal rationalities in developed countries strive to reduce the state's commitment to its welfare programs for families, older persons, and vulnerable groups. It is difficult to understand this role, however, without investigating more closely how social policies themselves are governmental and how political reason appears in them as a power of language. Along with the legacy of statistical and police technologies, the art of government identifies its communities and dependencies through social policies and, through the words and practices of their creators, bonds the public to the state. In the rest of this chapter we would like to look at how, in particular, saturation with detail in social policy discourse functions as a governmental technique—one that seeks to survey, occupy, and monitor social territory by linguistic means. To do so we must consider the ways in which political rationalities have been articulated by the rhetorics, scripts, and vocabularies woven into the textual designs of social policies. Our illustrative case is American social policies on aging.

The Government of Detail in Policy Reports

Reports and discussion papers on social policy routinely saturate the page (and the reader) with detail: details of law, administrative provision, statistical incidence of problems, previous actions, present discontents, and so on. This feature is accepted as generic for this type of text and skipped across without much reflection. The eye might be caught by an individual detail, made salient by textual design or readerly interest, but saturation itself is taken to be normal. All that normal reading registers is that the detail is dense and comprehensive, as expected.

By connecting this generic feature of policy discourse to the performance of government, we intend to reflectively replay this normally unremarkable feature so as to show its remarkable significance for the political process. We do this in light of a basic principle of critical discourse analysis that anything that immanently structures political communication should, for the sake of democratic community, be made a topic of discussion. (For an overview of some communicative factors relevant to democratic discourse, see Gastill, 1992.)

Our analytic guideline in this section is that government has to be signified in order to be made socially recognizable and palpably real. Saturation of policy writing with detail serves this significatory purpose, but the way in which it does so needs careful description.

The typical policy report conveys a textual mastery of detail through organizing facts, figures, organizational acronyms, program names, social narratives, legislative acts, group opinions, and so forth, into orderly arrays such as reviews, overviews, summaries, diagnoses, and prognoses. The actual disposition of these particular details at page surface level signifies government of that which they represent, namely society.

There is, however, something further signified by the textual performance of government, a second-order signified that can be called governmentality. The textual ordering of details, a first-order sign of government, becomes, in turn, the signifier of something more: access to a mastery of an infinitely extensive field of policy detail beyond whatever actually has been presented. The performed mastery of detail in a report or other document of government signifies prospective mastery of whatever detail—past, present, or future—might turn out to be relevant, simply by doing more of the same. Governmentality is thus assured.

Here the density and complexity of detailing become important. The more varied and dense the actual details, the greater is the saturation by detail, and the greater the saturation, the more strongly a policy text signifies governmentality. There is, then, a good semiotic reason for this generic feature and an equally good reason for its continued, cumulative reproduction.

The preceding argument can be given a more interactive and political cast by thinking in terms of rhetoric rather than semiotics. Considered from the standpoint of rhetorical contact between author and audience, the relation of the detail-saturated lay reader to the text is one of subordination and dependency: a relation of instructed to instructor, of recipient to designer, governed to governor. The sheer density of detail places the lay reader (for example, the democratic citizen) in the position of someone wanting instruction on what to notice and what to find. The saturated text is a rhetorical enactment of power to know, of power in knowing, relative to which the saturated reader is a governed subject.

With this preliminary bracketing of normal reading in mind, it is time to introduce some illustrative materials from the annual reports of the United States Senate Special Committee on Aging, *Developments in Aging*. For the sake of concise presentation, these will be confined to a single report, that of 1987, but it is typical of the entire series in the scope and density of its detail. The fact that it is longer and denser than the first of its kind (issued in 1963) is consistent with the idea that detail builds cumulatively in a policy area. The difference between earlier and later reports is, however, only one of degree. Every one of them is a good representative of the policy report genre.

Scope and Density of Detail in the 1987 Report of the Special Committee on Aging, United States Senate: Developments in Aging

The scope of detail in the report is readily apparent in its 14 chapter titles and the subordinate topics they include:

1. "Twenty Trends in Aging." The chapter summarizes statistical data on demographic trends, income levels, Social Security usage, residential status, marital status, and federal expenditures for older age groups.

2. "Social Security." An account of insurance provisions and benefits available to older people under Social Security legislation, in particular, OASI (Old Age and Survivors Insurance) and DI (Disability Insurance).[3]

3. "Employee Pensions." Separate discussions are provided of private pension schemes, state and local public employee plans, the Federal Civilian

Employee Retirement System, military retirement, and the Railroad Retirement System.

4. "Taxes and Savings." The chapter discusses provisions in the tax code that have particular relevance for older men and women.

5. "Employment." This chapter considers data, legislation, issues, and prospects for action regarding prejudice against older workers, retaining workers, and opportunities for part-time work in later life, mandatory retirement, early retirement, and the operation of the Age Discrimination in Employment Act of 1967 (ADEA).

6. "Supplemental Security Income." An account of the provisions, operations, and shortcomings of a program to provide a guaranteed minimum income to aged, blind, or disabled people. It details eligibility limits, benefits, and participation rates.

7. "Food Stamps." A detailed account of the Food Stamp Program, including its provisions to cope with malnutrition as well as hunger, problems in preventing abuse, and efforts to integrate the program with other welfare provisions.

8. "Health Care." The chapter deals with a variety of topics: Medicare costs to the federal government, the prospective payment system (PPS) to hospitals, health care use by older people, the Hospital Insurance Program, supplementary medical insurance within Medicare, supplemental health coverage in addition to Medicare, coverage for catastrophic illness, the definition of catastrophic, private-sector health care plans, government sponsorship of health research and training, and Congressional attention to the problems of Alzheimer's disease and osteoporosis.

9. "Long-term Care." A discussion of care in nursing homes, through community-based means, or at home; coverage and financing of the main types of care through Medicare, Medicaid, the Social Security Act, the Older Americans Act, private insurance, or out-of-pocket; the quality of care in nursing homes; the long-term care ombudsman program; and catastrophic health care legislation.

10. "Housing Programs." The chapter looks at federal housing assistance

to the elderly through public housing and subsidized rental housing, and the development of new housing arrangements for older people such as retirement communities, board and care homes, "granny flats," and elder cottage housing opportunity (ECHO) units.

11. "Energy Assistance and Weatherization." This chapter discusses the Low-Income Home Energy Assistance Program and the Weatherization Assistance Program in relation to the needs of older people.

12. "Older Americans Act." Passed in 1965, the act is the cornerstone of federal action to manage the lives of older people. It touches upon the various areas covered in the chapters of the report, also including federal support for gerontological research and education. The chapter focusses upon amendments to the act in 1987.

13. "Social, Community, and Legal Services." This, the most heterogeneous of the chapters, discusses the application of federal block grants for social services and community services to such activities as health programs, legal services, adult education, transportation, and the promotion of volunteer work by older people. Particular topics include services to the homeless, adult illiteracy, elder hostels, the foster grandparent program, the senior companion program, and transportation needs in the suburbs.

14. "Federal Budget." A short account of the impact of the Gramm-Rudman-Hollings Act of 1985, which mandated a schedule of annual budget deficit reductions, on Congressional legislative activity.

The sheer scale of detail managed in this policy report on aging is impressive and could be made even more so by adding topics considered elsewhere in the annual series, such as violence against the elderly and consumer frauds and deceptions, but enough has been said to make the point.

Regarding density of detail, the chapter titles and subheadings only skim the surface of what is compacted in the 1987 report. To sample the density of the detail it governs, here are seven passages found by random dipping into seven of the chapters:

A number of longstanding provisions in the tax code are of special significance to older men and women. These include the exclusion of Social Security and railroad retirement Tier I benefits for low- and moderate-income beneficiaries, the elderly tax credit for the elderly, and the one-time exclusion of up to $125,000 in capital gains from the sale of a home for persons at least 55 years of age. (Special Committee on Aging, 1987, p. 97)

An amendment added to H.R. 4154 in the House, passed by a majority vote, provided that public safety employees would be subject to the jurisdiction of States and local governments to determine whether or not they should be hired and whether or not they should be allowed to continue to work at any age. This amendment amounted, in effect, to a permanent exemption to the hiring and firing protections of the ADEA [Age Discrimination in Employment Act] for police and firefighters. (Special Committee on Aging, 1987, p. 126)

To qualify for SSI [Supplemental Security Income], an individual must be 65 or over, blind or disabled, and demonstrate a need for income supplementation. Need is determined through a means test .... In 1987, recipients' unearned income (Social Security and other benefits) could not exceed by more than $20 the maximum Federal SSI benefit ($340 for individuals, $510 for couples).

However, in calculating assets, the value of a person's home is not counted, nor is the first $4,500 in fair market value for an automobile and the first $2,000 in equity value for household goods and personal effects. Regulations also provide guidelines for determining the countable value of certain other assets, such as burial plots and life insurance polices. (Special Committee on Aging, 1987, p. 148)

Although 21 percent of food stamp households have at least one elderly member (age 60 or older), they make up only 8 percent of all food stamp recipients and receive 9 percent of food stamp benefits (an average of $31 per month) because of the typically small size of elderly households. (Special Committee on Aging, 1987, p. 159)

Short hospital stays by the elderly increased by more than 57 percent between 1965 and 1985. Since 1985, admissions for elderly patients have decreased. In 1985, a survey of non-Federal short-stay hospitals revealed that 10.5 million elderly patients were discharged from hospitals, 30 percent of all patient stays. Those 75 and older accounted for 15.7 percent of short stays. (Special Committee on Aging, 1987, p. 183)

To illustrate the extent to which Medicaid finances nursing home care, in fiscal year 1985, 21.8 million people received Medicaid benefits. Of that number 2.5 percent received skilled nursing facility care, and 3.8 percent received intermediate care facility services. Yet, of fiscal year 1985 vendor payments, 13.5 percent were for SNF care and 17.4 percent were for ICF services. (Special Committee on Aging, 1987, p. 273)

Medicare's Prospective Payment System (PPS) has placed increasing demands on transportation services. Under PPS, predetermined fixed payment rates are set for each Medicare hospital inpatient admission, based on the diagnosis-related group (DRG) into which that admission falls. This fixed payment is an incentive for hospitals to limit costs spent on Medicare patients either by reducing lengths of stay or the intensity of care provided. As a result many older persons are being released from the hospital earlier and in need of more follow-up care than before the introduction of PPS. Consequently, State and area agencies on aging now are spending more of their transportation funds to transport older persons to dialysis and chemotherapy and less for grocery stores and senior center transportation. (Special Committee on Aging, 1987, p. 387)

Governmental policy discourse shows an attention to fine detail that might be called compulsive, meaning an attention to detail seemingly beyond motives of adequate description, reasonable argument, sufficient demonstration, and clear communication. This is an excess of detail that seems gratuitous and *almost* defies comprehension. We must stress "almost" however, because reports are generically driven to signify the governmentality of their policy realms by linguistically grasping and, in that sense, comprehending the detail they present. They do so, for example, through devices like summary gist, where prolix detail is reduced to a compressed representation, yielding a rendered object of comprehension, and by using naming and renaming to organize multiple details into indices of the same object of knowledge—in this case, aging.

The reports of *Developments in Aging* create order in their heterogeneous detail, in fact, by means of a network of names derived from nominalizing the term "aging" and deploying variations of name across diverse topics, for example, the topics marked by chapter titles and subheadings, as illustrated above.[4] We take it that the placement of connected names around a policy object is simultaneously an exercise of government over the object and a signifier of the governmentality of the designated realm: an assurance that come-what-may in the form of detail and contingency, government can be extended over it. Signification of governmentality, of infinitely extendable rational rule, does not need dramatic spectacle; it can be achieved through "particles of verbal matter" in a "galaxy of trifling data" (Barthes, 1974, p. 22).

The 1987 report employs 226 different names to designate those who have undergone or are undergoing the process of aging. If we ask of this array what can be done with the names to organize discourse or what discursive uses they have, then four types of names appear:

1. Names that acknowledge [the aged] as others like ourselves, possessing personal identity and open to intersubjective forms of address, such as those used in conveying sympathy, understanding a status equality. Key semantic elements here are "people" and "individuals," as in "older people" and "aged individuals."

2. Names for [the aged] as fellow members of our national community, used to invoke solidarity and collective responsibility. Key elements here are "our," "nation," "citizen," and "America." Examples include "older Americans," "elderly Americans," "our Nation's seniors," and "senior citizens."

3. Names referring to institutional roles and organizational locations in society. Examples include "older workers," "retirees," "pensioners," "older taxpayers," "older patients," "elderly renters," "elderly residents," "veterans," "Medicare beneficiaries 65-69," "older spouse," "older Indians," "the older illiterate adult," and "the older suburban dweller."

4. Names of social groups defined by age include "the aged," "the elderly," "the oldest old," "the young elderly," "elderly whites," "the disabled elderly," "the healthy elderly," "the low income elderly," "the rural elderly," "the older population," and "the 65+ population."

Obviously, this is not a systematic classification, but it is sufficient to indicate the broad, flexible economy of the names as a textual governing device. The array covers the report like paths criss-crossing an open terrain and rendering it orderly. Wherever the reader is in the detail there is a name, a semantic pathway, leading back to the same policy object: aging. Just as physical pathways signify the ability to traverse a terrain, so do connected names signify the ability to know and, therefore, the ability to govern a policy area.

In this respect, it should be added that nominalization is especially useful in signifying governmentality because of the power with which it objectifies reality and makes "it" available for cognitive grasp and practical action. Gusfield (1981) has shown this with reference to the seemingly minor linguistic fact of transforming verbs of drinking and driving into the noun entity "the drunk-driver." Kitzinger (1987) examines the syntactic turning of certain acts into an entity called "the lesbian," allowing again for a more certain grasp of the noun designated reality than verbs permit. Killingsworth and Palmer, applying rhetoric analysis to Environmental Impact Statements, observe a preponderance of "noun style" over "verb style":

> The verb style pictures a world full of human actors performing purposeful actions upon objects in an ever-changing scene; it requires active verbs and human subjects…. By contrast, the objectivist syntax of the noun style—expressive of a world frozen into stasis and broken (analyzed) into its components—is dominated by features like passive voice, nominalizations, strings of noun modifiers, impersonality, and high levels of abstraction. (1992, pp. 172-73)

Noun style, we would say, is a more decisive way to govern detail than verb style, as is evident in its dominance of scientific, technological, legal, and bureaucratic discourses as well as policy reports.

Conclusions: Politics of Detail

In conclusion, it is important to stress that saturation with detail in policy reports is not the result of will, motive, or plan; it is generically produced. With reference to the particular case of the study of aging, this means that the phenomenon belongs to the structural environment of gerontological research, one of the givens of the field in which gerontologists work. Yet there is no transcendent decree saying that policy reportage must be done in just the way it has come to be done. Generic imperatives, like any other structural forces, can be turned from environmental givens to topics of study and action through the familiar dynamics of analysis, critical appraisal, and proposals for reinvention. To know what constrains social knowledge of aging is vital to gerontology, especially in its applied and political aspects, and generic conventions of policy reportage are among those constraints.

Saturation with detail signifies governmentality, but seems also to meet the formal liberal democratic requirement of openness, transparency, and full disclosure in government. The irony is that a surfeit of detail comes in practice to defeat the ability of laypeople—the democratic citizens—to process, decode, interpret, and judge the political significance of the flood of detail to which they are opened. Government of detail readily permits government by detail and, thus, reveals a vital literal dimension of Foucault's inventive plotting of modern political reason. On the surface, the 1987 *Developments in Aging* reports may seem simply to indicate how social problems that lead to the production of social policy are politically addressed. A deeper critical analysis fosters a different perspective, however, one in which such policy is understood as part of an ongoing assemblage of technologies that enfold the knowing and making of dependent populations into the art of government. As the prospects and problems of an aging population expand in the twenty-first century, these technologies certainly bear closer scrutiny.

Notes

Bryan Green is my recently retired colleague from the Sociology Department at York University. A few years ago he asked me to write the Preface for his book, *A Textual Analysis of American Government Reports on Aging*, published by the Edwin Mellen Press, 2001. As I read his manuscript I realized that we shared some similar interests, and I approached him with the idea of writing a joint paper on how textual "detail" in policy reports on aging could be viewed as a form of "governmentality" in the sense of the term used by Foucault. He agreed, and we wrote "The Government of Detail." The paper was submitted to and accepted for publication in *The Journal of Aging and Identity* 7(3), 2002, pp. 149-63. Bryan is a great writer, and I am grateful for the opportunity to collaborate with him. I also wish to thank Bryan's assistant at the time, Susan Rainey, for her seamless work in knitting together our various written sections. Permission to reprint the essay is granted by Bryan Green and Kluwer Academic/Plenum Publishers.

1. The version we are using is reprinted in *The Foucault Effect: Studies in Governmentality* (1991). The introductory essay by Colin Gordon is an excellent synopsis of the development of governmental rationality in modern societies. Foucault echoes his governmentality themes in two other important articles: "*Omnes et Singulatim*: Towards a Criticism of 'Political Reason'" (1981) and "The Political Technology of Individuals" (1988).

2. In this regard Paul Rabinow's writing on "The Third Culture" (1994) is instructive. Rabinow looks at Daniel Defert's work with persons with AIDS in France to show how the patient has become a "figure of social reform" by demanding an empowered involvement with drug experimentation and research. Here is a case where a political rationality based on "rights" and "freedoms," along with new rituals of care and dying, are utilized to contest a governmental rationality based on populational risk and medical authority. Rabinow also talks about the role of critical curiosity, that is, how the governed are motivated to become curious about their conditions of being governed, suggesting that the limits of liberal and neoliberal governance are tested not simply by their own weapons—rights and freedoms—but also by the reflexive forces such as *curiosity* that come from people being governed in a liberal way.

3. Acronyms will be filled out in parentheses or brackets. The practice in these reports is to give the full name and acronym at first mention but thereafter use the acronym alone, relying on the reader to recall the name. Acronyms contribute greatly to density of detail in a text.

4. Nominalization is the syntactic transformation of a verb into a noun form, turning the expression of an action or a process into an object. For example, "strikers picket university" becomes "picketing at university."

four

Reflections on the Gerontological Handbook

Handbooks are one of the most unique products of the evolution of books. As both commonsensical works of reference and innovative conceptual toolkits, their appeal has as much to do with their everyday usefulness as with their special status within academic traditions. This power of handbooks to span "high" and "low" literary cultures derives, in part, from their history. Known at first as "manuals" (from Latin *manualis* for "fitting the hand") handbooks began in the thirteenth century as portable, personal supplements to the Christian clergy's weighty medieval lectern and desk volumes. *Le Manuel des Péchés*, an Anglo-Norman penitential manual from the period, says of itself: "This is called a manual because it is held in the hand" (Bennett, 1988, p. 166).[1] Through the centuries, the handbooks and manuals of "high" culture were joined by guidebooks, primers, pamphlets, bulletins, readers, and brochures to form a constellation of utility texts written to teach and train ordinary people in the pragmatic arts of living. In a counter-movement emerging since the Enlightenment and growing during the nineteenth and early twentieth centuries, however, some of these popular texts became once again primary intellectual resources in those realms where the practical arts were transformed into secular professions. Handbooks on childcare, schooling, medicine—and eventually gerontology—became state-of-the-art purveyors of newly professionalized knowledges.

Gerontological handbooks, in addition to providing handy synopses of current research on aging and old age, can thus be seen as part of the wider cultural development of textual practices in Western society. As such they present us with two interesting questions about knowledge-production and scientific disciplinarity in gerontology. First, how is it that gerontological handbooks have become authorities on the myriad of issues and problems surrounding the aging process—especially in the United States? Secondly, outside of the handbook's constituent parts—chapters, themes, topics, and contributors—what other textual activities inherent in the handbook define and configure the field of aging studies as a professional enterprise? To address these questions, this chapter proposes a critical interpretive approach to gerontological handbooks that highlights their stylistic, literary, and rhetorical features.

Our approach begins with a look at the two editions of the *Handbook of the Humanities and Aging*. In the first edition, co-editor Thomas R. Cole remarks, "a 'handbook' in the humanities and aging certainly has its ironic side." On the one hand, gerontology handbooks are the fundamental texts by which the profession has identified itself as a scientific endeavour. On the other hand, Cole asserts that a humanities handbook on aging is different: It must be "less scientific and instrumental, more historical, more concerned with the limits and conditions of its own knowledge, and more focussed on questions of representation, meaning, and value than traditional handbooks in gerontology" (1992a, p. xii). Thus situated at some distance from mainstream gerontology, the first edition of *Handbook of the Humanities and Aging* promoted the methodological strengths of the humanities: interpretation, reflection, and criticism, along with an emphasis on experience, narrative, and dialogue. The double goal of the first humanities handbook, therefore, was to become "a standard reference for academic and clinical gerontologists, as well as a stimulus for future work in the humanities and aging" (Cole, 1992, p. xiv).

It is instructive to look back, therefore, from the viewpoint of the second edition of *Handbook of the Humanities and Aging* (2000), at the first edition's mapping of the conceptual encounters between the science of gerontology and the ingenuity of the humanities. The examination of gerontological textuality was central to this mapping, as the first edition's contributors explored the historical, spiritual, and literary dimensions of aging. Although the first edition did not include a study of handbooks, it did, in staking out its challenging position as a different kind of handbook with an "ironic side," imply a critique of the handbook genre itself. It is this implied but absent critique in the first edition, therefore, that this chapter addresses, as it appeared as an essay in the second edition. Specifically, I wish to introduce four overlapping reflections on the handbook as: (1) a genealogical document, (2) a gerontological standard, (3) a disciplinary practice, and (4) a public philosophy.

The Handbook as a Genealogical Document

A cursory check on the subject of handbooks in the *Sociofile* search catalogue produces 726 entries; the *Humanities Index* has 168 entries, which comprise handbooks themselves as well as critiques of them. They show that handbooks today are not limited to professional texts but also continue as popular guides to the art of living. The critical commentary embraces both streams: prosaic and largely forgotten handbooks are transformed into rich archival documents by researchers who trace the historical discourses through which human conduct has been shaped and regulated. For instance, Carol Auster's (1985) examination of twentieth-century Girl Scout Handbooks is a marvellous glimpse at the world of domestic expectations for girls in the period between 1913-84. Likewise, Yvonne Schutze (1987) looks at German medical handbooks to analyze the construction of "mother-love" and childrearing practices since the mid-eighteenth century. A broader cross-cultural impetus motivates Deborah Best and Nicole Ruther's (1994) astute survey of developmental psychology handbooks published between 1931-93.

These studies and others of supposedly minor and mundane texts have, in part, been influenced by the work of Michel Foucault and attest to one of the great strengths of his *genealogical* method (inspired by Nietzsche's *On The Genealogy of Morals*). By "genealogical method," its many users mean a multidisciplinary technique for discovering the contingent historical trends that underpin contemporary society's structures, discourses, and practices. For Foucault, the documentary history of Western cultures is not to be found in the "great" texts that various traditions have established as their canons. Rather, events are to be found, via the genealogical method, "in the most unpromising places, in what we tend to feel is without history." In Foucault's characterization, "genealogy is gray, meticulous, and patiently documentary. It operates on a field of entangled and confused parchments" (1977, p. 139).[2]

In using the genealogical method then, we are avoiding "the canons" and looking instead for the history resident in the "confused" archive of codebooks, rulebooks, underground writing, diaries, and handbooks that has been deposited in the present but which is routinely denied importance in reconstructions of the past. The genealogical method, in recovering this archive for historical analysis, enables us to ask via the archive's documents why certain discourses, vocabularies, and knowledges took on the status of truth at specific historical junctures, while others were marginalized or disparaged. As the next section shows, genealogy is an effective tool for uncovering the role of handbooks in establishing the truths of old age in the middle of the twentieth century.

I am suggesting that the ideas of Foucault generally, and of the critics of handbooks in other fields specifically, are valuable for a critique of the gerontological handbook archive, because they lead us to reconsider it as a body of historical documents that is socially significant in ways often overlooked by their authors and readers. In other words, it becomes possible to go beyond the overt purposes of the gerontological handbooks to discover them as chronicles of the development of the field's professional, multidisciplinary, and scientific codes. A genealogical approach also brings the handbooks into the interpretive realm of the humanities, where it is as important to understand the politics and practicalities of text making as it is to explicate the texts' contents and authorships.

The Handbook as a Gerontology Standard

The genealogical approach usefully frames an intriguing question: given the great variety of texts that can be written about aging and old age, why is the handbook a gerontological standard? Beginning with the publication of Edmund V. Cowdry's *Problems of Ageing* (1939; more fully discussed below), professional handbooks have assumed the dominant textual lineage in gerontology in a growing publication market. Cowdry's text went through two further editions, and by the time of the third edition in 1952 gerontological textbook production and research began to expand rapidly along the lines set out in his collections.[3] In the late 1950s and early 1960s the Inter-University Training Institute in Social Gerontology, under the directorship of Wilma Donahue at the University of Michigan, sponsored a trio of formative handbooks that emphasized the non-biological dimensions of aging in multidisciplinary formats (see Donahue, 1960): *Handbook of Aging and the Individual: Psychological and Biological Aspects of Aging* edited by James Birren (1959), *Aging and Society: Handbook of Social Gerontology* edited by Clark Tibbitts (1960), and *Aging in Western Culture: A Survey of Social*

Gerontology edited by Ernest Burgess (1960). These handbooks, in turn, stimulated further research, framed educational programs, and gave shape to the disciplinary discourse of gerontology, especially as it developed through the multiple editions of three predominant handbooks with James E. Birren as editor-in-chief: *Handbook of the Biology of Aging*, *Handbook of The Psychology of Aging*, and *Handbook of Aging and the Social Sciences*. These were published together with four editions each (1976/1977, 1985, 1990, 1996), the first two by Van Nostrand Reinhold and the latter two by the Academic Press. The handbooks' editors, all major figures in the field, largely remained the same through the different editions, while topics, emphases, and contributors have changed with the times.[4]

As these handbooks remain predominant, others have been published as well, especially since the 1980s as gerontology developed increasingly more subfields; for example, *Handbook of Geriatric Psychiatry* (E. Busse and D. Blazer, eds., 1980), *International Handbook on Aging* (E. Palmore, ed., 1980), *Handbook of Mental Health and Aging* (J. Birren, ed., 1992), *Handbook of Nutrition in the Aged* (R. Watson, ed., 1994), *Handbook on Ethnicity, Aging, and Mental Health* (D. Padgett, ed., 1995), *Handbook of Communication and Aging Research* (J. Nussbaum and J. Coupland, eds., 1995), *Handbook of Aging and the Family* (R. Blieszner and V. Bedford, eds., 1995), and *Handbook on Women and Aging* (J.M. Coyle, ed., 1997).

Supplementing gerontology's handbook corpus has been a host of book reviews and critiques from within the gerontological community. Often reviewers point out what is missing in a particular handbook, such as Elizabeth A. Kutza's complaint in *The Gerontologist* that the policy chapters in the final section of the 1996 edition of *Handbook of Aging and the Social Sciences* lack the theoretical rigour and political acumen developed in earlier chapters (1996, p. 828). Others cite handbooks as embodiments of the unimaginative, scientific rationalism that pervades gerontology. For instance, Haim Hazan, in his introduction to *Old Age: Constructions and Deconstructions*, disapprovingly observes that the Table of Contents of the second edition of *Handbook of Aging and the Social Sciences* (1985) "is a fine example of the attempt to preserve the distance of so-called scientific language from the categories enunciated by the subject of its study.... The calculated vocabulary is evident" (1994, pp. 9, 10). Likewise, in his philosophical analysis of subjectivity in aging studies, Ronald Manheimer invents a new category, the "handbook self," to poke critically at the empiricist, behavioural tradition in gerontological texts (1992).

Alan Walker, in an earlier review of the second edition of *Handbook of Aging and the Social Sciences*, made several penetrating criticisms that might apply to other handbooks as well. He wrote that many of the contributions make the text too advanced to be pitched at an introductory level (1987, p. 236). Walker's most telling criticism, however, was that the handbook is overwhelmingly American in content and approach, an ethnocentricism that belied the claim put forward by the title to general coverage of the subject. Walker asked: "what does the handbook reveal about the current state of gerontological research in the USA?" (p. 237). His stark conclusion was that the absence of critical structural thinking in the handbook reflected the lack of these features in American gerontology itself at that time. Although the next two editions of *Handbook of Aging and the Social Sciences* (1990, 1996) included more materials on structural relations, the political economy of aging, and international scholarship and authors, Walker's concern about the Americanization of aging studies remains an important point, but not necessarily because, as he suggested, "a handbook with a similar title produced in Europe would have a significantly different content" (Walker, p. 240).[5] Rather, Walker's critique points to the contextual nature of handbooks and the social relations of knowledge evident both inside and outside the text. Thus a progressive reviewer like Walker is criticizing the very embeddedness of the handbook genre in the specifics of American gerontological politics despite the genre's claim to transcend context and create a dispassionate science of gerontology.

More introspective reviews have been made by scholars who have themselves contributed to the handbooks. Edward J. Masoro, who wrote on "metabolism" for the second edition of *Handbook of the Biology of Aging* (1985), remarked that the 1996 edition of the handbook had several problems, amongst which was "the fact that each chapter is a free-standing review article" (1996, p. 828). This led Masoro to ponder two interesting questions: first, "why [are] collections of such articles ... published in books when their publication over time as review articles in the leading journals of biological gerontology would probably better serve the field?" (pp. 828-29); and second, "why doesn't a handbook on the biology of aging generate a consensus on what *aging* actually means as a biological phenomenon?" (p. 829). Appropriately, Masoro titled his review, "What Are We Talking About?"

W. Andrew Achenbaum, in his contributions to the second and fourth editions of *Handbook of Aging and the Social Sciences* (1985, 1996) and the first edition of *Handbook of the Humanities and Aging* (1992), and elsewhere (1995), has written extensively on the gerontological handbook. He has also been one of its most outspoken critics and on several occasions reviewed the biology, psychology, and social sciences handbooks in tandem (1991, 1993, 1996). Achenbaum criticized the handbook editions published in 1990 because, in his view, they provided no unifying themes, they typified the insularity of American gerontology, and their overspecialized chapters compromised their claim to multidisciplinarity (1991). He called "for more critical handbooks" (p. 134) that would also hark back to the spirit of innovation and dialogue that characterized Cowdry's classic volumes. Similarly, Achenbaum noted in his handbook reviews (1996) that a lack of cross-referencing to earlier volumes and bridge building amongst disciplinary communities meant that the "editors deliver fresh ideas, but leave it to readers to make connections" (1996, p. 826).

Achenbaum is right to have expected handbooks to fulfil gerontology's promise as a multidisciplinary, comprehensive, and accessible enterprise, one that provides its practitioners with state-of-the-art research and "gerontologic maps" to forecast the prospects of aging and the problems of old age. The limitations of the gerontological handbook may have less to do with the contents, the contributors, or the currency of the research, however, as the reviewers above suggested, than with the structure of the handbook genre itself. Rather than expect the handbook in all of its variations to accomplish the multidisciplinary ideals set forth by its mandate, perhaps we should detect in its lack of unity and thematic imbalances the patterns by which gerontological knowledge has been reproduced—a lack and an imbalance resulting from the handbook's nature as an "itinerant" text produced pragmatically to meet local shifting conditions. Judgements of gerontological handbooks based on positivist criteria of sufficiency and rigor or critical assessments of biases and scientism miss the point that handbooks are *productive* relays between authors, subjects, institutions, and worldviews. Further, such patterns involve more than just research models and data collections, however significant these may be, because the handbook also draws together the institutional practices of funding agencies, university programs, teaching curricula, relations of prestige, and the organization of expertise, as Walker's review above suggests. While the gerontological handbook's status as a standard appears to derive from its intellectual strengths, its real character comes from the burden placed on it to represent, in textual form, the disparate social and intellectual resources that have been brought to bear on the aging process. Gerontology's texts like gerontology itself, therefore, should be seen as part of a struggling, indeterminate, and ultimately incomplete project to make old age a knowable feature of modern life. Revisiting the gerontological handbook with these issues in mind, along with earlier reflections on the handbook as a genealogical document, moves us closer to the rhetorical aspects of gerontological knowledge and takes up the question of the handbook as a disciplinary practice with particular reference to Cowdry's foundational text.

The Handbook as a Disciplinary Practice in Gerontology

At a general level, scientific texts discipline knowledge; they not only organize research problems in professionally legitimating ways, but also enfold their historical contingencies and social values into narratives of progress and objectivity. Further, as Bazerman and Paradis put it, authors and texts are "produced by a complex of social, cognitive, material, and rhetorical activities"; in consequence, written texts both construe knowledge and represent it. As expressions of disciplinary practice, they also "dialectically precipitate the various contexts and actions that constitute the professions" (1991, p. 4). Thus, texts are practical events that do things beyond what their authors say they do and beyond their designated roles in academic fields. Thinking of texts as practical events also prompts us to discover that texts might rework what they supposedly represent and critically counteract their academic status. As Dominick LaCapra says, "The apparent paradox is that texts hailed as perfections of a genre or a discursive practice may also test and contest its limits" (1985, p. 141).

How might we reinterpret anatomy professor Edmund V. Cowdry's *Problems of Ageing* in this critical light? Thus reconsidered, it can be seen as not only an innovative text, but as a practical event and a complex of rhetorical activities around multidisciplinarity and state-of-the-art scientific thinking that set the stage for the gerontological handbooks that followed. Further, a critical interpretation of Cowdry's work may demonstrate its value as a resource to "test and contest" the limits of gerontology.[6] Specifically, as I shall show below, as a multi-authored, multidisciplinary text Cowdry's handbook proclaimed the scope of the enterprise. The prefaces and forewords of its various editions, and the featuring of authors' professional credentials in a textbook-style list of contributors, served to assert the existence, coherence, and scientific merit of a field of knowledge that was neither coherent nor scientific and was merely in process of coming into existence. And finally, in using the handbook as the textual vehicle for launching the enterprise, Cowdry established at the outset the hegemonic form of gerontological knowledge-production as scientifically accredited multidisciplinary research, framed as a practical guide for professionals, that has shaped the field ever since.

The idea of a multidisciplinary handbook in the early twentieth century was already central to other professions, especially child studies. Indeed, Cowdry had already published a handbook on the problem of arteriosclerosis in 1933 and a multidisciplinary text with the (irksome) title *Human Biology and Racial Welfare* in 1930. Within this context, Cowdry published the first edition of *Problems of Ageing* in 1939 and a second edition in 1942. In the Preface, Cowdry establishes the text's professional credentials: it was based on research presented at the Woods Hole Conference (Massachusetts) in 1937 (one of the first major scientific conferences on aging) and was sponsored by The Josiah Macy Jr. Foundation, the Union of American Biological Societies, and the National Research Council. Cowdry tells us in the handbook's Preface:

> Abstracts and complete manuscripts have been circulated widely among the contributors. Consequently, the opportunity to bring to bear on the problem the experience and points of view of many specialists, working together in a constructive way, has been unrivaled. But each contributor is personally responsible for his chapter. There are, as one would expect, some differences of opinion. These foreshadow progress since they will stimulate further investigation. The style is as simple as possible consistent with scientific accuracy. (Preface to first edition, reprinted in Cowdry, 1942, p. iii)

In the Preface to the second edition (1942) Cowdry adds "our principle of mobilizing and integrating the knowledge and experience of specialists in different fields has been widely followed as is evidenced by the arrangement of symposium after symposium on the subject of aging" (p. iv). He then follows with a list of symposia and new interventions by foundations and national agencies between 1940 and 1941. In the second edition's Foreword, Lawrence K. Frank, who would go on to become a leader in American gerontology, corroborates Cowdry's scientific optimism. He says, "It is evident that the problem of the ageing process is multi-dimensional and will require for its solution not only a multidisciplinary approach but also a synoptic correlation of diverse findings and viewpoints, toward which this volume offers a highly significant contribution of facts and of theoretical formulations" (p. xv). Here the multidisciplinary theme is fully enunciated as the solution to the "problem" of the aging process.

Hence, the prefaces and the Foreword in *Problems of Ageing* persuade the reader of the text's legitimacy by dissolving three tensions. (1) Although there are differences between researchers, they are united by a common disciplinary imperative as a community of scholars. (2) Although much more needs to be known about the aging process, the contributions stimulate further research. (3) Although the problems of aging are complex and hardly containable in one text, scientific methods can elaborate the reasonability of the aging process. American philosopher John Dewey, who further authenticates the multidisciplinary ambitions of the text, wrote the Introduction to *Problems of Ageing*. Dewey, elderly himself at this point, saw in the study of aging the opportunity to link biological and cultural explanations as a way of creating a new form of knowledge, where "science and philosophy meet on common ground in their joint interest in discovering the processes of normal growth and in the institution of conditions which will favor and support ever continued growth" (in Cowdry, 1942, p. xxxiii).

Following Dewey's introduction is a listing of the many contributors and their credentials, a feature of textbook construction designed specifically to strengthen the text's authority, through the rhetoric of the lists' entries. The bulk of the text consists of 34 chapters, each with standard summaries that illustrate how aging occurs in the evolutionary worlds from protozoa to humans. In their combination, the chapters of *Problems of Ageing* appropriate scientific modeling in their construction of old age. For example, they expand the usages of medicalizing terms such as "senile" to characterize a broad range of human behaviour. Book chapters are often organized according to anatomical models, comprehensive inventories and tables catalogue the special circumstances of old age, and the research pursuits of the book's contributors are legitimized through referral to work and authors in other already established scientific fields, such as pediatrics. The latter part of the second edition of Cowdry's text includes two chapters on the psychological aspects of aging. The first, by Yale psychology professor Walter R. Miles discusses perception, intelligence, motivation, and personal interests, thus enhancing gerontology's psychological profile. The second chapter by New York consulting psychologist George Lawton, on individual adjustment, endeavours to situate the psychology of aging as a rigorous analytical subject rather than a mere practical tool for eldercare. The author warns "all of us working in this field will do the science of gerontology an ultimate disservice if we confuse our desire to ameliorate with our desire to describe"; scientific gerontology must be separated from "pseudo-healing cults" and "quasi-psychological literature" (p. 791). In insisting that the psychology of aging is a science that must be separated from older pre-scientific knowledges about the aging process, Lawton makes a substantive contribution to the certification of gerontology as a scientifically grounded profession. Lawton predicts that in the future communities will have "schools for older people" and Old Age Centers (p. 792), while expert gerontologists would be "social engineers" of imagination, "who will manipulate community resources, and when necessary, devise new instrumentalities" (p. 808).

The last two chapters of the second edition of *Problems of Ageing* reiterate the importance of multidisciplinarity and professionalism to the project of gerontological knowledge-production. In the penultimate chapter medical professor Albert Mueller-Deham delineates the varieties of physical problems in old age, remarking that "the senile body is a pathological museum, an equation with not merely one, but several unknown quantities" (p. 863). In order to know this body, "geriatrics will develop by specialization within Internal Medicine, not as an isolated structure, but only as a central station where many cables meet" (p. 887). In the final chapter Edward J. Stieglitz, who as a physician conceived the idea of social gerontology, attempts to give a coherency to the concept of multidisciplinary gerontology via a metaphorical linkage between the human body and the "body politic." Dividing gerontology into three categories of problems—biological, clinical, and socio-economic—Stieglitz proposes that:

> As the cell is the unit from which the elaborate structure of the human body is constructed, so are individual men and women the basic units of collective society, the body politic. It is these socio-economic problems which have become so acute that now the need for knowledge in gerontology is a matter of true urgency. (p. 895)

The rhetorical practices of Cowdry's text—the contributors list, the authoritative Preface, the progressive chapter order, the multidisciplinary agenda, the emphasis on professional credentials, and the scientific vocabularies—bring the rationalities and aspirations of modern science to the problems of aging. In producing a text of this kind, Cowdry wedded the promise of gerontological knowledge to the handbook genre, and he has been praised by gerontologists for doing so ever since.[7] Indeed, if we look again at later handbooks, the same rhetorical practices are evident, and they continue to serve the same kind of disciplinary function, that is, to promote and shape the professional, multidisciplinary, and scientific status of gerontology. For example, in the first edition of the *Handbook of Aging and the Social Sciences* (1976), the Foreword and Preface remind readers that the text has a multidisciplinary focus, contains the work of the best available experts, and is to be used as a work of systematic reference by professionals, policy-makers, and students. Editors justify the publication of subsequent editions of the handbook because of the growth of gerontological research and the difficulty of containing such research in a single edition. This is quite a leap from the *Handbook of Social Gerontology* in which editor Clark Tibbitts claims that the book's 19 essays and critical reviews each deal with a separate topic "and thus, *in toto*" reflect the scope of the field (1960, p. x).

My point here is less to question the expertise of the research contained in these handbooks as it is to use such texts to reflect upon the interesting connections between the handbook as genre, science as truth, aging as knowledge, and gerontology as discipline. Furthermore, the exploration of the textual dilemmas of the gerontological handbook provides an opportunity for the humanities and the interpretive social sciences to apply their considerable critical capacities to the task of deconstructing the rhetorical means by which we have come to know our lives as aging.

Conclusions: The Handbook as a Public Philosophy

One of the first outcomes of the deconstruction I have just advocated may be to recover the promise of gerontology as a kind of "public philosophy" in the sense of the term used by Robert Bellah in his appendix to *Habits of the Heart* (1985) entitled "Social Science as Public Philosophy." Bellah's lament on the loss of the "public philosophy" tradition in the social sciences in the wake of their professionalization in modern institutions is particularly apt when applied to gerontology with its highly strategic professionalizing tendencies. In Bellah's view, this tradition merits restoration because professional social science has distanced itself from public concerns while harbouring a narrow vision of the social "whole" (p. 300). The transdisciplinary agenda of social science as a public philosophy, however, is to open up the "arbitrary boundary between the social sciences and the humanities" and to remake social science into "a form of social self-understanding" (p. 301). But how can we convert gerontology

handbooks—the dominant textual forum for gerontological knowledge—
to such purposes? And what role might handbooks, given their *raison d'être*
as professional development tools, play in furthering the public philosophical prospects of gerontology?

To cite Thomas R. Cole again, we should develop handbooks with a
"difference" (1992a, p. xii) and look to the humanities for guidance in
transforming the handbook genre. But this may be only a partial solution,
if, as I have argued here, the handbook's legacy as a scientific, disciplining
structure is left out of the critique of professional gerontology. A second
response would be to recall the original, historical purpose of the handbook as a nomadic and public text, a manual that linked scholarship with
commonsense and wisdom with instruction. Gerontology might be
reconstructed through the forging of these links as "a form of social self-
understanding."[8]

Reviewers of the first edition of *Handbook of the Humanities and Aging*
implicitly encouraged this more critical orientation by the very nature of
their backgrounds and commentary. Herbert S. Donow, a humanities professor, complains that in the handbook "humanistic study comes off looking fuzzy and confused," in comparison with the 1990 edition of *Handbook
of the Psychology of Aging*, which Donow considers to be better organized
and more intent on delivering what it promises (1993, p. 816). Chris
Phillipson, a political economist, praises the humanities handbook for
establishing "the case for a humanistic gerontology" and for being a har-
binger of a "new" gerontology (1996, pp. 364, 367). Finally, sociologist
Hans-Jürgen Freter warns that for interdisciplinary humanities texts on
aging to succeed, attention must be paid to overturning stereotyped
views held by some humanists that "mainstream" gerontology is "a static,
positivist monster" (1993, p. 258). These critics—a humanist writing in an
American journal about intelligibility, a political economist writing in a
British journal about a new gerontology, and a sociologist writing in a
Canadian journal about gerontological stereotyping—perhaps represent
some of the diverse voices that were stirred by the "public philosophy" of
gerontological thought.

Notes

In August 1997, Ruth Ray, one of the co-editors of the second edition of
Handbook of the Humanities and Aging, contacted me to ask if I would write a
chapter for the new edition. Since the first edition of the handbook, pub-

lished in 1992, had been such an influential text for me, I hardly hesitated in replying to Ruth, except to ask what to write about? Ruth, and later co-editor Thomas R. Cole, suggested I write something methodological about "critical gerontology." As I pondered what to do, I began to think about the handbook in gerontology as a genre deserving its own critical, reflexive treatment. Writing about handbooks for a Handbook became an exciting challenge, and the resulting essay emerged as "Reflections on the Gerontological Handbook." After several revisions, based on the much-appreciated close readings of earlier drafts provided by Victor Marshall and Teresa Mangum, the essay was published in *Handbook of the Humanities and Aging (Second Edition)*, edited by Thomas R. Cole, Robert Kastenbaum, and Ruth E. Ray (New York, Springer, 2000, pp. 405-18). The version here is slightly altered and expanded, but otherwise is reprinted with the permission of the Springer Publishing Company. I also thank Victor Marshall for letting me browse and borrow from his collection of gerontology handbooks.

1. *Le Manuel des Péchés* survives in several manuscripts, but the one Bennett discusses here is itself one example of the genre. I thank my colleague Professor John Andrew Taylor for pointing out these aspects of handbook history.

2. Accordingly, Foucault identifies numerous documents as genealogical expressions of the dilemmas of modernity, such as Jeremy Bentham's late eighteenth-century plan for the imprisoning *Panopticon* (1979), the memoirs of nineteenth-century hermaphrodite Herculine Barbin (1980b), and a "minor" periodical publication by Immanuel Kant in 1784 called "What is Enlightenment?" (1984a). An excellent example of a genealogical study of psychology is Rose (1989).

3. Birren and Clayton estimate that the literature on aging published between 1950 and 1960 equals all that had been published in the previous 115 years (1975, p. 74).

4. Besides gerontological handbooks, multiple editions are a feature of many other gerontological texts. For example, there are now five editions of *Later Life: The Realities of Aging* (H. Cox), six editions of *Social Gerontology: A Multidisciplinary Perspective* (N.R. Hooyman); eight editions of *Death, Society, and Human Experience* (R. Kastenbaum); and ten editions of *Social Forces and Aging* (R. Atchley).

5. Victor Marshall, editor of two distinguished editions of *Aging in Canada: Social Perspectives*, acknowledges the existence of national distinctions in gerontological scholarship by noting that "Canadian theory about aging is more structural, collectivist and historically grounded than the predominantly attitudinal, individualist and consensually oriented theorizing found south of the border" (1987, p. 4). Lawrence Cohen goes further to elaborate the international impact of Western gerontology texts with an illuminating focus on India (1998).

6. Historical gerontologists W. Andrew Achenbaum (1995), Thomas R. Cole (1992b), Carole Haber (1983), and David G. Troyansky (1989), amongst others, had pioneered the analysis of gerontological literature as a vibrant dimension of contemporary historical scholarship. See Richard Harvey Brown (1992) for examples of deconstruction and social science texts.

7. Why other texts did not become as foundational as Cowdry's is an important question. For example, psychology professor G. Stanley Hall's *Senescence: The Last Half of Life* (1922), written during his retirement from Clark University, is a *tour de force* that surveys not only the sciences of old age but also poetry, fiction, religion, ethnography, and autobiographies. In contrast to Hall's earlier influential work on adolescence, *Senescence* is regarded as too speculative, scattered, and unscientific. In his ambivalence about scientific explanations of aging (Achenbaum, 1993; Cole, 1993), however, Hall poses new questions in *Senescence* that gerontology is still challenged to answer.

8. I explore the possibilities of gerontological "undisciplining" elsewhere (Katz 1996). One interesting example of a traditional handbook format hidden within a modern one is *Handbook of Aging: For Those Growing Old and Those Concerned with Them* (1972), written by retired American academic Elliot Dunlap Smith. His promise in the Preface to make "the book short, partly to make it easy for elderly people to hold, but mainly because it is not a book of extensive particularization to be skimmed through quickly" (p. viii) is borne out in this slender volume which would not be out of place in the hands of an aging medieval cleric.

five

Critical Gerontological Theory: Intellectual Fieldwork and the Nomadic Life of Ideas

In the past two decades critical gerontology has grown as a vibrant sub-field blending humanities and social science ideas to challenge the instrumentalism of mainstream gerontology and broaden aging studies beyond biomedical models. This hybridized literature has provided an important critique of prevailing social policies and practices around aging, while promoting the rise of new retirement cultures and positive identities in later life. There are also numerous approaches within critical gerontology, outlined below, that create an internal debate regarding the subfield's constitution, accomplishments, and future directions. However, this debate has generally delimited criticality to research directly associated with radical theoretical traditions (e.g., Marxism, phenomenology, social constructivism) or radical social movements (e.g., feminist, anti-poverty, pension reform), thus overlooking the intellectual and discursive contexts in which critical ideas attain their position within gerontology. This chapter steps outside of these associations to locate gerontological criticality within the contextual dynamics of its own development.

In this spirit of reflexivity I begin on a biographical note. Several years ago at a social science conference, I participated in a session called, "After the Fall: New Directions in Critical Culture Theory." The "Fall" had several references: the fall of Soviet communist power and its many walls (both real and ideological), the fall of Marxism and socialism as world political platforms, and the fall of politically informed critical theory in the wake of postmodern skepticism. The invitation to present a paper on my area of research in gerontological theory inspired me at the time to reflect on three questions that were related to the session's theme. First, if Marxist political economy and affiliated critical discourses are *falling* by losing their prominent foundational and theoretical status in the social sciences, how is it that they are also resurfacing in rather unfamiliar places, such as gerontological studies of social aging? Second, in what ways does this resurfacing of major critical discourses serve to enliven professional fields, in this case, the constitution of a critical gerontology? Third, compared to other established areas in the humanities and social sciences, what are the institutional and intellectual means by which new critical elements in the professional fields are incorporated and promoted?

Since the conference these questions have continued to be of great interest, and here I would like to highlight their relevance to a discussion of critical gerontological theory.

In the three sections and conclusions of this essay I borrow from the theoretical work of French sociologist Pierre Bourdieu and philosophers Gilles Deleuze and Félix Guattari to address critical gerontology as a pragmatic and nomadic *thought-space* across which ideas flow and become exchanged, rather than as a kind of model, theory, or method. By depicting critical gerontology as a thought-space, a magnetic field where thought collects, converges, and transverses disciplines and traditions, I also wish to distance it from ongoing assumptions about multidisciplinarity in gerontology, especially the assumption that multidisciplinarity is a precondition for critical thinking. In many ways gerontology is unique because it has embraced the tenets of multidisciplinarity—diverse approaches, plural knowledges, and shared expertise. Indeed, these are seen as the fundamental intellectual resources by which gerontology grew as a profession since the early twentieth century (Achenbaum, 1995). It follows that much theoretical argument in gerontology today, concerned with the critical effectiveness of the field, questions whether or not it has become truly multidisciplinary. However, multidisciplinarity has also furnished mainstream gerontology with a rhetoric of criticality with which to articulate its objectives. As such, since the postwar period, multidisciplinarity has remained the critical hallmark of gerontology because practitioners draw upon its rhetorical appeal to shape their textbooks, curricula, journals, associations, funding organizations, and the overall cohesion of the field's "gerontological web" (Katz, 1996). As Bryan Green says,

> The unproblematic collection of multiple perspectives on aging and the aged into unitary handbooks, textbooks, and readers asserts the objective unity of what they are about. Maximization of variant perspective is indispensable to gerontology in ensuring the objectivity and coherence of its subject matter. (1993, p. 167)

Despite the critical ideals that characterize such studies, therefore, multi-disciplinarity can limit rather than enrich critical thinking about aging in professional and institutional practices. Hence, this chapter looks to other theoretical stories about gerontology, beginning with the one about its "data-rich but theory-poor" state of affairs.

Data-Rich But Theory-Poor: Theory and Critique in Gerontology

James Birren and Vern Bengtson introduced their 1988 text, *Emergent Theories of Aging*, by claiming that gerontology is "data-rich but theory-poor" (1988, p. ix). In the same text Harry R. Moody further states, "the paucity of theory in social gerontology is an embarrassment to academic students of human aging" (1988b, p. 21). Since that time, responsive gerontologists have enhanced the scope and quality of theories in aging in two main ways. First, they have revisited the development of gerontological theory in order to review or debunk its traditional knowledge claims. In the 1990s critical writers produced a series of instructive studies on the various schools of thought, "generations," "phases," or "periods" of theorizing that have emerged in gerontology especially since the postwar period (Bengtson, Burgess, and Parrott, 1997; Bengtson, Parrott, and Burgess, 1996; Bengtson and Schaie, 1999; Bond, Briggs, and Coleman, 1990; Hendricks, 1992; Lynott and Lynott, 1996; Marshall, 1999a). From these we learn how structural functionalism informed disengagement, modernization, and age-stratification theories; symbolic interactionism influenced activity and subculture theories; social constructivist theories of aging built on phenomenology and ethnomethodology; and life course studies combined macro-micro perspectives in the social sciences. Or, as Victor Marshall points out in his creative interpretation of the Kansas City Studies that produced disengagement theory, gerontological theory can be understood in terms of "stories about theories, theorizing and theorists" (1999a, p. 435).

Second, certain gerontological thinkers (discussed below) have introduced ideas from political economy, feminism, the humanities, and cultural studies into their work to establish their critical stance. In the process these thinkers have turned to structural models of social inequality, interpretive and deconstructive methodologies, and international and cross-cultural frameworks to contest gerontology's longstanding emphases on individual roles, masculinist life course models, biomedical frameworks, and liberal political agendas. The resulting books and papers produced through these critiques vary according to their authors' approaches to critical thinking within gerontology. For example, when Canadian gerontologist Victor Marshall first called for "radical" methods in gerontology in the late 1970s, he had in mind the adaptation of symbolic interactionist, phenomenological, and ethnomethodological sociologies (Marshall, 1978). In the early 1980s, when the decline of Marxism dominated the agendas of most of the social sciences, British writers such as Alan Walker (1981) and Chris Phillipson (1982), Americans such as Meredith Minkler and Carroll Estes (1984), and Canadians such as John Myles (1984) along with others (e.g., Olson, 1982) broke with traditional gerontological studies by establishing a political economy of aging. Specifically, their work focussed both on the history of capitalist production and the division of labour and on the political foundations of population aging and the welfare state. They criticized as well what Carroll Estes calls the "aging enterprise," that is, the conglomeration of experts, institutions, and professions that arose in the latter half of the twentieth century to cater to individual needs while neglecting their underlying historical and structural sources (Estes, 1979). However, the political economy of aging does not represent a meta-theoretical endorsement of Marxism; indeed, Marx is hardly referred to in the literature. Rather, the political economists merge selected aspects of Marxist theory with gerontological concerns in a creative bridging of theoretical discourse with professional practice.

In the late 1980s and 1990s the political economy of aging expanded by underscoring gender, regional, racial, and ethnic inequalities. This move gave gerontological theorists a wider foundation on which to build the parameters of a critical gerontology. An early example is the paper by Chris Phillipson and Alan Walker, "The Case for a Critical Gerontology" (1987), where the authors outline a number of feminist, discursive, and micropolitical issues typically neglected in formal political economy treatments. Two journals begun in the 1980s, *The Journal of Aging Studies* and *Journal of Women and Aging*, and later *Journal of Aging and Identity*, also radiated a widely critical approach. The influential text, *Voices and Visions of Aging: Towards a Critical Gerontology*, published in 1993, further established critical gerontology with a potent mix of philosophical, literary, postmodern, historical, and scientific commentary. In the text's "Overview," Harry R. Moody defines critical gerontology in the tradition of the Marxist-inspired Frankfurt School and its sustained critiques of instrumental reason, and "by its [critical gerontology's] intention of locating actual 'openings' or spaces for potential emancipation within the social order" (1993, p. xvii). This is also a direction Moody initiated in his earlier writings (1988a, 1988b) where he explored new critical directions in policy analysis by taking aboard Jurgen Habermas's ideas on the rationalistic colonization of the *life-world*. Habermas uses the idea of life-world in much of his work to indicate a vaguely traditional realm of human resources, communicative practices, and domestic spaces that has become subject to incursions by modern forms of "system" (Habermas, 1991). To support his thesis that modernity has been a process whereby rationalizing systems "colonize the life-world," Habermas points to new social movements whose leaderships use life-world issues such as human rights and environmental protection in place of labour demands for equitable economic distribution to resist global corporate domination. Thus, as Moody and others (Scambler, 2001) have discovered, Habermas's ideas have great value in the area of critical health studies.

More recently, the collection of essays in *Critical Gerontology: Perspectives from Political and Moral Economy* (1999), edited by Meredith Minkler and Carroll Estes, compels its readers to think politically and ethically about age-based inequality, poverty, and injustice as widespread structural problems. As with their former text, *Critical Perspectives on Aging: The Political and Moral Economy of Growing Old* (1991), here the editors fortify their political economy framework with E.P. Thompson's ideas on moral economy and include research papers that target the mostly American state agencies, health care systems, and social security policies that perpetuate these structural problems. In the "Introduction" to *Critical Gerontology* Minkler notes that it consists of two paths: the political economy of aging and the more "humanistic path" where the accent is on meaning, metaphor, textuality, and imagery in aging and old age. *Critical Gerontology* regards the second humanistic path as "an important supplement to political economy perspectives" (1999, p. 2; see also Minkler, 1996); hence, the text appeals more directly to those interested in how political economy research strengthens critical studies of age and gender, race, disability, and class. Students interested in humanistic studies must turn to approaches innovated by Kathleen Woodward (1991) in the United States, Mike Featherstone and Mike Hepworth in the United Kingdom (1991), and others who elucidate the new cultural processes redefining later life based on retirement lifestyles, cosmetic and body technologies, popular imagery, and consumer-marketing (Biggs, 1999; Blaikie, 1999; Cohen, 1998; Cole and Ray, 2000; Gilleard and Higgs, 2000; Featherstone and Wernick, 1995; Gullette, 1997; Hepworth, 2000; Hockey and James, 1993). Chris Phillipson's *Reconstructing Old Age* (1998) insightfully expands Minkler's synopsis of critical gerontology by identifying a third critical path or stream consisting of biographical and narrative perspectives that draw upon metaphysical humanist concepts of self, memory, meaning, and wisdom. In a parallel fashion, Achenbaum (1997), Brown (1998), Katz (1999a), Laws (1995a), and Ray (1996, 1999) discuss the co-development of critical and feminist gerontologies. I would also include within the critical gerontological fold those who, working in the area of Age Studies, explore the alternative, performative, artistic, fictional, trans-sexual, poetic, and futuristic conditions of aging and their radical contributions (Basting, 1998; Gullette, 2000; Squier, 1995; Woodward, 1999).

Studies of metaphorical development and terminology in gerontology have also been important in shaking up conventions about aging (see Kenyon, Birren, and Schroots, 1991). For example, metaphors-turned-concepts such as "male menopause" or "midlife crisis" signify how individual and social aging are intertwined. The term social or cultural "lag" is used by many gerontologists to indicate that negative social expectations of older people lag behind the more positive realities of aging (Riley, 1994). However, when Chicago sociologist William F. Ogburn came up with the idea of "cultural lag" in the 1920s he used it to discuss his observations on the lag between changing women's economic roles inside and outside the home (1957). Nevertheless, the metaphorical strength of "cultural lag" created a theoretical opportunity for gerontology to borrow and critically use the term for other purposes.

On the one hand, these kinds of organizational exercises and reflections reaffirm that gerontological theory is potentially more expansive, flexible, and inventive than the typically instrumental purposes to which it is put in research applications. Although, as Lawrence Cohen wisely remarks on critical gero-anthropology, the traditions of Habermas, Horkheimer, Marx, and others are often invoked in critical gerontology, but rarely engaged (1994, p. 139). Cohen warns that, "through the mobilization of anger and ambiguity, a disciplinary ethos emerges that envisions itself as mission practice against an empty past and writes itself through a mix of applied sociology and romanticized narrative" (p. 146). In other words, to account for its criticality gerontology cannot rely solely on its protective and positive mandate to liberate aging and older people from an ageist world, if it neglects to engage the theories and theorists it invokes in theoretically sophisticated ways. This not only romanticizes the narrative of gerontology's development but can also justify weak theoretical and historical approaches. Rather, we need to extend critical ideas to new areas in aging studies while being wary of relegating critical status to the scholarly politics of a benevolent "mission practice."

On the other hand, these exercises reveal that gerontological criticality is shaped by a destabilizing pattern unrelated to its horizon of critical positions. It seems that the more critical gerontologists attempt to discipline (or multi-discipline) the sub-field by refining its theories of stratification, exchange, social construction, feminism, and political economy, the less stable and more open critical gerontology becomes. In my view, it is this theoretical instability and indeterminacy that articulates gerontological criticality; that is, ideas become critical when they overflow their contextual boundaries, resist theoretical stasis, and accommodate emancipatory projects aside from professional pronouncements about their value and utility. Indeed, the critical force of ideas has much to do with the unpredictable life of the ideas themselves and the careers of those who conceive them, areas to which this chapter now turns.

Intellectual Fieldwork and The Life of Ideas

While social theory appears confined within the covers of texts, biographical or genealogical treatments depict a more contingent and political story about social theory as a form of practice, especially where professional and intellectual worlds meet. The crises and experiments that produce theoretical knowledge involve material contexts where ideas emerge, travel, and mutate. There are many examples in the theoretical traditions to which gerontologists look for inspiration. Antonio Gramsci's *Prison Notebooks* would not have existed without the covert work and risks taken by his partner Giulia and her sister Tatiania while Gramsci was imprisoned (de Lauretis, 1987). Max and Marianne Weber wrote and spoke in Germany about religious cults, race relations, the rights of women, and the moral dilemmas of democratic society after their transformative visit to America in 1904 where they met W.E.B. Dubois and William James (Scaff, 1998). Talcott Parsons's analysis of professional and institutional relationships in his *The Structure of Social Action* (1937) reflects the work of Elton Mayo and Lawrence J. Henderson, the two Harvard researchers in the 1930s with whom Parsons worked and whose Rockefeller-funded program on industrial hazards linked professional sociology to medical and industrial know-how (Buxton and Turner, 1992). Early twentieth-century urban sociology developed with Georg Simmel and Louis Wirth because Simmel lived in central Berlin, the largest metropolis in Europe, when he wrote "The Metropolis and Mental Life" in 1903 and other urban papers, and Wirth lived and worked in bustling, multicultural, and agonistic Chicago when he wrote "Urbanism as a Way of Life" in 1938.

Similarly, there is a great deal to learn about the making of gerontological theory from the lives of its leaders, for example, Bernice Neugarten's account of her career (Neugarten, 1988) or Nathan Shock's intellectual history (Baker and Achenbaum, 1992). Gerontological historians W. Andrew Achenbaum (1995) and Thomas R. Cole (1992b, 1993) also revisit the biographies of pioneering gerontologists Elie Metchnikoff and G. Stanley Hall to explain how they approached problems of aging with more intellectual curiosity, interdisciplinary boldness, and philosophical imagination than those who followed. The political lives of gerontological thinkers certainly play a role. For instance, Robert N. Butler, during a housing dispute in 1968 when he was Chair of the District of Columbia Advising Committee on Aging, introduced the idea of "ageism" to signal the widespread bigotry and injustices faced by older persons (Butler, 1969; 1990). While Butler went on to become the first director of the American National Institute on Aging in 1976, ageism has joined racism and sexism as a valuable critical sociological term.

These are not just biographical details; they illustrate the lived and practical realities behind the social and theoretical questions which we continue to ask today. In a related and very relevant sense sociologist Pierre Bourdieu claims that much of what he does as a theorist can be conceptualized as "fieldwork in philosophy," a phrase he borrows from philosopher John Austin (Bourdieu, 1990a). Philosophical fieldwork has two aspects. First, it is a way of discovering how sociological ideas are composites of different sources and sites. For example, Bourdieu admits his own notion of *habitus* echoes strongly in the works of Hegel, Husserl, Weber, Durkheim, and Mauss (Bourdieu 1990a, p. 12). *Habitus* is a complex mode of socialization that inscribes structural relations into the personal and bodily lifeways of different subjects. To write about it, however, Bourdieu deliberately takes a philosophical ethnographic path to see *habitus* as a compromise between phenomenology, Marxism, and structuralism. Second, for Bourdieu, the philosophical or intellectual fieldworker who traces ideas to the source-worlds of their thinkers also discovers the dynamic qualities of the ideas themselves. Thus, Bourdieu believes that studying theory as a practice and closing the gap between lived and abstracted worlds are crucial to understanding and using theory effectively, reflexively, and critically.

The work of Berkeley anthropologist Paul Rabinow is a good illustration. Rabinow combines aspects of Bourdieu's philosophical fieldwork with Foucault's ideas on the power/knowledge foundations of modern forms of truth. He then ethnographically traces the theoretical components associated with the Human Genome Project in his book, *Making PCR: The Story of Biotechnology* (1996). In an earlier historical text, *French Modern: Norms and Forms of the Social Environment* (1989), Rabinow sketches out the spatializing and professionalizing practices through which *reason* circulated in the making of French modernity in the nineteenth century. Here, along with the police and the state's bureaucracies, the philosophical enterprise of reason and related quasi-philosophical sociologies created the enduring political problems of "the social." Likewise, Barbara Marshall conceptually follows "the travels of gender" as a way of understanding sociology's sexualization of modernity (Marshall, 2001b, p. 98).

If we take Bourdieu's attitude of philosophical fieldwork back to explore critical gerontological theory, apart from the weaknesses of its multidisciplinary rhetoric, identification with radical traditions, and mission practices to liberate old age, what kind of alternative story about criticality might we find?

"The Gerschenkron Effect" and The Nomadic Qualities of Critical Gerontology

At first glance, the overall ethnographic story of critical thinking in gerontology would appear to be a case of what Pierre Bourdieu calls "The Gerschenkron Effect." Alexander Gerschenkron was the Russian economic historian who explained that capitalism was unique in Russia because it arrived so late relative to Western Europe. By analogy, Bourdieu suggests that the social sciences "owe a great number of their characteristics and their difficulties to the fact that they too only got

going a lot later than the others, so that, for example, they can use con-
sciously or unconsciously the model of more advanced sciences in order
to simulate scientific rigour" (1990b, p. 37). For Bourdieu, sociology's characteristics are due in part to the "lateness" of its advancement as a discipline and its problems in translating the precision and (assumed) consistency of the hard sciences into the social field. Similarly, one can see that
the gerontological study of aging, in its embrace of Marxist political
economy and related critical models, has theoretically lagged behind the
other major human sciences which had long ago elaborated such models
only to repudiate them during the 1980s and 1990s in favour of other perspectives. Indeed, an advantage gerontology has had in developing half a
century behind the major social sciences, and thus trailing in critical and
theoretical maturity is that it can recuperate their theoretical innovations
unburdened by their disciplinary constraints.

However, as social gerontology enters its critical phase, it is only partially in the time warp of the "The Gerschenkron Effect" since such an
effect is really a feature of "before-the-fall" rather than "after-the-fall"
theories, to return to my earlier discussion. In other words, "before-the-
fall" theories such as Marxism are still very much with us, but they are
based on the general project of disciplinary progress, unity of knowledge,
and universality of representation. By contrast, "after-the-fall" theoretical
formations derive their criticality less from a cohesive disciplinarity than
from the creative tension effected by the interplay of plural and dislocat-
ed discursive fragments. In this sense, contemporary criticality has been
structured in the shadow of the postmodern fracturing of the moral and
intellectual foundations of modern knowledge formations. This postmodern fracturing features in a number of intellectual contexts, such as
François Lyotard's attack on modernity's "master-narratives" (1984), feminist critiques of biased "malestream-ism" across intellectual traditions,
Foucaultian subversions of institutionalized knowledges as stratagems of
power, and university programs that engage in poststructuralist renuncia-
tions of Western canons and methodologies. Social gerontology's theoretical transformation, in its political economy and critical developments
during the last two decades, therefore, may be an interesting case of how
critical theory in general operates in an "after-the-fall" sort of way. In
brief, the discourse of critical gerontology pragmatically recombines
"before-the-fall" fragments to recast formerly uncritical ways of knowing.
And this process, rather than through multidisciplinary studies alone, is
how and where critical gerontology is becoming a promising new genre
that challenges mainstream gerontology.

To refine and speculate further on the dynamics of critical gerontology in the terms presented above, the discussion shifts to the work of French philosophers Gilles Deleuze and Félix Guattari, in particular their ideas about *nomad science* and *minor literature*. Deleuze and Guattari are members of the wider poststructuralist camp that has celebrated the fall of Marxist and psychoanalytical meta-theory (which Deleuze considers to be an "intellectual bureaucracy"). However, their own way of radicalizing critical thinking is germane to our concerns with gerontological criticality.

Nomad science is a term developed by Deleuze and Guattari in *A Thousand Plateaus*, where they envision distinct "nomad" and "state (or royal)" sciences, separated by a "constantly moving borderline." State science perpetually appropriates the contents of nomad science, while nomad science "continually cuts the contents of royal science loose" (1987, p. 367). State science reproduces state power through the formalization of universal laws and the separation of intellectual from manual labour, as was the case of Gothic architecture. In contrast, nomad science, "which presents itself as an art as much as a technique" (p. 369), is heterogeneous, flowing, discontinuous, indefinite, ambulatory, and potentially radical in its undoing of state science, as was the case of the practices of medieval building associations and guilds. Deleuze and Guattari define the two kinds of science by way of historical example. For instance, differential calculus,

> had only parascientific status and was labeled a "Gothic hypothesis"; royal science only accorded it the value of a convenient convention or a well-rounded fiction. The great State mathematicians did their best to improve its status, but precisely on condition that all the dynamic, nomadic notions—such as becoming, heterogeneity, infinitesimal, passage to the limit, continuous variation—be eliminated and civil, static, and ordinal rules be imposed upon it. (p. 363)

Another case is bridge building in eighteenth-century France, where roadways (royal science) "were under a well-centralized administration while bridges [nomad science] were still the object of active, dynamic and collective experimentation" (p. 365). Hence, bridge building became subordinated to the State and subsumed under its architectural and administrative authorities. In these and their other historical examples, Deleuze and Guattari maintain that:

In the field of interaction of the two sciences, the ambulant [nomad] sciences confine themselves to *inventing problems* whose solution is tied to a whole set of collective, nonscientific activities but whose *scientific solution* depends, on the contrary, on royal science and the way it has transformed the problem by introducing it into its theorematic apparatus and its organization of work. (p. 374)

The distinction between state and nomad science is parallelled by one between *major* and *minor* languages, which Deleuze and Guattari formulate in their work on Franz Kafka (1986, 1990). Major language is homogenizing and tries to stabilize the relationships among meanings, grammatical structures, literary figures, and national subjects. Minor language disrupts major language by creatively using non-major terms and forms of expression, politicizing literature, and inventing new genres. In turn, minor writing becomes revolutionary because it allows marginalized peoples to articulate their contradictory relationship to major cultures in a collective fashion. Hence, Kafka, in mixing Czech and Yiddish with German, develops a minor language in his writing that challenges the major status of German. In theorizing Kafka's work, Deleuze and Guattari praise the minoritarian status of his writing, saying that "there is nothing that is major or revolutionary except the minor" (1990, p. 67) since minor writing provides an escape for language. The authors advise their readers not to "dream" about major writing, but to "create the opposite dream: know how to create a becoming-minor" (p. 68). Furthermore, according to Ronald Bogue, minor languages act "as a literature that has an immediately social and political function; that fosters collective rather than individual utterances; and that uses a language 'with a strong coefficient of deterritorialization'" (1989, p. 116). Hence, a language or a theoretical discourse whose sources are nomadic and minor, and whose form is incomplete and lateral, gains in criticality what it loses in stability and majoritarian legitimation (see Patton, 2000).

The Deleuzoguattarian (Bogue's term; Bogue, 1989, p. 108) position on nomadic and minor discourses is unique because it suggests that "after-the-fall" theoretical ideas and fragments can be critically empowering without resorting to their reorganization along the disciplinary lines of "before-the-fall" schools of thought. Such ideas and fragments can be brought to bear on new investigative areas traditionally regarded as minor and peripheral to dominant fields and can enhance their critical stature and social importance. Examples have been the study of accounting, nursing, the history of statistics, and urban planning. Social gerontology is also such an area because it developed its critical incarnation first through its openness to Marxist political economy and feminism, and later by adding other theoretical fragments to open a critical thought-space for the study of age. But what continues to fill this space does not follow any particular agenda since the nomadic filling of this space *is* the agenda. Thus, critical gerontological projects and texts appear rather messy (Katz, 2000b; Weiland, 2000). They are amalgams of seemingly multidisciplinary but fragmented collections of often unrelated research. Their chapters range from empirical biological and psychological studies, to basic political economy investigations, to cultural speculations on the postmodern life course. This was clearly the case in the development of critical gerontology during the 1980s and early 1990s. For example, *The Journal of Aging Studies* in its editorial policy announces that "it highlights innovation and critique—new directions in general—regardless of theoretical or methodological orientation, or academic discipline." In *Critical Perspectives on Aging*, editor Carroll Estes says that the political economy perspective draws on "all varieties of neo-Weberian and neo-Marxist theoretical developments" (1991, p. 21). The critical work begun in the humanities also took aboard plural and heterogeneous theoretical elements from cultural and literary studies in order to portray the plural and heterogeneous realities of the human life course.

Hence, arguments levelled at framing the constitution of critical gerontology as a special theoretical intervention are difficult to make. Jan Baars, in his paper "The Challenge of Critical Gerontology: The Problem of Social Constitution," tries to introduce a formal sense of critical gerontology by stating:

> Critical gerontology can be understood as a study of aging that takes methodological problems seriously but doesn't *restrict* its criticism to such issues. It includes in its critical analyses normative questions, material interests, the functioning of gerontology itself and other factors that are regarded by the mainstream as only of "contextual" importance. (1991, p. 221)

But Baars misses a point, which is that critical gerontology's criticality does not derive from the coherent, disciplinary, and scholastic attributes characteristic of "before-the-fall" paradigms. Rather, and despite the haphazard and eclectic textual organizations of critical gerontology, criticality is an accumulative effect of deterritorialized political economy, cultural theoretical, and related remnants, which are fractured, diluted, transfigured, and reordered to create a critical resonance within geronto-logical studies.

Bourdieu, Deleuze, and Guattari offer an active theoretical model where ideas live, mobilize, and nomadically congregate in minor dis-courses to produce radical critiques of state and major systems of repre-sentation. Their work implies that the fragmentation of meta-theory need not be apolitical, ineffective, or permanently and postmodernly crisis-rid-den, and that the "fall" of major social science theories can also theoreti-cally revitalize other minor areas. In the process, peripheral areas such as gerontology can and do become important critical zones through which new ideas flow against the grain of scientific tradition and the status of theory itself (see Gubrium and Wallace, 1990) and where new theoretical inquiries into the social construction of aging in late capitalist society are raised. In our case the demographic changes effected by growing aging populations in Western society are set to transform every social institu-tion from the family to the state and resonate through every social and political register. Sorting out the prospects and problems caused by these changes will require both critically powerful theoretical ideas and a strong sense of how they can be sustained in the gerontological field. In the same way that G. Stanley Hall in writing *Senescence: The Last Half of Life* (1922) struggled to understand old age by combining elements from poetry, fiction, psychology, religion, ethnography, and autobiographies, critical thinking today continues to be an open exchange between fields of thought, practice, and imagination. When Simon Biggs explains social policy from a narrative perspective (2001), Julia Twigg examines eldercare "bodywork" and bathing by way of cultural studies of the body (2000), Russell, Hill, and Basser question health promotion programs through critical discourse analysis (1996), and Victor Marshall rethinks the con-cept of "case study" from a reflective and interpretive position (1999b), they along with the other critical gerontologists discussed in this essay join Hall's legacy in making gerontology an inventive thought-space where theoretical solutions to the complexities of an aging society can be identified and advanced.

Conclusions: The Gerontological Imagination

W. Andrew Achenbaum agrees that "'critical gerontology' shapes some investigations of ageing-related problems," but he cautions, "its influence thus far has been marginal" (1997, p. 17). The reasons behind this marginality are not simply intellectual. The predominance of biomedically driven funding policies, the privatization of health care resources, the priorities of corporate and pharmaceutical research, and the popularity of an alarmist demography that blames growing aging populations for the fiscal collapse of social programs—all these contribute to the marginalization of critical thought. At the same time, much gerontological research is increasingly affiliated with governmental projects to *responsibilize* a new senior citizenry to care for itself in the wake of neoliberal programs that divest Western welfare states of their health, educational, and domestic life course commitments and extend their political power to new areas of micro-social management and community affairs (Katz, 2000a). Examples are certain health promotion and risk-management campaigns, lifestyle and activity regimes, and self-improvement and lifelong learning programs. The HMOs (Health Management Organizations) in the United States are the most obvious illustration of these forces, but they are also becoming more influential in countries with more socialized public service traditions as well, such as the United Kingdom (Bunton, Nettleton, and Burrows, 1995; Gilleard and Higgs, 1998) and Canada (Broad and Antony, 1999). Thus, social conditions challenge gerontological criticality today just as they did ten years ago when Carroll Estes wrote that "academic gerontology is in danger of 'selling its soul' to mindless, theory less positivism without retaining or regenerating the reflexivity that is essential to the resurgence of the 'gerontological imagination'" (1992, p. 60).

This chapter has argued that, to counter the "danger" of a soul-less, mind-less, and theory-less gerontology, we need to recognize gerontology's critical and practical configurations and spaces (however marginal and minor) and link them to the boundary-crossing nomads, knowledge-hybridizing practitioners and intellectual fieldworkers who would imagine new forms of expertise and advocacy for a new age. Understanding the internal strengths of critical gerontology as a resourceful thought-space is key to accomplishing this task and tackling the political and ideological forces that govern aging and old age in the twenty-first century.

Notes

This essay first appeared in *The Need for Theory: Social Gerontology for the 21st Century*, edited by Simon Biggs, Ariela Lowenstein, and Jon Hendricks (Amityville, New York: Baywood Publishing, 2003, pp. 15-31). It is reprinted here with the permission of the Baywood Publishing Company.

Working on this project also gave me the opportunity to get to know Jon Hendricks and become the beneficiary of his legendary mentorship. I also wish to thank Trent University's Committee on Research for its support of this research. A preliminary essay exploring some of the ideas in this essay appeared in *The Discourse of Sociological Practice* 3(1), 2000.

six

Creativity Across the Life Course? Titian, Michelangelo, and Older Artist Narratives

Stephen Katz and Erin Campbell

Studies of aging have always posed artistic creativity as an enigmatic problem. On the one hand, creativity is considered a facet of maturity and life course development; accordingly, artistic productions are interpreted in relation to the age, biography, and cultural milieu of the artist. On the other hand, the creative impulse is seen to be ageless, or at least adaptable to the pitfalls and impediments of later life. Professional and popular gerontological research has addressed the enigmatic nature of artistic creativity through two opposing narratives. The first looks to statistically ordered comparative data to argue that there are "peaks" to creativity; in particular, there are mid-life peaks after which creativity either declines into unimaginative aesthetic expressions or hardens into static stylistic conventions. Thus, peak-decline patterns are assumed to be observable within the lives of artists and the inventories of their work. The second narrative asserts that creativity continues, grows, and renews itself across the life span and throughout an artist's life in immeasurable ways. As the illustrious careers of Michelangelo, Rembrandt, Picasso, Yeats, Verdi, Goya, Titian, Bertrand Russell, Georgia

O'Keeffe, Stravinsky, Alfred Lord Tennyson, and many other older artists demonstrate, there is no shortage of exemplary creative biographies to support this narrative and enrich the gerontological texts which use it to bolster anti-ageist models of the life course.

The tension between these two narratives is significant to the gerontological humanities because of how it has structured the field's inquiries into aging, artistic production, and late-life style. In other words, by being cast into opposing negative/ageist versus positive/anti-ageist positions, these narratives have come to discipline the gerontology of creativity as an area of major debate. This study examines the discursive dynamics behind the structuring of the debate and focusses on the possible alternative narratives offered by critical studies in the history of art. In so doing we aim to rethink the intellectual, cultural, and historical conditions under which a recognizable older, mature, or late-life artistic style can be said to exist and question what this might mean to our understanding of age and creativity. Our examples are the Renaissance artists Titian and Michelangelo and the final stages of their careers and creative styles. Not only did these artists live long lives, practise their art until the end, and produce fascinating self-reflexive poetry, letters, and self-portraiture, they are also central to modern art history and art-historical notions of old-age style. Indeed, since the inception of art history as an academic discipline, Titian and Michelangelo have remained idealized figures in the canon of "genius" promoted in both current scholarship and the popular imagination about great art. Furthermore, our interest in these artists as elderly public figures is inspired by the marked divergence between the reception of their final works by artists, critics, and collectors in Renaissance and Early Modern societies and the aesthetic standards and heroic biographical accounts by which such works are judged today. By placing these artists and their art more accurately in their specific historical and cultural contexts, the study probes this divergence in order to suggest a different vision of the strategic representations of the aged genius artist in gerontological thinking on creativity.

Narratives on Age and Creativity

Measuring Peak and Decline

Harvey Lehman's *Age and Achievement* (1953) is often cited as the epitome of the peak-and-decline narrative about creativity. Based on research done in the 1930s, Lehman claimed that the greatest scientific, artistic, and philosophical discoveries were produced by creative individuals in their youth. Using exhaustive statistical tabulations slanted towards stereotypical great scientific inventions, works of art, and athletic records, *Age and Achievement* projected a series of "performance age-curves" that consistently showed the greatest achievements to have occurred during mid-life, usually before the age of 45 but peaking in the 30s. Decline inevitably followed peak. Lehman was a developmental psychologist who began researching children and was not considered a major psychological figure. However, as Simonton states, Lehman's study "can be considered a minor classic in adult developmental psychology" (2002, p. 71) because of the controversy it sparked about age and creativity. Wayne Dennis (1956, 1966) was the first to attack Lehman, pointing out his methodological flaws and the gerontophobic biases built into his standards of measurement and choice of cultural achievements. Other critics eagerly lined up to castigate *Age and Achievement* as an example of a negative discourse on aging which tethered creativity to a limited stage model of life course development.[1]

In narrative terms, Lehman's work was a reinstatement of an older problem about the possibility of correlating creativity with age in a methodological rigorous way. This problem goes back to Adolphe Quételet's (1796-1874) historic statistical survey, *A Treatise on Man and the Development of His Faculties* (1842), which developed the norms and variations of the "average man" and situated the onset of old age between 60-65 years. Quételet also affixed patterns of achievement and decline in age variations to what he considered to be the laws of demographic probability. Francis Galton, taken by Quételet's statistical approach, likewise introduced his idea of artistic genius in *Hereditary Genius: An Inquiry into its Laws and Consequences* (1869), where he tried to measure creative genius in terms of hereditary distribution models. In the United States, the influential physician George Miller Beard contributed to the peak-and-decline narrative with his text, *Legal Responsibility in Old Age* (1874). Ostensibly writing in response to concerns about the circumstances under which elderly persons could be held legally responsible for their actions, Beard begins his study by listing the highest cultural and intellectual achievements according to the age of their creators, concluding that "seventy per cent of the work of the world is done before 45, eighty per cent before 50" (p. 7).[2] Dying in 1883 at the age of 44, one year before he claimed that creativity peaks, Beard never got to experience the old age he so vehemently condemned nor correct the methodologically flawed research by which he plotted productivity inversely against age (see Cole, 1992b, pp. 162-70).

The peak-and-decline narrative resonated in the many treatises, texts, and surveys throughout the nineteenth and twentieth centuries whose authors sought to create a science of calculability around the creative capacities of human productivity. The person most faulted for publicizing the decline ideology, however, was the renowned Canadian physician, William Osler. In his famous "The Fixed Period" speech to the medical school at Johns Hopkins University on February 22, 1905, Osler claimed that the most productive years of life were between 25 and 40, after which time creative accomplishments were few and insignificant in comparison. "The Fixed Period" was the title of Anthony Trollope's novel (1881) about an imaginary society where people over the age of 67 years would be painlessly chloroformed to death. In Osler's words: "The effective, moving, vitalizing work of the world is done between the ages of twenty-five and forty—these fifteen golden years of plenty, the anabolic or constructive period, in which there is always a balance in the mental bank and the credit is still good" (Osler, 1926, p. 398). Yet, even more useless than men over 40 were men over 60. Despite the fact that Osler was reflecting satirically on his own prestigious career (he had come to Baltimore at age 40 when creativity supposedly peaked and was leaving at age 55 close to the age of being utterly useless), the newspapers quoted his words as if he were literally recommending Trollope's ironic solution to the ailments of twentieth-century industrial society. Flooded with critical responses, Osler tried to remain above the controversy from a safe distance at Oxford.

Contrary to the virulent ageism evident in the popular, political, and professional images of modern life, the sciences of geriatrics and gerontology in the early twentieth century aspired to promote a more enlightened understanding of the aging process. Two prominent early gerontologists were Elie Metchnikoff (1845-1916), the immunologist who worked at the Pasteur Institute, and American psychologist G. Stanley Hall (1844-1924). Both men turned their attention to the problems of aging in the latter part of their careers. It was Metchnikoff who coined the term *gerontology* and devoted a large section of his text, *The Prolongation of Life: Optimistic Studies* (1907), to artistic achievement by praising Goethe as a model of long-living active creativity. Meanwhile Hall organized his text, *Senescence: The Last Half of Life* (1922), as a vehicle to explore the human resources with which older persons could forge new and creative roles in the American progressive era. Despite his view that old age was a unique and degenerative stage of life, Hall produced most of his major work after the age of 50, including *Senescence*, which he wrote two years after retiring from Clark University.

While these more positive directions in gerontology would expand in the latter twentieth century, they did not necessarily still the legacy of Quételet's challenge to measure creative genius and limit it to a peak-and-decline model. Research in developmental psychology, with its over-whelming focus on individual achievement, continued to chart life course curves, career trajectories, and probability distributions. Perhaps the best representative of this line of thinking is the work of Dean Keith Simonton (1994, 1997, 2002). Both critical of and sympathetic with Lehman's work, Simonton has promoted a quantitative approach to measuring creative genius according to multi-factored biographical diagrams configured by birth orders, parental loss, siblings, family status, educational levels, mar-ginality and distance to mainstream culture, physical disabilities, etc. He also gives age and creativity a more flexible and interactive relationship, opening up the possibilities for both peak and decline at various points along the life course. To the critics, Simonton still operates within a peak-and-decline narrative because this is seen to be the essential life pattern dominating instrumentalist approaches to creativity. Charting peaks and decline in individual careers to the neglect of historical and cultural circumstances is at the heart of the authoritative rhetoric of mea-surement and predictability. In our view, however, Simonton's work is important because it raises the issue of late-life artistic style. One of the advantages of engaging with the biographical limitations of a peak-and-decline narrative is that it permits Simonton to wonder if "in many late-life styles we can sense the artist expressing deeper thoughts and feelings with more economy of means" (1994, p. 209). In other cases he notes that there is a "last-chance syndrome" (p. 211) whereby artists take on some-thing new before they feel it is too late to do so. Thus, Simonton poses an insightful question about understanding age and creativity through *style*, a question to which we return after reviewing the second gerontological narrative characterized by an embrace of creativity across the life span.

Creativity Across the Life Span

Betty Friedan, reflecting on her experiences attending a major American gerontology conference, describes her impression of the field as belittling of the humanities and dismissive of the possibilities of late-life creativity and personal change (1993, p. 123). She asks "why do we feel such a need to diminish or disparage the very possibility of continued or new creativity in age?" (p. 125). Friedan is right about the humanities not figuring predominantly in scientific gerontology, but it would also be rare today to find a gerontologist from any background who would not agree with her that the image of diminished creativity with age deserves to be contested. Indeed, as we argue, one of the more delicate problems faced by those of us in critical age and art studies is the tendency for the gerontological community to *gerontologize* creativity. By this we mean that the *gerontologization* of creativity effectively reduces artistic achievements to the strategic assumption that, if artists live and work into old age, then their work should be viewed as both unquestionably creative and obviously evincing of the wisdom and power of aging. Contemporary gerontologists and grey activists, with their roots in the optimism of Metchnikoff and Hall, have justifiably attacked negative medical, cultural, and political portrayals of aging that reduce it to problems of illness, decline, and dependency. In their place, they have promoted more positive images around activity, independence, resourcefulness, and creativity. As the essays in this book repeatedly stress, however, this positive vision of aging has created new problems, among them the equating of positive aging with successful aging and anti-ageism with anti-aging (Cole, 1992b; Gullette, 1998; Hepworth, 1995; Katz 2000a; Katz, 2001; Laws, 1995b). Thus, when gerontological conferences, texts, and programs introduce the topic of creativity, they often do so within a narrative of *creativity across the life span* that supercedes individual differences, artistic traditions, and historical contexts.

Specifically, this narrative's focus on creativity shifts it from artistic products and collections to the adaptive human capacity for imaginative problem-solving and coping with the physical and cognitive challenges of aging. For example, in their examination of successful aging and creativity, Bradley and Specht interview older artists and observe, "creative activity is less about the products resulting from the process as it is about the process itself" (1999, p. 467). Artwork, when defined as an expression of self, means that older artists are "less afraid of challenges and the associated frustration" (p. 469) and thus become "role models of successful aging" (p. 470; also see McLeish, 1976). Other researchers agree that artistic creativity builds life skills such as "fluid intelligence" (Moody, 1998) and the ability to respond to adversity (Cohen, 2001). Furthermore, in those cases where the lives of the great artists are considered, the narrative veers into rumination on how their late styles represent an inner flourishing, depth of perspective, and retreat from external constraints. "It is as if the older artist is able to discard mere technical achievement in favor of some essential and elemental quality of art" (Moody, 1998, p. 405). Thomas Dormandy, a medical pathologist and historian, looks at painters who continued to work after the age of 75 and states that "all the case histories point in one direction—the extraordinary flowering of artistic genius in old age" (2000, p. 181). Longevity, in Dormandy's view, brings with it "a slow and mysterious but extraordinarily powerful shift in the inner forces which impel men and women to create" (p. 197), and in later art there "is a commitment to truth" (p. 316).[3]

Clearly the narrative on creativity across the life span pitches a more nuanced and subjective approach to creativity and age in contrast to the quantitative profiles characteristic of the peak-and-decline literature. At the same time, this narrative overlooks how the terms of reference of its humanistic approach are shaped and restricted by the promotional and gerontologizing mandate of positive aging; hence, it shares two crucial problems with the peak-and-decline narrative despite their conflicting frameworks. First, both narratives tend to isolate artistic creativity from its material and often contradictory conditions of production and the historically situated lives of the heroic artists themselves. Second, the structure of the debate imposed by the two narratives provides little room for a critical treatment of the issue of late-life or old-age artistic style. Where gerontological and historical writers on age and art venture beyond these narratives on creativity, they offer new interpretative directions (e.g., Murphy and Longino, Jr., 1998; Kastenbaum, 2000). A notable direction is the work of Amir Cohen-Shalev who considers artistic old-age style and late works of art from a life-span approach (1989, 1993, 2002). While Cohen-Shalev focuses more on the artist than the art, his writings suggest a common ground for art history, the gerontological humanities, life span and human-development creativity theories, and artistic models of old age style to intermingle productively. This is the ground which the second part of the paper sets out to explore by tracing old-age style and artistic biography as cultural problems.

Problems of Old-Age Style and Artistic Biography

The Problem of Old-Age Style

Late artistic or old-age style (OAS) appears to be an inherent and durable essence of the "great works" or "masterpieces" of "old masters"; thus,

OAS adds enormous prestige to the commercial and cultural exhibitions, museums, auctions, and collections in which such works are circulated (see Galenson, 2001). Upon closer scrutiny, however, the idea of OAS is less a manifestation of intentional artistic creativity than a discursive product of art history. In fact, since the emergence of art history as a specialized discipline, OAS has been one of its most influential ideas for interpreting the later-life creations of artists (Clark, 1972; Einem, 1973; *Allen Memorial Art Museum Bulletin*, 1977-78; Held, 1987; Rosand, 1987; Soussloff, 1987). Old age was first associated with a style marked by specific formal qualities with the advent of the formalist approach to the study of art in the late nineteenth century, which coincided with the development of Impressionism and Post-Impressionism. Significantly, one of the earliest studies to devote a chapter to old-age style (*Altersstil*) is entitled *Der Impressionismus in Leben and Kunst* (*Impressionism in Life and Art*) (Hamann, 1923). In the text the author considers the late works of Rembrandt, Goethe, and Beethoven in the context of a broader study of Impressionism as a cross-media stylistic phenomenon.

The formalist impulse to associate old age with precise stylistic qualities received systematic treatment in Heinrich Wölfflin's pioneering theories of the development of form. In *Kunstgeschichtliche Grundbegriffe* (*The Principles of Art History*) (1923), Wölfflin's goal was to systematize the qualities of period late style (*Spätstil*). According to Wölfflin, late style represented a "baroque" elaboration of a preceding "classic" phase of style. He anatomized these changes in the formal vocabulary of style as part of what he believed to be a "history of form working itself out inwardly" (1923, p. 248). For the study of personal OAS, his most consequential suggestion was that the formal changes which he ascribed to period late style were parallelled and reflected in the development of personal style, an idea subsequently tested in Albert Brinckmann's *Spätwerke grosser Meister* (*Late Works of the Great Masters*) (1925). Brinckmann refined the Wölfflinian qualities of late style with the concept of *Verschmolzenheit* (the blending of form and subject), which he arrived at through a study of the final works of artists, musicians, and writers. In succeeding studies, interest shifted to the articulation of a psychology of the formal qualities of OAS (Tietze, 1944; Clark, 1972); for example, Hans Tietze argued that the forms in artists' late works expressed a fundamental difference in the spiritual outlook of old age (Tietze, 1944).

In current research on artistic development, the concept of OAS continues to exert a significant influence (*Allen Memorial Art Museum Bulletin*, 1977-78; Munsterberg, 1983; Held, 1987; Rosand, 1987; Joannides, 1992;

Courtright, 1996). Yet, as David Rosand observes in an editorial statement for the issue of *Art Journal* devoted to the subject: "while apparently a commonplace in art-historical thought, old-age style is hardly a concept that has been subjected to sustained serious examination, nor is it a phenomenon that has been adequately defined" (Rosand, 1987, p. 91). To be more precise about the notion of OAS, Rosand suggests case-by-case empirical studies of the style and physiology of individual artists. With reference to Monet's late works he argues, "we must be able to isolate, define and interpret as students of art the special qualities of brushwork and color and pictorial structure that make relevant the question of the old artist's physical deterioration" (Rosand, 1987, p. 91). Rosand's empirical approach to the late works of artists offers one way to consider the question of creativity in elderly artists, but it also brings to the fore how unreflexively the idea of OAS has been used. In short, the idea of OAS is part of an historical vocabulary of art criticism struggling to classify later works of art. Similarly, the related idea of artistic biography needs to be addressed as a problem of historical discourse.

The Problem of Artistic Biography

The discursive importance of artistic biography in aging studies was mentioned above in the review of professional narratives on aging and creativity. Legends of artistic genius, or what Ernst Kris and Otto Kurz originally called "artistic anecdotes" (1979 [1934], p. 10), also provide a framework in which biographies of older artists' lives come to permeate the understanding of their work and its place in the history of art. This critical problem can be traced back to the tradition inspired by Giorgio Vasari's *Lives of the Most Famous Painters, Sculptors and Architects* (1966) initially published in 1550, the first literary survey blending art and artist within the same grid of interpretation. According to Catherine Soussloff, Vasari inspired the later Romantic notion of artistic genius in the early eighteenth century, followed by German philosophies of cultural production in the nineteenth century (Soussloff, 1997). Hence, "the figure of the artist moves unimpeded through the discourse of art history because he is embedded in the genre of the biography and the assumptions in art-history writing, such as origin and originality, that rely on interpretations of the genre" (1997, p. 109). The artistic biographical genre, therefore, tends to trap older artists in ahistorical, presentist notions about genius, originality, and the problem of old age in general.

Our case study of Titian and Michelangelo attempts to illustrate how late-life artistic style might better be seen apart from the unreflexive notion of OAS and the ahistorical genre of artistic biography. In their place we look to the socio-cultural values associated with *artistic judgement* that situate these artists' final works within the shifting and contingent constructs of aging and old age in the Early Modern period.

Titian and Michelangelo in Early Modern Culture

Old Age, Artistic Judgement, and Early Modern Cultural Production

As this critical survey has argued, the cultural moment of the elderly artist must be part of any account that seeks to use late works as evidence for creativity in old age. Indeed, we hope to show that the modern obsession with creativity masks the social, intellectual, and economic currency of OAS during the Early Modern period. To demonstrate how old age inflects in historically specific ways the value of this currency, this part of our study focusses on Early Modern perceptions of the elderly Titian and Michelangelo, whose final works help define notions of masculine artistic creativity in old age during this period. Our emphasis here is on the reception of artistic judgement, since Early Modern conceptions of artistic creativity sharply differ from those formulated in Modern criticism.

In Early Modern discussions of the creative process, the faculty of judgement was accorded the central role in the creation of art works (Summers, 1987; Cropper, 1984; Summers, 1981; Klein, 1979; Kemp, 1977; Dempsey, 1977; Kemp, 1976). At the simplest level, judgement was the ability to discriminate (Summers, 1987). Such discrimination occurred at the levels of sense and intellect, serving a broad range of judgements from the operations of sense to moral decision. If the act of judgement enabled one to make distinctions on the basis of a standard or mean, then, with respect to Early Modern art, that mean was provided by nature. At the levels of both sense and intellect, judgement was thought to govern all the faculties involved in the process of artistic creation, including imagination, memory, perception, and execution. As the sixteenth-century Italian artist and art theorist Armenini explained, judgement was required at all stages of creativity from conceiving the "invention" (i.e., the story or narrative of the work), to arranging the composition to suit the invention, and, ultimately, to improving upon the model of nature itself through selection (Armenini, 1988 [1587], pp. 15-16).

Artistic judgement could also be expressed at the level of practice via the skillful exercise of the "judgement of the eye." The highest manifestation of judgement in practice was the seemingly spontaneous creation of gracefully proportioned figures, without recourse to laborious measurements. We have to remember that the mastery of the human figure was the central goal of Early Modern art.[4] The consummate display of the judgement of the eye was thus achieved in the execution of foreshortened figures, which brought judgement close to artistic ingenuity or *ingegno* (the Early Modern precursor to the modern notion of genius), so that the creative force of the artist became equivalent to the workings of nature itself (Klein, 1979, p. 165). Such figures made it possible to create the illusion of a three-dimensional figure on a two-dimensional surface, which was the basis for the entire art of painting. The ability to create figures with proportions seemingly beyond measure was proof of the nobility of artists, separating them from the ranks of mere craftspeople. The notion of the judgement of the eye could also be understood in broader terms, as the source of visual pleasure in painting and sculpture achieved by adjusting form not only according to the principles of art, but also to please the eye of the beholder (Vasari, 1962, II, pp. 39-40). It was through such adjustment based on the eye of the artist that personal style emerged (Summers, 1987, p. 30).

If, for the Early Modern artist, the historically specific aesthetic faculty of judgement was the basis of the creative process, there was no actual concept of a distinct OAS in the modern sense. Instead old age was a phase of life to be universally feared by artists as a period of diminished powers, reputation, and earnings.[5] The perception of old age as a problematic time in the artist's career first emerged during the sixteenth century within the increasingly important genre of artists' biographies, in writings by artists, and in the burgeoning discourse on the qualities of artistic styles where the physical and mental decline of old age became a constant theme (Campbell, 2002). It was a critical axiom from the sixteenth through to the eighteenth centuries that an artist's career rotated through periods of youth, prime age, and old age, with prime age or maturity representing the best age followed by the inevitable decline of old age. Indeed, the stigma of stylistic decline in old age was so great that aging artists were advised to retire from practice (Campbell, 2002). Collectors did allow for the deterioration of an artist's mature style in old age to be compensated by a pleasing formal effect, thus according some respect to the possibility that the limitations imposed on artistic style by old age could be transcended. However, unlike both the gerontological narratives of the late nineteenth and twentieth centuries, the primary consideration for Renaissance art critics was neither the chronological age of the artist nor the waning of individualistic creative vitality, but the maintenance and decline of stylistic integrity according to conventional cultural standards. If an artist's style did not change with aging, then old age was not a problem. Age, style, and the power of artistic judgement thus had a special relationship in Renaissance society as can be seen in the different receptions of the later works of Titian and Michelangelo.

Titian and Michelangelo as Older Artists

The challenge that old age represented to the creative process, status, and livelihood of Early Modern artists is forcefully illustrated in Vasari's biography of Titian, first published in the 1568 edition of the *Lives* (Vasari, 1966). Vasari's critique of Titian's final works demonstrates the opprobrium levelled at artists who continued to paint in old age despite the perception of stylistic decline (Campbell, 2003). Traditionally, Vasari's description of the works for Philip II of Spain has been the *locus classicus* for establishing the stylistic qualities of Titian's late style (Vasari, 1966, VI, p. 166). Here, Vasari does not establish the signs of old age in the works for Philip II, which he praises highly; instead, the problematic paintings appear to be the Church of S. Salvatore's (Venice) *Annunciation* and *Transfiguration*, or the even later ones about which Vasari tersely notes that they lack the "perfection" of the artist's earlier works (Vasari, 1966, VI, p. 165). Not only does Vasari express the wish that Titian had never painted them, but he also remarks that it would have been better if Titian had painted merely to pass the time in old age. Implying that the aged Titian should have relinquished his brushes before the onset of physiological decline impaired his ability to paint and even perhaps his judgement, Vasari hints that the artist was motivated by greed in his final years (Vasari, 1966, VI, p. 169). Furthermore, Vasari's disapproval of the aging Titian is thrown into relief by the example of other artists in the *Lives* who are commended for practising their art purely for recreation in old age. Luca Signorelli, for example, is characterized as working "more for pleasure than for any other reason" in his old age (Vasari, 1966, III, p. 638), and Michelangelo's final sculptures are presented, at least in part, as works done "to pass the time" (Vasari, 1962, I, pp. 82, 99). Underscoring the principle that artists should not continue to work in old age, Vasari also quotes Michelangelo to the effect that painting and especially fresco are artistic activities not suitable for the elderly (Vasari, 1962, I, p. 82).

Vasari's criticism of artists who continue to work in old age simply for the market and his corresponding encouragement to artists to retire before the onset of physical deterioration both signal the pressure put on the professional image of the artist by the public spectacle of stylistic decline. Given the prevailing conviction that old age was a period of stylistic deterioration, we suggest that the public display of physical decline drew attention to the manual basis for art, which in turn put into crisis the learned image and identity of the artist. Vasari's censure of Titian's final works in the *Lives* indicates an important critical response to the threat of old age. In addition, Vasari maintained that the Venetian art typical of Titian lacked a foundation in the discipline of *disegno* or design, the method of artistic creation that he believed formed the basis for the intellectual claims of the visual arts. In his theoretical definition of design, Vasari equates judgement with intellect and with *disegno* as both the internal concept (*concetto*) of the artist and the outward expression of the *concetto* "with the hands" (*con le mani*). Vasari does not explicitly state in his criticism of Titian's final works that the decline in style was due to a lack of a proper grounding in the principles of art; however, the belief that old age provided a particular threat to those styles, which were not based on the true principles of art, appears in later sources. Hence, there is a corresponding sentiment that the principles of art, expressed both as theoretical study and *disegno*, are the potential means to ensure the transcendence of old age, a sentiment very clearly represented in the reception of Michelangelo's later works.

In contrast to Titian, Michelangelo was recognized as an elderly artist whose artistic judgement, nurtured in the discipline of *disegno*, resisted the effects of decline with age. The physician and art connoisseur Giulio Mancini, in his unpublished treatise on art written in the first decades of the seventeenth century, developed this theme. In the biography of the artist Tommaso Laureti, (who was *principe* of the art academy in Rome, the Accademia di S. Luca, in 1595), Mancini uses the example of the elderly Michelangelo to argue that aged artists retain the power of rational judgement (Mancini, 1956-57, p. 233). According to Mancini, the decline of the senses and manual dexterity make it difficult for aging artists to practise the figurative arts; however, since elderly artists still retain the power of rational judgement, they may cultivate the abstract art of architecture.

Mancini's text seems to make a virtue out of necessity by promoting the idea that elderly artists retain rational judgement in old age. By contrast, Vasari represents the disparity between judgement and execution in the elderly Michelangelo as a sign of the perfection of artistic judgement. This idea is developed in his account of Michelangelo's inability to complete the Florentine *Pietà* in the 1568 edition of the *Lives* (Vasari, 1962, I, p. 99). Initially, Vasari offers technical reasons for Michelangelo's failure to complete this work. He also acknowledges the problems posed by Michelangelo's old age. Thus, he uses Michelangelo's biography to portray the consequences of aging for artists in general (Vasari, 1962, I, p. 82), and he presents the Florentine *Pietà* in part as work performed by the aging Michelangelo, again, "to pass the time" (Vasari, 1962 I, pp. 82, 99). He even reproduces letters by Michelangelo and the sonnet "*Giunto è gia' l corso della vita mia*" ("The Course of My Long Life Hath Reached at Last") to refer directly to the artist's difficulties with the aging process (Vasari, 1962, I, pp. 94-95, 97, 98, 101). Nonetheless, Vasari also suggests that Michelangelo broke the sculpture because his judgement had become so perfected that it could not meet his artistic expectations, and as a result the artist's concepts simply could not be materialized in sculpture.[6] Hence, in contrast to Mancini's emphasis on physiological decline as the inspiration for Michelangelo's pursuit of architecture, Vasari represents the gap between execution and judgement in the aged Michelangelo as a sign of great genius.

To understand the significance of Vasari's praise of the elderly Michelangelo's judgement in the context of the artist's development, it is helpful to recall Leonardo da Vinci's comments on artistic judgement (Summers, 1981, pp. 226-27). According to Leonardo:

> When one's work is equal to one's judgement, that is a bad sign for one's judgement; and when one's work surpasses one's judgement, that is worse, as happens when a painter is amazed at having done so well; and when judgement exceeds the work, that is a very good omen and a young man so endowed will without doubt produce excellent work. He will compose few works, but they will be of a kind to make men stop and contemplate their perfection with admiration. (Leonardo da Vinci, 1965, pp. 74-75)

In Leonardo's terms, therefore, when judgement surpasses execution it is a sign of artistic genius, and this appears to be Vasari's perception of Michelangelo's judgement. Vasari, however, elaborates Leonardo's observations by placing judgement within the developmental context of the artist's career. Vasari implies that the gap between Michelangelo's judgement and execution begins to develop after the works of his youth, and he alludes to this gap to account for the unfinished works of his maturity. Ultimately, in the context of Vasari's description of Michelangelo's difficulties with the Florentine *Pietà*, the sense is that in Michelangelo's final years his judgement was so developed through experience and age that it far surpassed the ability of the hand to execute.

Conclusions: Towards a Gerontology of Creativity

What does it mean, therefore, that the reception of Titian and Michelangelo's final works is strikingly different? Titian's style was perceived to suffer a decline, and he was criticized for his lack of judgement because he continued to work in old age, while Michelangelo was praised for the quality of his artistic judgement in old age, and his final works were construed as proof of his consummate perfection. This divergence of critical opinion is due to the representational means employed by each artist. Titian's artistic practice was based in the art of colour (*colorito*), which Renaissance critics and theorists claimed relied purely on sensual experience and hence was more susceptible to decline in old age as the senses deteriorated. By contrast, Michelangelo's art was thought to be resistant to decline since, ultimately, his art resided in the intellect and the mental work of artistic judgement. The intellectual basis for Michelangelo's art was provided by the discipline, again, of *disegno* or design, which was the foundation for his training in the arts of painting, sculpture, and architecture. This is why the form of artistic judgement to which Vasari refers in the case of the elderly Michelangelo is of the highest order. It is artistic judgement developed through profound knowledge of the principles of art and through experience, which elevates such judgement to the level of theoretical knowledge in its highest sense. It is close to the "universal judgement" (*giudizio universale*) that unites the arts of architecture, sculpture, and painting with the underlying order of nature itself, which Vasari refers to in the preface on painting in the second edition of the *Lives* (Vasari, 1966, I, p. III). Hence, as David Summers has argued, the portrayal of Michelangelo's artistic conceptions and judgement as resistant to material expression was in fact the greatest form of praise Vasari could offer the elderly artist (Summers, 1981, pp. 226-27), with the unfinished state of the Florentine *Pietà* as the ultimate demonstration.

We propose that this chapter, with its focus on artistic judgement and associated aesthetic values, offers three insights to gerontological research on creativity in old age and older artist narratives. First, by viewing the final works of Michelangelo and Titian through the lens of Early Modern criticism and its divergent receptions, we glimpse something meaningful about the historical articulation of age, art, and the cultural imagination. Second, we might think more critically about the roles played by aging, biography, late works, and OAS, along with artistic production itself and the social relations that confer lasting value on it. Here Pierre Bourdieu's notion of "the field of artistic production" is useful because Bourdieu claims that "'the subject' of the production of the art-work—of its value but also of its meaning—is not the producer who actually creates the object in its materiality, but rather the entire set of agents engaged in the field ... who confront each other in struggles where the imposition of not only a world view but also a vision of the artworld is at stake" (Bourdieu, 1993, p. 261). Lastly, the importance of the late works and lives of older artists goes beyond the strategic uses to which they have been put in popular narratives of peak-and-decline and creativity across the life span precisely because they beckon us to look intensely into the stone and pigment of Titian, Michelangelo, and many others, and behold in their historical dilemmas a deepening of our own questions about the arts of life and the passage of time.

Notes

The ideas for this chapter emerged through an ongoing dialogue over several years with Erin Campbell, assistant professor of European Renaissance Art in the Department of History in Art at the University of Victoria. Erin is one of the few art historians to research aging and artistic representations of older artists. This essay is published here for the first time, and I thank Erin for permission to include it.

1. A fascinating area related to the peak-and-decline narrative concerns the mid-life crisis, especially in the case of the male life course. This idea, developed originally by Elliott Jaques (1970), has been critiqued subsequently in the work of Mike Featherstone and Mike Hepworth (Featherstone and Hepworth, 1982b; 1985a; Hepworth and Featherstone, 1998) and Margaret Morganroth Gullette (1997, 1998).

2. A common feature of the peak-and-decline literature is its ethnocentricism in that the great achievements of the "world" or "civilization" or "humankind" are inevitably restricted to those of Western industrialized societies or their classical

antecedents.

3. Here we are not considering an important and emergent research focus on the relation between older artists, creative style, and dementia. For example, Pia Kontos considers the late work of Willem de Kooning, who died at the age of 92 in 1997, but who suffered from Alzheimers disease through a long period of his later life (Kontos, 2003). Anne Davis Basting also highlights the special creative outcomes possible in cases of dementia in her *Time Slips* storytelling project (Basting, 2001, www.timeslips.org).

4. Also of great importance is what Michael Baxandall, in *Painting and Experience in Fifteenth Century Italy* (1988), discusses as the common experiences of perceptive sensibility on the part of the public who viewed Renaissance art, often based on their knowledge of other kinds of artistic skills such as geometrical dancing, narrative forms, or gauging proportions.

5. As to the age an artist would be considered old in the Renaissance, this is difficult to answer since age boundaries were subject to a wide diversity of opinion. In his classic article, "When did a Man in the Renaissance Grow Old?" (1967), Creighton Gilbert presents a wealth of Renaissance sources to determine the chronology for the onset of old age. However, he fails to acknowledge both the diversity of opinion on the stages of aging and the rhetorical role of age chronologies within his sources. For competing chronological schemes and their rhetorical roles, see Burrow (1986) and Shulamith Shahar (1993, 1997, 1998), who argue that cultural texts variably set the onset of old age at 35, 45, 50, 58, 60, or 72.

6. There has been extensive scholarship on this work; for example, see the bibliographies in Leo Steinberg's two articles (Steinberg, 1968; 1989). His Freudian reading of the sculpture has attracted the most attention; however, here we are dealing with contemporary reception rather than psychological motivation.

PART TWO: LIFESTYLE AND THE FASHIONING OF SENIOR WORLDS

seven

Busy Bodies: Activity, Aging, and the Management of Everyday Life

The association of activity with well-being in old age seems so obvious and indisputable that questioning it within gerontological circles would be considered unprofessional, if not heretical. The notion of activity, a recurring motif in popular treatises on longevity since the Enlightenment, today serves as an antidote to pessimistic stereotypes of decline and dependency. Indeed, Francis Bacon's nostrum that older individuals should "live a retired kind of life" but that "their minds and thoughts should not be addicted to idlenesse" (1977 [1638], p. 180), would not be out of place as a credo of modern gerontology and associated health care professions that promote activity as a positive ideal.[1] Activity in old age appears to be a universal "good," therefore. And to prove it, a host of gerontological studies convincingly demonstrates the benefits of physical and social activities to those who must cope with illness, loneliness, disability, and trauma. Out of the many examples in the literature, Patterson and Carpenter (1994) show how greater participation by widows and widowers in leisure activities helps maintain higher morale, while Misra, Alexy, and Panigrahi (1996) examine the positive relationship between physical exercise, self-esteem, and self-rated perceptions of health among a group of older women, the majority of whom lived alone.

However, activity is also a relatively recent conceptual and ethical keyword that has helped to shape gerontology and our understanding of later life. For these reasons, reflecting upon activity's unique intellectual status and practical importance within the field is a worthwhile exercise, apart from elaborating the gerontological nexus connecting activity, health, and successful aging. More specifically, in this chapter I wish to explore some of the critical intersections between activity and regimes of care and lifestyle with a focus on the management of everyday life in old age. In so doing, I seek to raise three questions: (1) what does the concept of activity reveal about the theoretical and empirical means by which gerontological knowledge and gerontological subjects are brought together; (2), how have researchers and professionals formulated activity as an instrument to administer, calculate, and codify everyday conduct in institutional and recreational environments; and (3), what role might activity also play as a resource for those who contest the normalization of old age through activity regimes. Conclusions ponder the wider contexts of activity where the declining welfare state has encouraged neoliberal policies and market-driven programs to "empower" older individuals to be active in order to avoid the stigma and risks of dependency.[2]

But what is activity? Despite the pervasiveness of the term in gerontological research, there is no universal definition or standard science of activity. There are certainly different forms of activity referred to by gerontologists, in particular, activity as physical movement, activity as the pursuit of everyday interests, and activity as social participation. While these forms are studied and promoted both separately and jointly, it is apparent that the idea of activity courses through a gerontological web of theories, programs, and schools of thought whose influence and status are based less on *what* activity means than on *where* it is utilized (which is everywhere). Thus, mapping the circuitry of activity within a field of practices—as a gerontological theory, an empirical and professional instrument, a critical vocabulary for narratives of the self, a new cultural ideal, and a political rationality, among other things—might better account for its widespread appeal in discourses on aging than simply tracing the progress of formal activity models within gerontology. Nevertheless, such models provide a point of departure from which to consider how the idea of activity first entered gerontological thinking and practice.

Activity as a Gerontological Theory and the Problematization of Adjustment

In the postwar period mostly American gerontologists adapted social science perspectives to the study of aging to expand it beyond medical and social welfare models. Two important formations in this undertaking were the Gerontological Society in 1945 and *The Journal of Gerontology* in 1946. The American Social Science Research Council had earlier established the Committee on Social Adjustment in Old Age in 1944. Under its auspices, Otto Pollak published the influential *Social Adjustment in Old Age* (1948). A second text, *Personal Adjustment in Old Age*, by University of Chicago researcher Ruth S. Cavan and her colleagues, followed in 1949. It was an equally significant indicator of the new convergence on *adjustment.* Why adjustment? Not, it seems, because it was developed as a rigorously theoretical concept. The definition provided by Cavan *et al.* that "personal adjustment finds its context in social adjustment" and that "social adjustment" facilitates "personal adjustment" (1949, p. 11) hardly seems to break new intellectual ground. Rather, adjustment was a complex problem that encouraged researchers to explain new social issues of aging and retirement according to the dominant paradigms of the time, such as functionalism, individualism, and role theory. For example, research on adjustment consolidated data on individual adaptation, attitude, satisfaction, morale, and happiness into quantifiable indicators of the problems of aging.

In order to revisit adjustment as a focal point for a wide array of professional ideas and social contexts, it would be useful to consider it as a *problematization* in the sense of the term used by Michel Foucault. For Foucault, a problematization involves a set of practices that transforms a realm of human existence into a crisis of thought. Foucault stated:

> For a domain of action, a behavior, to enter the field of thought, it is necessary for a certain number of factors to have made it uncertain, to have made it lose its familiarity, or to have provoked a certain number of difficulties around it. These elements result from social, economic, or political processes. But here their only role is that of instigation. They can exist and perform their action for a very long time, before there is effective problemization by thought. And when thought intervenes, it doesn't assume a unique form that is the direct result of the necessary expression of these difficulties; it is an

original or specific response—often taking many forms. (1984b, pp. 388-89)

Hence, problematizing practices discipline everyday life by transforming ordinary and sometimes arbitrary aspects of human existence—such as adjustment to retirement—into universal dilemmas that call for administrative and professional interventions buoyed by a politics of "thought." Indeed, Foucault summarized his life's work as a series of studies about how normalizing practices problematized madness and illness (*Madness and Civilization, The Birth of the Clinic*), punitive practices problematized crime (*Discipline and Punish*), and practices of the self problematized sexuality (*History of Sexuality* series) (Foucault 1985, pp. 10-12). In his work on ancient aesthetics and "the arts of existence," Foucault asked: "How, why, and in what forms was sexuality constituted as a moral domain? Why this ethical concern that was so persistent despite its varying forms and intensity? Why this 'problematization'?" (1985, p. 10). Following Foucault we might also ask how, why, and in what forms was active adjustment to old age constituted as an ethical domain, and why has this ethical form become so persistent despite its varying forms and intensity? Addressing this question leads to our tracking the persistency of activity and adjustment in relation to the social problems to which they appeared as fitting conceptual, ethical, and practical solutions, as well as in the professional discourses that framed them as such.

Foucault also argues that the power/knowledge arrangements that arise out of a particular problematization often endure beyond its initial crisis to supplement other political movements. In a related way, the academic focus on individual adjustment eventually lost its prominence as social gerontologists proceeded to cultivate sociological notions of social role, social status, subculture, senior citizen, stereotype, generation, class, ethnicity, and gender. As an intervention by "thought" into the dilemmas of the new labour, welfare, and retirement cultures of the postwar period, however, adjustment, with its cluster of theoretical, practical, ethical, and professional issues, became a benchmark problematization that gave rise to the ideal of activity within aging studies. This emerged most clearly in the University of Chicago's Committee on Human Development's influential project in Kansas City in the 1950s, the *Kansas City Study of Adult Life* that, in turn, led to some of gerontology's first social science theories. The two most consequential were *disengagement* (Cumming and Henry, 1961) and *activity* theories, the celebrated debates with which gerontologists are all too familiar and that do not warrant repeating here, except to note the following developments of activity theory.[3]

On the one hand, activity theory predates disengagement theory. In the 1950s, gerontologists emphasized the importance of activity to the process of healthy adjustment in old age. Havighurst and Albrecht (1953) insisted that old age can be a lively and creative experience and that idleness, not aging, hastens illness and decline. They also targeted for support those services and programs that stressed active participation and integration. On the other hand, during the 1960s and 1970s, critics of disengagement theory consolidated prevailing ideas about activity into a *theory* of activity that jelled with popular and philosophical writing in championing retirement life as busy, creative, healthy, and mobile. For these reasons, the activity position emerged as the winning formula to the problem of adjustment, while disengagement theory was drummed out of the gerontological field and condemned for advocating that disengagement from lifelong activities could have certain advantages. Those who have courageously revisited disengagement or related theories, particularly in connection with research on very old age or death and dying, have proceeded defensively even as they critique the original theory's functionalist limitations (Johnson and Barer, 1992; Kalish, 1972; Marshall, 1980; Tornstam, 1989).

Criticisms made of the activity position and affiliated frameworks are also well known within gerontology. During the 1980s political economists such as Carroll L. Estes (1983) and Meredith Minkler (1984) castigated activity theorists for their narrow focus on individual adaptation and satisfaction to the neglect of larger structural issues and differences in old age based on class, race, and gender. The critical legitimacy of activity theorists that derived from their censure of passive or disengagement models of old age did not extend to a concern with social inequality in areas such as housing, health care, and social security. Cultural critics have also pointed to the kinship between positive activity models of aging in gerontology and consumerist ideologies. For example, David Ekerdt saw the construction of an active "busy ethic" in retirement to be a form of moral regulation akin to the work ethic: "It is not the actual pace of activity but the preoccupation with activity and the affirmation of its desirability that matters" (1986, p. 243). Likewise, what Harry Moody calls the "frenzy of activity" in old age can actually mask, rather than diminish, the emptiness of meaning (1988a, p. 238). Martha Holstein has gone farther to illustrate the sexist implications of gerontological models of "productivity" (1999).

Despite the criticisms, however, the enduring legacy of activity theory is that it provided a conceptual space for the ideal of activity to emerge and circulate expansively within aging studies and among those professions where new roles in recreational counselling, health promotion, and rehabilitation therapy were being created. In other words, activity survives activity theory as a core discourse within gerontological studies for two practical reasons. First, as intellectual capital, activity continues to extend the disciplinary flow between gerontology and old age by coordinating sociological theories, research subjects, academic expertise, and ethical concerns. Second, as professional capital, activity continues to frame the relationships between the experts and the elderly because of what it connotes: positive, healthy, independent lives. In short, activity expands the social terrain upon which gerontologists and related professionals who work with the elderly can intervene while addressing the problematization of adjustment from multiple vantage points. The chapter now turns to this terrain by examining activity's practical utility within institutional and leisure environments.

Activity as an Empirical and Professional Instrument

Ignatius Nascher, the American physician who coined the term *geriatrics*, stated in his formative text *Geriatrics: The Diseases of Old Age and Their Treatment* that while "mental stimulation is the most important measure in the hygiene of the aged" (1919, p. 488), "a walk through an unfamiliar forest path will not alone give physical exercise but will stimulate the brain and cause continual mental exhilaration. Nothing, however, equals a few hours of fishing when fishing is good" (p. 492). Nascher's commonsensical advice seems to advocate contemplative as well as physical forms of stimulation. Likewise, G. Stanley Hall, another pioneer in aging studies, reports on his visits to old age homes in his seminal book *Senescence: The Last Half of Life* (1922). In response to his question, "To what do you ascribe your long life?" residents list a number of reasons: heredity, physical activity earlier in life, good habits, and absence of overwork (pp. 324-25). "One determined early in life to make the mind rule the body" (p. 325). There is no talk in Hall's research, however, of activity schedules or lifestyle standards. In fact, Hall says that his subjects "all praise early retiring and insist that a generous portion of the twenty-four hours must be spent in bed, even if they do not sleep" (p. 327). Again, meanings associated with contemplation and rest are given some priority over meanings associated with continual activity.

As the problematization of adjustment and the ideal of activity emerged in the postwar period, leisure in old age became less associated with contemplative pursuits. This shift was reflected in the work of activity researchers who devised empirical methodologies to measure the aging process in terms of ranked and static categories of behaviour and conduct, often infused with culturally laden values around individualism, family, and senior citizenry. For instance, in *Personal Adjustment in Old Age* (1949), authors Ruth S. Cavan *et al.* create an "adult activity inventory" (pp. 137-42) that classifies activities into five groupings: leisure (including organizations), religious activities, intimate contacts (friends and family), and health and security (p. 142). The activity inventory, together with the attitudes inventory, is supposed to provide the researcher with a methodology to gauge *how* older individuals are adjusting to old age. Again, the fact that terms like adjustment and activity are vague and imprecise takes nothing away from their authority or gerontology's claim to objectivity. The main point, as Cavan *et al.* stated, is that "one general criterion of adjustment is the extent and degree of the person's participation in a wide range of activities such as work, recreation, having friends and visiting with them, family association, membership and status in organizations, and church membership and religious behavior" (1949, p 103). We see here an early rhetorical pattern bound for elaboration and duplication in activity studies. Elements of everyday existence are converted into activities; then activities are classified as scientifically observable facts; these facts in turn become the bases upon which other calculations, correlations, and predictions are constituted.

Another influential study by Bernice Neugarten and colleagues in 1961 attempted to measure life satisfaction by rating and scoring types of activities. In one category, "Zest vs. Apathy," the high scorer is one who "speaks of several activities and relationships with enthusiasm. Feels that 'now' is the best time of life. Loves to do things, even sitting at home. Takes up new activities; makes new friends readily, seeks self-improvement. Shows zest in several areas of life" (Neugarten *et al.*, 1961, p. 137). In the middle is the person who "has a bland approach to life. Does not seem to get much pleasure out of the things he does. Seeks relaxation and a limited degree of involvement. May be quite detached (aloof) from many activities, things, or people" (p. 137). At the bottom is the person who lives "on the basis of routine. Doesn't think anything is worth doing" (p. 137). Thus, the aged subject becomes encased in a social matrix where moral, disciplinary conventions around activity, health, and independence appear to represent an idealized old age (see also Hepworth, 1995).

More recent studies and applications of activity regimes further illustrate this form of subjectification. For example, Tinsley *et al.* (1985) feature a classification of leisure activities that takes the simple and once impulsive act of picnicking and reassigns it to a "compensation" cluster of activities,

> ... the most salient characteristics of which were the high level of compensation and low level of security experienced by picnickers. This suggests that picnicking satisfies the elderly person's need to experience something new, fresh, or unusual. The low score on security suggests that elderly persons do not perceive themselves as making a long-term commitment to the activity but as engaging in it to experience temporary escape from their daily routine. (p. 176)

Tinsley *et al.* also hope that their approach to picnicking and other clusters of conventional activities would be "cost effective in that a leisure program can be developed that provides the broadest array of psychological benefits from a relatively small number of leisure activities" (p. 176). Hence, activities are not just classified but also rationalized as part of a "leisure program."

Key to the management of old age through activity is the reinvention of activity itself. But again, what exactly constitutes an activity in gerontology is more elusive. In *Activity and Aging: Staying Involved in Later Life* (1993), editor John R. Kelly opens his introduction with a straightforward definition: "In this book, *activity* refers nontechnically to what people do" (p. vii). Meanwhile, the chapters that follow correlate increasingly technical types of activities and typologies of leisure with taxonomies of cognitive functioning and life-satisfaction factors. For example, one study organizes activities in bluntly economic discourse (Mannell, 1993). In it there are "high-investment activities" that involve "commitment, obligation, some discipline, and even occasional sacrifice" (p. 127); "serious leisure" activities where "leisure may be no fun" (p. 130); and "flow" activities where skills and personal satisfaction match the activity (p. 132). This study was carried out with 92 retired adults who carried electronic pagers for one week and, upon receiving signals that were given at a random time within every two-hour block between 8 a.m. and 10 p.m. daily, stopped to complete a survey on their experiences (p. 135). Based on the 3,412 self-reports that were produced, the overall message Mannell gives us is that virtuous commitment to high-investment activities wins over pleasurable less-committed pursuits. Also, so-called volunteer/home/

family activities are considered both freely chosen and highly satisfactory with no reference to gender differences.

The *Activities of Daily Living* (ADL) is another standardized framework through which specific physical competencies necessary to maintain an independent life are measured. In turn, ADL indicators are linked with other indices, such as *quality of life* (Lawton, Moss, and Duhamel, 1995). Researchers who articulate and operationalize a variety of local concepts and problems that determine successful aging further use ADL studies. However, there is much more to ADL as the following broad explanation from *The Encyclopedia of Aging* illustrates:

> ADL is central to any assessment of level of personal independent functioning. Information on ADL activity capacity has been used more extensively, and for a greater variety of purposes, than has information from any other type of assessment. It has been used to indicate individual social, mental, and physical functioning, as well as for diagnosis; to determine service requirement and impact; to guide service inception and cessation; to estimate the level of qualification needed in a provider; to assess need for structural environmental support; to justify residential location; to provide a basis for personnel employment decisions; to determine service change and provide arguments for reimbursement; and to estimate categorical eligibility for specific services (e.g., attendant allowances). Accurate assessment of ADL is probably one of the most valuable of measures. (Fillenbaum, 1987, p. 4)

The influence of empirical activity frameworks such as the ADL reaches beyond individual assessment to encompass housing, financial, and service provisions. Thus, activity is not simply something people do, but a measurable behaviour whose significance connects the worlds of elderly people to the largesse of expertise.

Where problems and limitations in the measurement of activity exist, these can become exacerbated when activity is used to schedule and organize life in institutional settings.[4] James R. Dowling, an activity specialist at the Alzheimer's Care Center in Gardiner, Maine, writes in *Keeping Busy: A Handbook of Activities for Persons with Dementia* that while "a good activity program restores a sense of purpose, identity, and control," activity directors "still find some participants who are sleeping, some are wandering, one or two are shouting, and one who is absorbed in disassembling her soiled diaper—but few who join in a carefully planned activity or show evidence of being enriched by it" (Dowling 1995, p. vii). One way to deal with such problems is for "behavior management" to keep the individual constantly occupied: "In a prosthetic, dementia-appropriate environment, behavior management generally means keeping the individual occupied. This, in turn, means being busy enough without being too busy, without becoming overly tired" (p. 4). According to Dowling, group programs may last an hour, but with the rest between often less than 15 minutes and "quiet hour" itself rarely lasting 60 minutes. Although I appreciate that Dowling and others who work with persons with dementia certainly face special challenges, often with limited resources, their exhaustive approach to scheduling also reinforces the point that bodies, to be functional, must be busy bodies.

Activity work is also central to the success of care institutions. As Gubrium and Wallace (1990) pointed out, activity programs provide professionals and activity specialists with a way to measure their own resourcefulness and account for their productivity:

> Fieldwork in several nursing homes and rehabilitation facilities also suggested that there could be an ideological aspect to ordinary theorising. Theories were used that coincided with particular interests. For example, in speaking to activity therapists in several nursing homes, they mentioned the "pressure" they could be placed under if they did not show evidence of participation by patients and residents. According to the director of one department, they "had" to see things in terms of patients being active or they would eventually lose their justification for being, not to mention their jobs. (pp. 139-40)

I have used the representative examples above to argue that activity is utilized to manage everyday life in old age where professionals coordinate the following techniques: empirical classification tables of activities, applications of activity checklists, correlations of activities with other factors in successful human functioning, persistent monitoring of bodily conduct, and unyielding time scheduling. However, management by activity can also inspire resistance to it through anti-activity activities.

Anti-Activity Activities

In reality the totality of life's activities in old age, as with any age, is immeasurable even in institutional contexts. Activities overflow the boundaries of scheduled environments and disrupt the stability of standardized calculations. For example, the activities checklist used in a study by Arbuckle *et al.* (1994) was chosen to predict cognitive functioning in the elderly. According to the researchers, for some activities such as "napping" there is little expectation of a relation with cognitive functioning, but napping is included in order for the checklist to "provide a reasonably comprehensive list of daily activities" (p. 559). On the one hand, napping falls out of the classification system because it does not correlate with anything in particular; on the other hand, there is no way of disregarding napping because it is such a prevalent part of people's lives. In related research, ambiguities also surface because the distinction between passive and active behaviours is often constructed according to the diversity of local circumstances and the interpretive criteria of the researchers. For instance, in their investigation of impaired elders and their caregivers, Lawton *et al.* classified television watching along with resting as a passive category, yet they also admitted that "some portion of television watching is unquestionably active and stimulating" (1995, p. 163).[5]

While the methodological difficulty with translating and codifying everyday behaviour into activity lists presents one problem, the omission of particular activities from the lists presents another. Activity studies are often moored to traditional moral virtues; sex, drinking, and gambling, for example, are rarely registered. Indeed, what many activity checklists indicate as appropriate, normal, and healthy activities for older individuals are those which coincide with middle-class moral and family-oriented conventions. Most neglected are the activities of people who resist normalizing activity practices and inflexible scheduling. In this sense senior centres, which provide activity programs full of tours, hobbies, and reports, can double as the sites where elderly clientele challenge the activity-driven management of their lives (see Hazan, 1986). An ethnographic treatment of the active "social worlds of the aged" invisible to social science research (Unruh, 1983) and a penetrating study of aging political activists in the United Kingdom (Andrews, 1991) also demonstrated that older people engage in a variety of socially productive activities not necessarily limited to the measurable individual activities promoted by gerontologists and professionals in research journals such as

Activities, Adaptation, and Aging (launched by The Haworth Press in 1980) and mostly linked to minimizing the risks of dependency.

Equally significant and overlooked are the *conceptual* activities of elderly persons who construct their own analytical models of later life based not on gerontological theories or activity schedules, but on the lived experiences routinized in their everyday environments (Gubrium and Wallace, 1990). In particular, as Gubrium (1992), and Gubrium and Holstein (1993, 1997, 1998) have shown in a number of insightful studies, people theorize their lives by translating professional vocabularies into personal narratives. We all extract pieces and elements from standard psychological, medical, and sociological vocabularies and fit them into our daily discourse in order to explain ourselves to others and to address problems that seem to demand some kind of familiarity with professional knowledges. People discussing grief or chronic illnesses, for example, inevitably talk about "stages" of coping. Although such stages are originally a product of academic scholarship, they become embellished, emplotted, and moulded to everyday contexts through social interaction and narrative discourse. Thus, people fracture and recombine the conceptual, practical, and ethical aspects of professional vocabularies in ways that shed new light on both the vocabulary and its embeddedness in everyday life. With these points in mind, in the next section I consider the relation between vocabularies of activity and narratives of active living.

Narratives of Active Living

Narrative gerontologists seek to understand what Kenyon, Ruth, and Mader call "the inside of aging" (1999, p. 54).[6] They show that narratives are more than just biographical stories: they are practices that connect the contents of stories and the circumstances of storytelling to the art of rendering lives coherent and meaningful. What happens to activity as a professional vocabulary when it enters the narrative practices of older people and the inside of aging? Further, if the problematization of adjustment and the theories, ideals, practices of, and resistances to activity management were powerful elements in situating older people in the postwar social order, then how might stories of becoming active senior subjects in this order illustrate the incongruities of activity as the hallmark of responsible living? Inspired by these questions, I recently supervised a project involving interviews with retired individuals who live part of each year in a trailer-home resort on Lake Ontario near Toronto.[7]

When questioned about their plans and ideas for retirement, the respondents frequently referred to activity and activities as key elements in their lives. While they incorporated the professional vocabulary of activity into their stories of retired living, they also demonstrated a keen theoretical understanding of activity as a plural term riven with contradictory meanings. Specifically, as the following examples suggest, older people are sharply aware that the usefulness of activity as a concept is limited by its regulatory and instrumental connotations. And even though they freely participate in a wide range of new and continuing activities, they also understand the potential for activities to be imposed and spliced into a larger ethical regime of self-disciplining in later life.

Agnes, aged 62, worked as a teacher and librarian. Reflecting on her past, she says that: "At first I thought I have to keep going—got to make a contribution—make sure your life is worthwhile. And now I still have to struggle with days when I feel I'm not doing anything." However, she also believes that people are "conditioned" to feel this way and that living in retirement communities can often bolster this conditioning. "If you live in these places [retirement communities] and don't participate you are pressured into taking part. People with the best intentions want you to participate." Speaking of her own community, Agnes says: "I don't feel compelled to be on any of the committees [at the trailer-home resort], but I could be on this committee in town which these [resort] people don't know about and don't care about."

On the one hand, Agnes rightly understands how activity and participation are professional and cultural ideals that condition and pressure elders. On the other hand, she asserts that activities are things which one can choose to do against the grain of overly managed retirement living, as in the case of her joining the committee in town instead of the one at the resort. Agnes refers to this situation again when asked to comment on how lifestyles have changed.

I think, say twenty or thirty years ago someone sixty years [old], especially a woman dressed in browns, navies, blacks and wearing oxfords, stayed in the background and kept her mouth shut, unless you were really weird, like a bird watcher or a mountain climber or something (laughter). [Seniors] still have an interest in life [and want] to be active. Seniors don't just sit in the background and observe, they participate and they are encouraged to participate. Now we see seniors in pastel jogging suits … the "white fluffies." The whole emphasis is not just for seniors, but also for everyone to

be active and participate. This sounds like a contradiction to what I
said earlier, when I said I don't want to take part in activities. It isn't
that I want to be nonactive, though, it is that I want to choose.

While seniors want to be active they are also encouraged to be so,
along with "everyone." The question for Agnes, therefore, is not whether
to be active or inactive, but whether to be active in directed but personal-
ly delimiting ways or in ways that open up her life to new possibilities.

Another discussion with a retired couple, Joe and Dorothy, revealed
how activity was a vital element in their decision to move to Florida
where more year-round outdoor activities are available. Joe's philosophy
of life is also activity oriented: "Busy hands are happy hands. You have to
generate your own energy ... if you are doing something you enjoy, you
seem to find the extra energy to do things. If something happened like
you had a stroke, you could find things. Like if I could play chess or read
a book and that's all I could do, I would still be active." Meanwhile,
Dorothy recounts her perception of their retirement community in
Florida:

We live in a community in Florida and some of the people there
are what I call institutionalized. Now this is what I call the
thing. They tell you we're going to have a pancake breakfast at
eight o'clock on Wednesday, now all you little seniors have
nothing to do. Everyone gather here at eight, see.... We live
there, we hardly do anything in there, we have a lot of lovely
friends and we enjoy their company at home. I went to school
as a child, I don't want to go back to that as a senior. [Laughing]
Now we're going to clap our hands and going to go like this.

   That is what this lifestyle [referring to the more organized
communities] communicates to me, because that's what they call
them down there [Florida]. There are people who have been in
that park for eight years that cannot believe that we know the
mayor down in our town there, that we know people at the
country club, that we know the poorest people on the street.
They say, "How do you meet them?" You just get out of this little community here and you go. That is the awful part about
this.

Joe interjects: "You see some of the parks down there [Florida], they have
Recreational Directors and they have programs set up for every day of

the week whether it be bingo, shuffle board, or dance." Dorothy adds,

> You have no idea, exercise, it's just like you were back at school, as if
> you're such imbeciles you couldn't think of a thing to do yourself.
> When people say, oh you should take line dancing; I say oh, I'm not
> old enough. Inside this body, that may look like it's aging to you, is
> still a fourteen-year-old screaming to get out.

Joe and Dorothy are obviously critical of regulated activity programs
that transform communities into school-like institutions (according to
Dorothy). Yet the couple also agrees that being active in retirement is
progressive. When asked about generational relations, Dorothy replied,
"Sometimes I see the next generation being even more active than we are,
and then I see some of them revert back to when granny was in the rocking chair." Joe and Dorothy understand themselves as part of a transitional generation in a changing demographic and increasingly aging society.
The challenges they face in avoiding scheduled environments while
experimenting with new activities require a dynamic conceptualization
of their lives as active.

A final example is Harriet, who comments on the idea of an "active
senior lifestyle":

> You have to decide what a "senior citizen" is. Do you want to be
> told what to do, when you should go and play golf, when to join a
> group, or do you want to do things because you enjoy them? For
> example, in senior citizen retirement homes your meals are planned
> for you and your company is planned for you. You see it right here
> too, that is, what we would call a senior citizen or active retired
> "lifestyle." I think some people need this retirement lifestyle,
> because they are insecure. They want to have their meals planned;
> they want to be told what to do. This is a good, comfortable way of
> life, but it's not for everybody.

Harriet also remarks that the idea of an active retired lifestyle is attractive because it provides a break from handling children, especially since
she had small children around her up to the age of sixty-five.

> What we liked most was, number one, it was an active retired
> lifestyle. This means that I didn't need all the little kids around, but
> I like to sit out on the deck and hear them in the park. I like to walk

down there and see them with their bikes and everything. I didn't want to be placed in a portion of the park where you never heard a young child again. I just didn't want them crawling around the trailer. So for us it was the best of two worlds.

Hence, an active retired lifestyle in this case has no one set of meanings, but includes ways of life that intersect along lines of being freed from certain activities, such as caring for children, while possibly being tied to other activities, such as having planned meals and social events.

When the retirees speak of activity, therefore, they narrate and qualify its meanings and images in personal terms even as they adapt it as a keyword in an authoritative vocabulary on lifestyle. Thus, their narrative practices also become theoretical practices as they translate their experiences of activity and social participation into critical reflections on contemporary social aging. In so doing, Agnes, Joe, Dorothy, and Harriet also touch on a larger political issue, which is the association between their negotiated identities as active senior citizens and their participation in an emergent "active society."

Conclusions: Busy Bodies in an Active Society

Most gerontological and policy discourses pose activity as the "positive" against which the "negative" forces of dependency, illness, and loneliness are arrayed. However, retired and older people understand that the expectations for them to be active present a more complex issue than that suggested by the typical positive/negative binarism inherent in activity programs and literature. Specifically, this issue is that, as neoliberal anti-welfarist agendas attempt to restructure dependency through the uncritical promotion of positive activity, they also problematize older bodies and lives as dependency-prone and "at risk." It is not just the medical and cultural images of an active old age that have become predominant, but also the ways in which all dependent non-labouring populations—unemployed, disabled, and retired—have become targets of state policies to "empower" and "activate" them. The older social tension between productivity and unproductivity is being replaced with a spectrum of values that spans activity and inactivity. To remain active, as a resource for mobility and choice in later life, is thus a struggle in a society where activity has become a panacea for the political woes of the declining welfare state and its management of so-called risky populations.

Mitchell Dean (1995) and William Walters (1997) have already discussed the impact of the "active society" on unemployment policies. With reference to Australia, Dean argues that income support for those at risk of long-term unemployment now requires "activity tests" and the monitoring of a person's attitudes, conduct, and social networks. Becoming "job-ready" is a project demanding self-discipline as well as bureaucratic supervision. Yet, the positive spin put on training, entrepreneurship, volunteer work, job clubs, and so forth transforms an involuntary dependency into an imaginary opportunity for career empowerment and self-improvement. Perhaps in a related way we are witnessing today a new mandate to encourage people to be "retirement ready" and "retirement fit" by allying their active, subjective efforts at maintaining autonomy and health with the wider political assault on the risks of dependency.

Again, Foucault's notion of problematization is useful here, especially in his analysis of how the professional knowledges associated with disciplinary forms of power problematized the human body in the nineteenth century. In his text *Discipline and Punish*, Foucault's critique of the "control of activity" (1979, pp. 149-56) focussed on the deployment of scheduling in the pursuit of regulation, productivity, and efficiency. While the older use of timetable "was essentially negative," says Foucault, "discipline, on the other hand, arranges a positive economy; it poses the principle of a theoretically ever-growing use of time: exhaustion rather than use; it is a question of extracting, from time, ever more available moments and, from each moment, ever more useful forces" (p. 154). Furthermore, the new "positive" investment of time in the body also constitutes a new kind of body, "the body of exercise" (p. 155). Thus, exercise is not simply natural but a construction of the *natural in the body*.

Applied to the context of aging and old age, Foucault's critique neatly encapsulates much of what I have been arguing in this chapter. In particular, activity is part of a positive economy that shapes aged subjects within gerontological knowledge and research as knowable and empowerable and inside care and custodial institutions as predictable and manageable. The production and celebration of an active body in old age is a disciplinary strategy of the greatest value. Indeed, it is the construction of the body as active that allows it to become such a productive transfer point in the circulation of intellectual capital and professional power.[8] It is within this disciplinary constellation of knowledge, power, health care, and lifestyle industries and practices, where nonstop activity is meant to take the place of personal growth in later life, and where those "who prefer their inner worlds to the external world" (Kalish 1979, p. 400) are considered problem persons, that many elderly persons find themselves today. Hence, their struggle, as the interviews with retired individuals above suggest, is not simply for better pension plans, housing, and care facilities, but also to reclaim their bodies, subjectivity, and everyday lives from their management by activity. Perhaps we can anticipate, therefore, that the strongest opposition to the political and marketing rationalities governing today's "active society" will come from older, rather than younger, cohorts of people because it is they who are experiencing and critically reflecting upon the professional, practical, and ethical circuitry that links social success to human activity.

Notes

This essay first appeared in *Journal of Aging Studies* 14(2), 2000, pp. 135-152 and is reprinted here with permission of the publisher, Elsevier Science Publishers. I am grateful to E. Suzanne Peters for her assistance in conducting the research interviews and data collection.

1. For synopses of longevity literature see Cole (1992), Freeman (1979), and Gruman (1966).
2. The idea of empowerment as a governmental strategy has been developed by Barbara Cruickshank in her analysis of the American "war on poverty" (1994) and by Chris Gilleard and Paul Higgs in their examination of consumerist discourse in British health care policy (1999).
3. Here and elsewhere (Katz, 1996) my interest is how problematizations in old age, rather than schools of thought, determine the prominence of gerontological theories. However, intellectual history in gerontology is an important and often undervalued aspect of gerontological research (see Achenbaum, 1995). Of the many overviews of the disengagement/activity debates, the most theoretically inventive are by Marshall (1994, 1999a) for his linking the debates to wider disciplinary developments in the social sciences.
4. Critiques of ADL measurements also exist within the empirical gerontological literature because the application and contexts of such measurements are constantly changing. For example, Sinoff and Ore (1997) report that the validity of the Bartel Index for assessing ADL may be limited amongst people over 75 years old because of discrepancies between self-reports and actual ADL performance scores for this age group. In another study Rodgers and Miller (1997) point out that measurement errors in ADL surveys contribute to apparent changes in functional health data.

5. The question of whether or not "passive" behaviours are also activities is an interesting one. Lawton (1993) notes that in cases of physical decline, for chronically ill people house-bound or in institutions, "behavioral space is greatly restricted, but continuity may be maintained through such means as looking at photographs or iconic representations of past behavior, watching the activity of others, or recounting one's past achievements," so that "continuity of meaning may be maintained in the face of behavioral decline. Such mechanisms as fantasy, reminiscence, onlooker behavior, and passive social behavior may supplant the more active forms" (1993, p. 38). In other words, the active production and continuity of meaning can be maintained by rather passive means.

6. See also the special issue of *Journal of Aging Studies* 13(1), 1999, devoted to narrative gerontology.

7. Names of participants are fictionalized.

8. I have not ventured here into the relationship between activity and consumer economies, but the critical literature on travel, cosmetic, leisure, and real estate "gold in grey" markets has been growing (Laws, 1995b, 1996; Minkler, 1991; Sawchuk, 1995). How these markets exemplify aspects of a new "ageless" and "postmodern life course" is also significant (Featherstone and Hepworth, 1991; Featherstone, 1995; Katz, 1999b; Turner, 1994).

eight

Exemplars of Retirement: Identity and Agency Between Lifestyle and Social Movement

Stephen Katz and Debbie Laliberte-Rudman

Critical perspectives in gerontology consistently fault Western welfare states for constructing later life and retirement as negative stages of decline and dependency. Current cultural theorists point to the emergence of a "new aging," described as "positive," "successful," and "productive," and represented by images of independence, social mobility, and agency. However, the "new aging" is built on the ethics and responsibilities of self-care, creating a contradictory culture of aging in the process. While middle-aged and older people are encouraged to develop active and healthy lifestyles to protect them against dependency, where they fail to do so they fall prey to being socially stigmatized as vulnerable and dependency-prone. In probing this contradiction, this chapter raises several important questions about the relation between agency and identity in later life by examining two cases: first, the individualized images of the *retired worker* and *opportunity-seeking consumer*, as exemplars of retiree identities, are drawn from a Canadian newspaper; second, the image of the

Third Age learner in the historical development of the British Universities of the Third Age (U3A) movement is taken up to argue that agency is a potent social force if it is experienced and negotiated as a collective identity. Thus, the promise of the "new aging" and the resolution of debates about agency, identity, and resistance lie beyond the bounds of the privileged site of individual subjectivity to more collective forms of action.

Agency, Structure, Identity, and Lifestyle

The field of sociology, despite its diverse intellectual heritage and divisive schools of thought, articulates its coherence with a tense and durable vocabulary of dualisms—individual/society, macro/micro, positivist/ interpretive, and qualitative/quantitative, among others. As Stephen Fuller comments, "what this does is to confer on sociology a spurious sense of internal divisions, one due more to lack of communication than genuine disagreement" (1993, p. 137). Of these, the most salient dualism in recent years is the one connecting "agency" and "structure," along with the social problems, political bearings, and analytical areas which each circumscribe. While agency refers to subjectivity, resistance, action, reflexivity, empowerment, and mobilization, structure evokes constraint, socialization, power, domination, and social reproduction. Furthermore, social thinkers look to identity and lifestyle as the most obvious theoretical connection points between agency and structure. Thus, sociological perspectives addressing identity can also be typified according to their position along an agency-structure continuum (Baber, 1991; Marshall, 1996). At one end of this continuum, structural perspectives such as role theory or functionalism or certain variants of political economy propose that structural features determine the conditions of identity ascription, over which individuals have little control. At the other end, theories based on the interpretive traditions of symbolic interactionism or phenomenology or ethnomethodology emphasize that individual agents engage in a continual process of negotiating and recreating their identities by drawing upon the social practices and rituals of their everyday worlds (Blaikie, 1999; Marshall, 1996).

This mix of perspectives on identity has inspired many researchers to approach the agency-structure dynamic by addressing individuals and collectivities as social actors who both shape and are shaped by existing social structures (Baber, 1991; Layder, 1994; Lee, 1990). For example, Gubrium and Holstein propose that although individuals constructively narrate "selves" using local and meaningful resources, "features of narra- tive practice may also be formally designated or constrained, especially in a contemporary world replete with formal organizations, interest groups and bureaucracies" (1998, p. 173; see also Gubrium and Holstein 1995). Sociologist Anthony Giddens, best known for his work on structuration theory, has written extensive critiques of dualistic thinkers and their ten- dency to privilege either the action of human agency or the dominance of social structures. Central to Giddens's theory is the concept of lifestyle (1984, 1990, 1991, 1999), a sociological problem first identified by Max Weber and Georg Simmel (see Cockerham, Rutten, and Abel, 1997; Veal, 1993). According to Giddens, the cultural contexts of late modernity and self-identity have become increasingly indeterminate, future-oriented, internally referential, and reflexive. Hence, human agents respond to these contexts by engaging in a "reflexive project of the self," a continu- ous ordering of self-narratives and lifestyle practices within the widening subjective possibilities of post-traditional society. While lifestyle prac- tices appear to flow from individual choice supported by various forms of expertise, Giddens also maintains that such choice is constrained by the structural resources and social systems that configure life chances. The relationship between agency, identity, and lifestyle, therefore, is bound by the animation of choice and reflexivity as social processes.

The theories of reflexivity which Giddens and his French counterpart, the late Pierre Bourdieu, and their associates advance, have also been criticized especially by feminist thinkers for overlooking those areas where post-traditional gendered identities reinstate, rather than disen- gage from, traditional patriarchal relations (Adkins, 1999, 2001; Jamieson, 1999; McNay, 1999). Indeed, in the context of gender the politics of the body refigure how lifestyle and identity bridge agency and structure (e.g., Gardiner, 1995; McNay, 2000). Unfortunately, few feminist theories of agency and structure have crossed over into aging studies (see Bury, 1995; Tulle-Winton, 1999), nor has the work of Giddens, Bourdieu, and others, who highlight lifestyle as a self-reflexive project or an embedded *habitus* through which individuals maintain identity, been systematically applied to post-traditional aging and the life course. Giddens does suggest some starting points, however, by stating,

Self-identity for us forms a *trajectory* across the different institution- al settings of modernity over the *durée* of what used to be called the "life cycle," a term which applies much more accurately to non-modern contexts that to modern ones. Each of us not only "has," but *lives* a biography reflexively organised in terms of flows of social and psychological information about possible ways of life. (Giddens, 1991, p. 14)

Thus, "the lifespan becomes more and more freed from externalities associated with pre-established ties to other individuals and groups" (p. 147). Gilleard and Higgs concur, noting that "only in the late twentieth century has the idea emerged that human agency can be exercised over how ageing will be expressed and experienced" (2000, p. 3).[1] These ideas have been further developed by the pioneering work of Mike Featherstone and Mike Hepworth (as our references throughout this study indicate) who investigate the life course as a focal point for the increasingly powerful role of the cultural sphere in late capitalist society. How critical gerontologists have reflected upon the theoretical and cultural conditions of the new aging is briefly discussed below.

Aging and the Critical Impulse of Social Gerontology

Over the past three decades the critical impulse within social gerontology has targeted the political and structural regulation of aging populations. "Structured dependency" theories, the type of political economy framework that dominated critical gerontological discourse throughout the 1970s and early 1980s, described how state policies and institutional practices, ostensibly designed to improve the lives of older people, at the same time reinforced their dependent, marginalized, and disempowered status (Estes, 1979; Minkler, 1984; Phillipson, 1982). Thus, solutions to the problems of aging were sought at the level of structural change and political resistance. The critics also rebuked micro-sociological and interpretive traditions for their neglect of the macro-constraints, ageist economics, and social inequality inherent in capitalist life course regimes.

Despite the weaknesses of their theoretical perspectives, however, these micro-traditions expanded the domain of human agency within studies of aging. For example, during this period several gerontological theories arose from research on individuals who maintained their personal integrity while coping with decreased physical capacity or the loss of social roles (Breytspraak, 1984; Matthews, 1979). Robert Atchley applied his continuity theory to show that older adults, within socially structured limitations, still employed information management and social strategies to maintain a sense of continuity of identity throughout the life course (1989, 1991). Today we also have exciting developments in narrative and related qualitative gerontologies that further strengthen the subjective dimension within critical gerontology (Basting, 1998; Cole and Ray, 2000; Deats and Lenker, 1999; Kenyon, Clark, and de Vries, 2001; Twigg, 2000).

Clearly the tension between structural and interpretive theories in gerontology reiterates the dualism between agency and structure across the social sciences. Thus, leading gerontologists tackle identity in later life by examining the relational and co-constituting interplay of social forces between agency and structure (Birren, 1995; Hendricks, 2003; Marshall, 1996; McMullin and Marshall, 1999). For instance, Sharon Kaufman's theory of the "ageless self," while posing agency in terms of the symbolic construction of identity through themes of meaning, also asserts that identity development is a dialectical process between self and culture (1986, 1993). Kaufman contends that the ideational aspect of culture, which consists of shared meanings and symbols, provides an interpretive framework upon which aging individuals selectively draw in order to create a viable and ageless self. Cultural gerontologists have gone further to call for a re-conceptualization of critical gerontology itself in order to take account of the changing culture of post-traditional aging (Andrews, 1999; Blaikie, 1999; Cole et al., 1993; Gilleard and Higgs, 2000; Jamieson, Harper, and Victor, 1997; Katz, 1995, 2003; Phillipson, 1998; Tulle-Winton, 1999). They look at the shaping of new aging identities in the context of the fragmentation of the social institutionalization of retirement, advances in life expectancy and longevity technologies, the expanding affluence of aging groups, the blurring of fixed chronological boundaries, and the shift from production-based to consumption-based economies. In particular, what critical gerontology adds to the structurative framework of Giddens and other sociologists who track post-traditional social forms is the unique contradiction between personal freedom and structural constraint engendered by contemporary aging. At the heart of this contradiction lies the superseding of ubiquitous images of decline and negative social roles by new positive ideals of activity, independence, and self-care (Hepworth, 1995; Katz, 2001).

The Contradictory Identities of Consumer Society

If, as cultural gerontologists argue, aging persons are increasingly expected to fashion rewarding identities through lifestyle and self-reflexive
practices, then we find growing evidence of this development in popular
gerontological, biomedical, marketing, leisure, media, and health promotion discourses (Ekerdt and Clark, 2001; Featherstone and Hepworth, 1991;
Generations, 2001; Hepworth, 1999; Laws, 1996; Ylanne-McEven, 1999). In
related academic texts, four common themes feature prominently: (1) a
critical attack on the belief that aging is essentially a disease; (2) a focus
on activity as crucial to individual happiness and health; (3) a celebration
of the possibilities of stretching midlife and postponing old age; and (4)
an emphasis on adaptation skills that reduce dependency on public
health care systems (Featherstone and Hepworth, 1995, Fisher and
Sphect, 1999). According to Kevin McHugh, "to be active in aging has
now attained the status of a societal mantra. The so-called 'third age' of
life is viewed as limitless. Productive activity is the route to happiness
and longevity; to live otherwise is tantamount to a death wish" (2000, p.
112). Applied gerontological research also underlines the social conditions
and individual behaviours that contribute to the attainment of "successful
aging." Thus, a composite professional/popular knowledge has emerged
that elaborates the kinds of productive, physical, ethical, and socially
interactive activities appropriate for aging lifestyles (Holstein, 1999; Katz,
2000a).

A deeper problem with this knowledge is that it appears to support a
"tyrannical" positive aging culture that overshadows the difficulties and
challenges experienced by many older individuals (Blaikie, 1999, p. 209).
Indeed, for those individuals who lack the requisite economic resources,
personal skills, and cultural capital to participate in consumer culture in
successfully agential ways, or for those who suffer irreversible bodily
decline or dependency on others, the new era of aging creates a profound
sense of personal failure and social marginalization (Featherstone and
Hepworth, 1991; Holstein, 1999; Hopflinger, 1993; Minkler, 1990, 1991). At
the micro-level of personal identity, the cultural emphasis on "new
aging" may also heighten the tension between self, identity, and the body
for those who live through deep old age and long periods of frailty
(Turner, 1995). In these cases "the outer body and face can become a rigid
alien structure of imprisonment which can mask forever the possibilities
of the self within" (Featherstone and Wernick, 1995, p. 2).[2]

Thus, the agential freedoms and arts of lifelong learning, financial planning, and retirement fitness assumed by the bearers of new aging identities come with a moral edict to live risk-aversion and self-caring lives. This paradox is evidently part of late twentieth and early twenty-first century neoliberal politics, where empowered communities and agential identities are made to subsidize the de-structuring of the public sphere. The social spaces through which agency, structure, identity, and lifestyle are conjoined have been rationalized along the lines of what Nikolas Rose calls "powers of freedom" (Rose, 1999). In short, power works through freedom as well as against it. For this reason, several critics have conceptualized the "new aging" as a form of governmental rationality, a neoliberal geometry that maximizes individual responsibility in the service of meeting political goals of minimizing dependency and universal entitlements. While the scope of this chapter prevents a fuller discussion of the Foucaultian-inspired governmentality school of thought that informs this kind of critique, we can use two of its basic concepts—*technologies of government* and *practices of the self*—to refine our observations about the contradictory features of new aging identities based on our cases of "exemplars of retirement" outlined in the next section.[3]

Technologies of government describe and make practicable those ideal identities that best express the fit between political and personal goals (Burchell, 1993; Dean, 1999; Rose, 1992). Such technologies operate through the *practices of the self* around consumer and psychological behaviour so as to "autonomize and responsibilize" individuals potentially at risk of dependency and recast them as active entrepreneurs of the self (Rose, 1993, 1999). For example, technologies of government, through consumer campaigns about the need for individuals to secure their future, promote practices of the self that engage in risk-preventive measures such as acquiring insurance or adopting healthy lifestyles (Castel, 1991; Rose, 1999). At the same time, psychological and behavioural skilling, disseminated through instructional courses, self-help manuals, community programs, and the media, reframe the problems of everyday life into manageable episodes and "growth experiences" that require regimes of conduct commensurate with the norms of an autonomous self. Thus, problems previously (and accurately) understood as social and political issues become transmuted into personal challenges articulated by the therapeutically "empowering" discourses of professional expertise (Cruikshank, 1999). As our examples below illustrate, aging and retirement cultures have become rich environments in which technologies of government and practices of the self operate to idealize prudential human agents who take responsibility for their destinies, lifestyles, and projects of self-discovery.

Exemplars of Retirement in the *Toronto Star*: The *Retired Worker* and the *Opportunity-Seeking Consumer*

The following section critically describes, in our terms, two "exemplars of retirement"—the *retired worker* and the *opportunity-seeking consumer*—from a sample of 138 newspaper articles about retirement life published between 1999 and 2000 in the *Toronto Star*, Canada's largest newspaper in terms of readership (on-line *NADBank Survey*, 2000).[4] We are using the term "exemplar" to signify how personal profiles or biographical narratives are transcribed into neoliberal, positive-aging parables about accomplished midlife and older identities.

The *retired worker* is a person who chooses to forego or delay a traditional leisure-based lifestyle by refusing to retire from work upon retirement age. Instead, she or he selects to continue in a midlife job, find a new job, or change jobs in midlife in order to establish a retirement career for later life. The sample articles are filled with anecdotal testimonials to the psychological, physical, and social rewards of working past retirement, while the retired worker is heroized in glowing terms that appeal to readers considering post-retirement work options. For example, work offers "a rhythm and structure to one's life, a sense of identity and purpose, social contacts, and an opportunity to be creative" (*Specials*, 25 September 1999).[5] Post-retirement work is also linked to a youthful mind, body, and lifestyle, epitomized by a photo caption included in an article describing an 84-year-old office courier which states: "FOREVER YOUNG: Born during World War I [and] fought in WWII [this man] vows not to surrender to retirement. He keeps busy now as an office courier" (*News*, 12 December 1999). In these stories happy, busy, and self-fulfilled retired workers are referred to by their "new" successful work roles, such as the "supermarket man" (*Life*, 25 March 2000), the "ageless composer" (*Specials*, 28 October 2000), the "performer" (*Life*, 28 October 2000), and the "entrepreneur" (*Business*, 22 March 2000). This kind of vocabulary emphasizes the freedoms that await the entrepreneurial spirit in retirement who overcomes restrictive age-based identities through productive lifestyle choices.

The *opportunity-seeking consumer* is a person who chooses specific lifestyle options in the consumer market that promise to transform retirement into an opportunity and a "second chance" for self-development and social success; these include, for example, lifelong learning courses, retirement "fitness" skills, Internet classes, and leisure travel. Prominent in the newspaper articles are learning and exploring opportunities because these appear to have multiple rejuvenating benefits whereby retirees can "find a new focus for life after work" (*Business*, 26 November 2000), get "another chance in life" (*Specials*, 25 September 1999) and realize the "joys of opening up to new friends and becoming one of the group" (*News*, 14 October 1999). Texts that feature the opportunity-seeking consumer stress repeatedly the need to match lifestyle choices with personal desires. For example, an article on "mature" learners begins: "Bingo and quilting bees are not for [a 71-year-old woman who says,] 'the drum I beat now is there's more to life than quilting.' 'I don't believe in the old stereotype of retirees'"... (*Specials*, 25 September 1999).

Both the retired worker and the opportunity-seeking consumer are exemplary identities which fit the "new aging" emphasis. On the one hand, they are used to promote different lifestyle agendas and possibilities for agency in later life. For the retired worker a production-based identity is central, while for the opportunity-seeking consumer engagement in learner-focussed and leisure activities are essential. On the other hand, both identities convey to the public how success in later life is an attainable individual responsibility. Readers are provided with the supposedly sad facts about the risks and consequences for those who disregard retirement expertise, choose not to acquire appropriate decision-making skills, and delay the consumption of financial and lifestyle products. Hence, there are penalties and the threat of social censure for those who become "unfit" retirees. In an article entitled "Ambition needs redefining," a clinical psychologist advises readers to change their work attitudes:

> There is this sobering thought: one recent U.S. study showed that eighty per cent of baby boomers believe they'll be working right through their so-called retirement. In other words, it's no longer a sprint, it's a marathon. If somewhere along that race route, you don't redefine your ambition, you're in trouble. (*Business*, 7 October 1999)

Another article about retirees warns that "forty per cent were dissatisfied with retirement." Hence, readers should seek "retirement happiness" by participating in retirement workshops and developing "a plan that will meet your needs and your skills" (*Business*, 26 November 2000).

In addition, we find in these texts that persons who triumph as retired workers or opportunity-seeking consumers are regarded as instant public authorities. For example, in an article entitled "No age limits when it comes to learning," a 66-year-old woman who recently graduated from a college program states, "'You are never too old to give yourself a second chance in life,' she says. 'But you have to take responsibility for yourself and have a self-generated desire to do something new'" (*Specials*, 25 September 1999). A 58-year-old "social whirlwind" who divorced late in life advises readers that there are "101 places to go" in order to "meet your match" (*Specials*, 17 April 1999), and a 62-year-old retiree who recently learned how to use the Internet advises readers to "have a little confidence in your ability" (*Specials*, 19 June 1999). Such expertise also extends to providing guidance on the risks of poverty, a decreased standard of living, inactivity and dependency, and social marginalization, all conceptualized as personal rather than collective problems. The aging individual at risk of inadequate finances is reconstructed as a retired worker who proactively plans a retirement career in a quest to maintain personal financial health, as well as a range of other personal benefits.

One article on the advantages of post-retirement work glibly states, "Here's a way to reduce the risk of outliving your money: Don't retire" (*Business*, 19 November 2000). With respect to social marginalization and inactivity, one man who set up a business after retiring indicated that it is "nice to know that you're wanted or needed. I didn't understand that until I found myself retired" (*Specials*, 28 October 2000). A recently widowed woman who learned how to use a computer in her eighties suggests that "the computer has been her salvation by keeping her connected" (*News*, 29 April 2000). The real success for retired workers and opportunity-seeking consumers, however, is to avoid the risk of aging itself by not succumbing to negative attitudes or behavioral traits that could be interpreted as "old." The articles provide readers with a quasi-sociological forum about expanding positive social trends anchored by the truism that one is never "too old" to do anything: "it's never too late to learn" (*News*, 14 October 1999), "you're never too old to surf ... the net" (*Specials*, 19 June 1999), and age is "no barrier for venture in cyberspace" (*Specials*, 29 April 2000).

From these newspaper articles and their characterization of successful aging identities we can make three important observations.

First, such identities exercise their agency in self-reflexive ways. The first step for the opportunity-seeking consumer is to identify "emotional and work-related needs" (*Business*, 26 November 2000); and the retired worker needs to assess "strengths and weaknesses" (*Business*, 19 November 2000). The mature lifelong learner should first consider how a "lack of confidence" could be overcome through "drive" and the right learning opportunity (*Specials*, 25 September 1999). And retirees of all backgrounds must "work on some feel-good improvements" (*Business*, 26 November 2000) in order to open "up a whole new world" and satisfy their "yearning for knowledge" (*Specials*, 19 June 1999).

Second, as our examples above illustrate, successful aging, good health, activity, independence, mobility, and self-support appear to be the results of responsible individual choice unencumbered by structural or political constraints. At the same time, risk becomes the inevitable consequence of an individual's irresponsible choice or a refusal to become retirement-fit. Numerous articles provide case examples where good choices make for a good life. A 90-year-old variety store owner is described as keeping "a schedule that would tire a person half his age" (*News*, 21 January 2000), a 101-year-old music composer does not have "much to worry about. A cane given as a gift collects dust in a corner" (*Specials*, 28 October 2000), and a 75-year-old Elderhostel participant recently completed "five days of canoeing, swimming, hiking, rock-climbing and 'wolf-howling'" (*City*, 1 October 1999).

Third, the exemplars of retirement embody the contradictory practices of the self that encompass freedom and power, discussed earlier. Aspiring to be a retired worker or an opportunity-seeking consumer appears to be an attractive personal exercise, capable of liberating people and the aging process itself from the negative ageism of retirement conventions. However, such an exercise also intersects life course and lifestyle in ways that satisfy neoliberal technologies of government that reduce dependencies through enforced individual responsibility without recourse to structural resistance. Just as aging Western populations are growing on an unprecedented scale, governments are decreasing the availability of financial programs to retirees (Battle, 1997; Cheal and Kampen, 1998; Kalisch and Aman, 2001; Kemp and Denton, 2003). Just as the retired worker in Canada is promoted as an exemplar identity, policy reform is contracting the use of public pension systems as support to "early" retirees, while favouring an increase in the retirement age and removal of incentives for early retirement (Kalisch and Aman, 2001; Redvay-Mulvey, 2000; Walker, 2000). In Canada, just as the economic status of retirees in general has improved since the 1980s (Hauser, 1999; Statistics Canada, 2000), large numbers of workers in key economic sectors continue to face mandatory retirement regulations and Old Age

Security "clawbacks." In the case of particular groups such as retired widows, there is also a greater likelihood of living in poverty (Klassen and Gillin, 1999; McDonald, 1997; Pulkingham and Ternowetsky, 1999).

Thus, we see that agency in later life, while it is a human quality that is judiciously invested in positive and culturally mandated practices of self-reflection and self-fulfillment, is also an instrument of investment in governmentalized forms of senior and retired citizenry attendant upon such practices. Through their liberating identities and proactive lifestyles our retired exemplars strengthen, rather than resist, the bonds that hold between agency, structure, consumerism, and neoliberalism in the context of new cultures of aging. The next section looks to a different example, therefore, to question whether these bonds can be better challenged if agency becomes a quality of collective rather than individual action.

The British U3A Movement: Agency and Identity in a Collective Context

The preceding discussion suggested that the exigencies of neoliberal cultures are narrowly represented through individual exemplars of retirement, whose later life agency is reduced to market ideals around choice and the "powers of freedom." Thus, agency, structure, and lifestyle function to turn identity inside out, so that the internal biographies of selected retired individuals have become the externalized heroic cultural narratives of successful aging, or in some cases the anti-narratives of failing individuals who neglect or refuse to become accomplished retirees. The discussion below looks at a different context whereby agency, structure, and lifestyle assemble within a context of collective identity and shared lifestyle. This comparative exercise is worthwhile because it proposes that collective agential identities in aging cultures can negotiate structural relations with different kinds of resources and orientations. In other words, perhaps the agency-structure problem is due to the heavy focus of its theorists on privileged, self-reflexive, individual identities to the disregard of collective identities and actions geared to social change.

To clarify this point further, this section of the study looks at *Universities of The Third Age* or U3As as they are called in the United Kingdom. Part mutual-aid society, part social movement, part educational facility, and part lifestyle culture, U3As are a unique organization that give new definition to the "Third Age" itself, a rapidly changing and expansive life course space which, as Blaikie notes, "the term 'retirement' does not wholly elucidate" (1999, p. 70). Indeed, the age markers of the third age, recognized as beginning sometime after 55 or 60, are less relevant than the freedoms and accomplishments that are assumed to distinguish it from younger second and older fourth ages. Part of the uniqueness of the U3As is that they constitute a *new* social movement in the sense that they bear little relation to traditional "grey lobby" or protest movements based on pension reform, social security entitlements, and health benefits.[6] In this sense the senior power behind the U3A movement shares many of its characteristics with that of other contemporary groups who use local and diverse strategies to connect political goals with lifestyle practices in an era of diminishing social supports.

Third Age movements in general have also demonstrated that older populations do not necessarily constitute an unified "interest group," "voting bloc," or "senior citizenry" (Street, 1999), and political participation is often a result of a lifelong interest in all aspects of public culture rather than simply the onset of older age (Jirovec and Erich, 1995; MacLean, Houlahan, and Barskey, 1994). Group memberships crosscut by existing gender, ethnic, regional, and class differences are as consequential in shaping collective identities as those based on age. Most importantly, the politics and agency of older people are not necessarily socially progressive or critical of state policy, as Robert Kastenbaum's poignant account of retired senior voters in Arizona who opposed the creation of a Martin Luther King Jr. holiday in the United States demonstrates (1991, 1993). "Chances are that gerontologists will continue to find employment in exposing and combating ageism for a long time to come. But one never reads or hears about older adults as themselves practitioners of bigotry, racism, discrimination" (Kastenbaum, 1993, p. 166). Thus, agency is not as an essential condition of being aged; rather, agency is exercised in various ways because it is an effect of how older groups of people utilize the contingencies of social life as practical resources.

British Universities of the Third Age may or may not be based in a university. They are programs organized by and according to the interests of people usually over the age of 55. The first U3A or *Université du troisième age* was established in Toulouse, France in 1972, followed by the establishment of The International Association of Universities of the Third Age (AIUTA). The first British U3A, inspired by the French model, began at Cambridge in 1982. Unlike Universities of the Third Age in Europe and in North America associated with university facilities, the British groups are uniquely built on a self-help, mutual aid ethos recalling a more traditional concept of sociality (Midwinter, 1984, 1996; Swindell and Thompson, 1995). Branches are self-governed, decisions are collectively made, and sessions are held in local community spaces and members' homes. No pre-requisite experience or educational qualifications are required for membership, nor are credentials, certificates, or degrees offered. Since the initial U3A was established in Cambridge, the movement has expanded rapidly and currently stands at 540 groups consisting of 141,514 mostly female members, who study, teach each other, and discuss their interests in thousands of courses, which span hundreds of topics ranging across disciplines and cultural experiences.

At first glance U3As seem to be an unequivocal success not only as an opportunity for an inventive and inexpensive adult education, but also as a forum for local social reform. They are a fascinating example of how identity and agency meld as participation in them creates the conditions under which one becomes a Third Ager, a character in a new stage of life where, as the late Peter Laslett and founder of the British U3A movement says, "blanket phrases, which include 'the Elderly,' 'Senior Citizens,' 'The Retired,' and so on, have ceased to be appropriate now that the vital necessity of recognizing differentiation during that lengthy phase of life has become apparent" (1995, p. 10). For these reasons, Laslett (1989) and other key figures in the movement such as Michael Young (Young and Schuller, 1991) have been accused at times of advocating "Third Ageist" cultural and lifestyle priorities over economic and political issues and for glorifying the positivity of the Third Age at the expense of the Fourth Age (see Blaikie, 1999, pp. 184-87; Biggs, 1997; Gilleard and Higgs, 2000, pp. 38-42). Haim Hazan's ethnography, *From First Principles: An Experiment in Ageing* (1996), elaborates the interpersonal discourses and rituals through which Cambridge U3A participants rethink their identities as a kind of "buffer zone" between middle age and old age (p. 33). Members are encouraged to experiment and "abandon conventional parameters of time, space, and meaning and to reconstruct their own" (p. 51). For Hazan, this experimentation also encourages an anti-aging and death-denying atmosphere so that agency leads away from social realities, historical time, and educational enlightenment to a symbolic culture based on "the code of the existential state of the speakers" (p. 148).

Despite the criticisms made of Third Ageism, few studies examine how the establishment of a Third Age identity within the U3A enterprise has been a process of ongoing negotiation and change and how agency emerges as an overall property of collective action. To illustrate these points the remaining part of this chapter outlines three tensions through which identity, agency, lifestyle, and structure dynamically interacted during the U3As' formative years of development. These tensions are:

central vs. local politics, research vs. non-research activities, and commercial vs. educational interests. Most importantly, these tensions, rather
than limiting U3A organizers and participants, have inspired them to conceive of new solutions to the demands for lifelong learning in an aging
United Kingdom where it is estimated that 19.8 million people are aged 50
and over (www.statistics.gov.uk). Thus, we see the U3A learner as less of
an individualistic exemplar of retirement than as a person contending
with life course continuity within a social movement aimed at rattling
second ageist educational systems.

Central vs. Local Politics

In February 1981, Cambridge scholar Peter Laslett, Lord Michael Young
(who was also instrumental in establishing the United Kingdom's Open
University) and Eric Midwinter (talented writer and director for the
Centre for Policy on Aging) met at Cambridge for a seminal discussion of
U3As. Later that year in July, Midwinter publicized in a BBC radio broad-
cast the U3A idea of local groups of retired and elderly people meeting to
teach and learn from each other. He asked for responses, and he immedi-
ately received 400 letters. On the basis of this enthusiastic reaction and
Laslett's drafting of a formational document, "Objects and Principles,"
the U3A founders established a National Committee, secured a Nuffield
Foundation donation, began an experimental "Easter School" at
Cambridge with 75 participants, and initiated a newsletter in 1982. By 1983
The Third Age Trust, to which all U3As belong, was registered as a chari-
ty with eight U3As. It was still a low-key organization, with the first meeting of the National Committee taking place in Michael Young's car in
1982 (on the road from Cambridge to London) and the first executive sec-
retary, Dianne Norton, running the organization out of her home office.
As the movement grew throughout the 1980s, administrative challenges
ensued. For example, struggles for financial support led to the need for
members to contribute modest membership fees. The expanding numbers of U3As also required a permanently staffed, central coordinating
office, and a small London office was founded in 1988.

In 1989 a general meeting was called to revise the Constitution of the
Third Age Trust, with the result that the Cambridge U3A along with
three other groups withdrew from the national organization. Concerned
about the centralization and bureaucratization of the U3A movement and
vexed that the planned expansion of The Third Age Trust would have
few benefits for the largish Cambridge U3A, its then Chair, David Clark,

wrote to the Third Age Trust outlining the Cambridge decision to separate. After that, the Cornwall U3A Forum also fell outside the national
organization's trajectory. These separations signalled that the U3A movement, as with other social movements, had matured to the point where it
was being shaped by the tension between central and local politics.
Hence, locality began to play a key role in determining what kind of
structural form the U3As would take and how memberships could be
identified. In the late 1980s and early 1990s, the National Office moved to
larger premises, launched a Travel Club, and established new sub-com-
mittees on services, conferences, and finance. Today the U3A has expanded its informational and organizational programs through the Internet
(www.u3a.org.uk).

As the U3A movement continues to grow and becomes, no doubt, one
of the largest universities in the world, will this development require
more centralization or create more tension with certain local U3As? How
can the movement, premised as it is on self-help communitarian and popular democratic principles, continue in its accelerated growth to meet a
multiplicity of visions and directions without risking groups opting out?
These issues lead to a second tension about U3As as research units.

Research vs. Non-Research

Peter Laslett's seventh U3A objective from his founding "Objects and
Principles" document is "to undertake research on the process of ageing
in society" (in Cloet, 1993, pp. 16-18). Laslett believed that U3A members
are in an ideal situation to undertake research and publishing that would
counter not only the predominance of second age-generated literature on
the aging process, but would also conform to one of his initial objects to
"assail the dogma of intellectual decline with age." True to his word,
Laslett helped to write the first piece of U3A research at Cambridge in
1984, the text *The Image of the Elderly on TV*, which looked at the negative
effects of TV ageist stereotyping (Lambert, Laslett, and Clay, 1984). Later
in 1990 the Harpenden U3A members undertook a similarly critical project to scour daily newspapers for images and references to old age and
later analyze the results (Midwinter, 1996, p. 37). One of the most interesting research projects occurred in early 1985, when the Centre for Policy
on Ageing and the Community Education Development Centre advised
the BBC on its 12-part series of Dickens's *The Pickwick Papers*. Sixteen U3A
discussion groups organized by Eric Midwinter agreed to watch and evaluate the series. They drew up documentation that the BBC took very

seriously, and while the groups enriched their education in Victorian drama, the BBC learned something new about images of aging by working with some sharp Third Age media critics.

Other research efforts that have come out of the U3As include local historical projects documenting village antiquities and joint programs with the former *DesignAge* of London's Royal College of Art that ran competitions for product innovations geared to elderly consumers. However, most groups produce no research. After all, they are seeking an education apart from formal accreditation institutions, and Laslett's mandate to create an alternative, Third Age research base appeared to be daunting. As David Clark, former Chair of the Cambridge U3A admitted in an interview, research "means going through an awful lot of papers and counting things and messing around with adding machines ... and we're not going to do that sort of hard work."[7] Research, for Clark as well as for others, remains an academic career activity and not something that should be foisted on those learning for pleasure, at leisure. (For Hazan, 1996, this anti-research stance is another example of the U3A ideological denial of the objective realities of aging).

Hence a second tension has emerged between those groups and leaders who promote scholarly production and political engagement and those who do not. Part of this tension hinges on how the U3As envision both their impact on the wider society and their role in representing the Third Age as a social-demographic force. These issues point to a third tension between commercial and educational interests.

Commercial vs. Educational Interests

On the one hand, with the growth of the U3A movement the concept of the Third Age has become respectfully popular as a signifier of a new literate citizenry. The multivolume *Carnegie Inquiry into the Third Age* (1992-93) did much to publicize the cultural, health, and economic profile of this citizenry and, according to the Inquiry, "was prompted by one of the great social achievements of the 20th century—for the first time people have 20 or 30 years of active life ahead of them after finishing full-time work, rearing a family, or both" (*The Carnegie Third Age Programme* brochure). A more telling illustration was the story about then 80-year old Lord Michael Young's new baby in the British newspaper *The Independent* headlined by "Father of the Third Age" (20 January 1996) without further explanation of the term. On the other hand, the concept of the Third Age spread into commercial categories as Third Agers were presumed to constitute a homogeneous and prosperous market group. For the U3A groups, there also developed a number of enterprising activities such as a volunteer-run translation service (The Int/Tran Service) begun in 1992, Dianne Norton's establishment of The Third Age Press in 1994, and a widening network of international leisure, travel, and skills-exchange programs.

U3A members who felt increasingly vulnerable to their redefinition as a marketing target did not always desire such networking. For example, in 1994 Saga Insurance offered the National Committee a deal whereby the company would take on the costs of running and updating the newsletter, *Third Age News*, in return for free advertising space. The deal was decided by a membership vote that favoured the Saga offer for a two-year trial period. Nevertheless, the incident triggered a widespread debate and internal division between those who wanted to keep U3As free from commercial interests and those who saw productive partnerships with the private sector as beneficial to the growth of the movement. In the words of Marion Bieber, one of the founding organizers of the London U3A:

> When you've worked for ten years without ever even considering payment, when you sweated to do everything on a shoestring, and have done it successfully, and when you know that there are the skills and abilities out there in U3A that could run that newspaper standing on their heads … why do we suddenly have to have paid journalists to write articles? We should always limit ourselves to what we can do within the philosophy which we represent. If we can't do it then let's not try.[8]

While the "Saga saga" (as it was called) was eventually resolved, and since 1998 there has been a new U3A bulletin called *Sources*, Marion Bieber's "philosophy which we represent" is still a relevant indicator of the kind of agency/structure tensions upon which the U3A identity was being forged.

To the three U3A tensions we have been describing—central vs. local politics, research vs. non-research activities, and commercial vs. educational interests—one could add others, for example, political vs. non-political actions, or homogeneous vs. heterogeneous memberships. In all these cases agency and identity derive from an expansive set of collective practices riven with the internal tensions of defining a Third Age way of life as well as resisting those external structures that would marginalize it. In a rapidly aging country like the United Kingdom, we have the exciting opportunity to observe how the problems and prospects of British U3As, with their modest origins and having celebrated their twentieth anniversary, are part of a reordering of the relationship between demographic, social, educational, and experiential spheres and a rethinking about what aging and learning can mean to each other. Criticisms are acknowledged; as Eric Midwinter notes, there is "a muted flat note among the melodious songs of praise for U3A. It may be that its very success has allowed the perilous thought to permeate that it is *the* answer" (1996, p. 15).

Conclusions: The Contingencies of Age and Identity

This chapter began by reflecting on the theoretical fit between agency and structure, identity, and lifestyle within the practical context of retirement and Third Age cultures. By examining two illustrative cases, Canadian "exemplars of retirement" and British U3A lifelong learners, we can suggest that this theoretical fit is multidimensional, relational, uneven, and contingent. In the first case, the layering of neoliberal technologies of government with idealized practices of the self creates identities stretched between anti-conformist, inventive lifestyles, and the "powers of freedom" that constrain them. In the second case, the making of identity through collective struggle and local educational politics has resulted in a new social movement whose growth and success overrun the bounds of individualism set by such technologies and practices of the self. From both cases we learn that this new stage of life—retirement or third age or "fresh map of life" (Laslett, 1989)—is an indeterminate identity-zone, where the tension between agency and structure can be observed anew in a society that remains largely hostile to the emergence of genuinely meaningful and empowering older identities. As Chris Phillipson remarks,

> ... the secure place on which to make one's stand may depend, not on the shifting sands of consumer identity, but through the creation of a protected inner core and an external environment that provides both an adequate material base while remaining sufficiently secure to allow experiments with social identity to emerge. (1999, p. 165)

If the coexistence of security, material adequacy, and experimentation is the ground upon which the contradictions of aging identities are to be worked out, then, as sociologists of aging, we have an obligation to contribute our critical skills to this new stage of life where already political, cultural, scientific, commercial, professional, and biographical enterprises are staking claims.

Notes

This essay was written with Debbie Laliberte-Rudman in response to an invitation from Emmanuelle Tulle for a chapter contribution to her edited book, *Old Age and Agency*, (New York: Nova Science Publishers, 2004). At the time, Debbie was completing her Ph.D. thesis at the University of Toronto on the construction of images of retirees in Canadian newspapers. She is now an assistant professor at the School of Occupational Therapy, Faculty of Health Sciences, University of Western Ontario. The project gave both of us a chance to think about the contradictory nature of identity and aging as it arose in our applied work. I am grateful to all the staff and members of U3A organizations whom I met in England prior to writing this essay who generously offered their time and assistance, especially the late Peter Laslett, a true elder-leader. I thank Debbie and the publishers for permission to reprint the essay here in a slightly altered form.

1. Giddens's ideas have some resonance with the substantial gerontological literature on human agency in developmental and life course studies and the role of individual action and choice on the trajectories and transitions across the lifespan (see Settersten Jr., 2002). The prolific work of Glen Elder Jr. (1974) is strongly associated with these studies, beginning with his research on cohorts during the Great Depression in North America. Other gerontologists have specified how human evolution itself would not have been possible without the constant intervention of human action (Dannefer, 1999). As both a social and a biological species "we" have made "ourselves," therefore. While this is a significant literature, our study more narrowly focusses on identity and lifestyle as critical agency-structure problems.

2. Many of these issues are related to the postmodern remaking of midlife identities and "midlifestylism" as vital yet indeterminate categories. Biggs (1999), Gullette (1998), and Hepworth and Featherstone (1998) provide excellent discussions of these developments.

3. Foucault's concept of *governmentality* or "the art of government" (1991, p. 90) and his essays on the genealogy of liberal rule (1981, 1988) have inspired an exciting subfield of governmentality studies (Burchell, Gordon, and Miller, 1991; Barry, Osborne, and Rose, 1996; Dean, 1999; Rose, 1999), as discussed in Chapter Three.

4. This research is part of Debbie Laliberte-Rudman's Ph.D. dissertation, *Active, Autonomous and Responsible: A Critical Discourse Analysis of Canadian Newspaper Constructions of Retirees*, Department of Public Health Sciences, University of Toronto, 2003.

5. References to "Specials," "News," "Life," "Business," and "City" indicate bundled sections of the *Toronto Star* newspaper, not separate magazines or papers.

6. Grey lobby movements and pension politics have a complex international history and impressive record of debates about the making of aging identities (Clifford, 1990; Haber and Gratton, 1994; Orloff, 1993; Pratt, 1993; Vincent, 1999).

7. Interview with Stephen Katz, 18 January 1996. On the academic role of older researchers in a non-British University of the Third Age and other programs, see Glanz and Neikrug (1997) and Lemieux (1995).

8. Interview with Stephen Katz, 14 November 1995.

nine

Forever Functional: Sexual Fitness and the Aging Male Body

Barbara L. Marshall and Stephen Katz

Where old age is the cause of impotence, there is, alas! no remedy, except to submit as gracefully as possible to the decrees of fate, and by carefully husbanding the sexual resources to prolong the usefulness of the genital organs, as far as possible. (F.R. Sturgis, *Sexual Debility in Man*, 1931)

Remember, the norm is that you should be getting it and enjoying it for a long time to come; and if you aren't you should be wondering why. In the great majority of cases, whatever is stopping you can be remedied. (O.J. Seiden, *Viagra: The Virility Breakthrough*, 1998)

To Michel Foucault we owe particular gratitude for shaking human sexuality loose from its familiar historical and intellectual contexts and grounding it in the political and cultural uncertainties of modernity. According to Foucault, sexuality is "an especially dense transfer point for relations of power" and "capable of serving as a point of support, as a linchpin, for the most varied strategies" (1980a, p. 103). Foucault did not include in his captivating reconstruction of sexuality and its bodies, populations, and strategic deployments, that other great somatic resource, human aging. Indeed, Foucault said little about age and one can only speculate as to the ingenuity of his insights on the subject had he lived into elderhood himself.[1] In this he joins other theoretical and historical inquiries that address the different cultures and discourses in which age and sex figure prominently, but generally fail to consider their areas of intersection. Rather, most academic and professional fields, critical and otherwise, accept either the biological tradition, claiming that sexual decline is a natural consequence of the aging process, especially after the reproductive years, or the cultural tradition that favours sexual activity as a prerogative of youth and middle age, but regards it as unhealthy, if not unscrupulous and certainly unsightly, in later life. And while we may have left behind the historically patriarchal, sexist, and gerontophobic values underlying these biased traditions, our new era of feminist and enlightened gerontological consciousness continues to problematize the relation between age and sex via a hackneyed mutual negation that still says: no sex with aging; no aging with sex.

However, if we return to Foucault's inspired ideas on sexuality and elaborate them in relation to human aging, then we can critically extend the inquiry into sexual technologies of embodiment to include the dynamics of bodily time. For example, the critique of modern gendered identities and sexological discourses can be complemented by one that tackles modern life course regimes and human development discourses. Thus, we can expand upon Foucault's thinking and that of his associates on how sexuality was made to operate as points of "transfer" for relations of power and "support" (for the most varied strategies), by understanding sexual bodies also as aging bodies. This would cast new light on that range of human sciences, political rationalities, and moral regulations through which the life of the embodied subject, as both sexed and aged, became a problem of truth. Informed by this broader challenge, we wish to focus in particular on male sexual "fitness" as a pivotal sex/age problematization, around which nineteenth-century patriarchal politics of life (regeneration, population, nation), and later twentieth-century cultures of lifestyle (health, activity, agelessness) coalesced.

We focus on men here for several reasons. First, relatively little attention has been paid to male bodies *qua* male bodies, in contrast to that paid to problematizing women's bodies through, for example, research on the menopause and hormone replacement therapy (Bell, 1987; Harding, 1997; Kaufert and Lock, 1997; Lock, 1998; Oudshoorn, 1994; Palmlund, 1997).[2] Second, the accelerated medicalization and technologization of sexual function in the late twentieth century have been premised upon discoveries about the mechanisms of penile erection, the functionality of which is defined by its ability to penetrate a vagina.[3] More recent work in sexual medicine on female sexual function/dysfunction has developed subsequent to, and in direct relation to, the work on men (and often conducted by the same scientists). For example, there has been an outpouring of research on vascular flow to the female genitalia, which has taken as its blueprint the earlier research on the vascular mechanisms of penile erection and which has created corollaries for "erectile dysfunction" in the form of "vaginal engorgement and clitoral erectile insufficiency syndromes" (Goldstein and Berman, 1998). The concern here is clearly "insufficiency" for penile-vaginal intercourse, evidenced by lack of vaginal lubrication among other reasons.[4] Third, the clinical and market success of Viagra appears to have secured a medicalized understanding of male sexual function entirely outside of reproductive concerns, and its cultural take-up has been proclaimed as nothing less than a "sexual revolution" (Hitt, 2000). As Palmlund (1997) has suggested with respect to the marketing of oestrogens to menopausal and post-menopausal women, drugs are social products, and "much capital, both economic and cultural, is vested to move the products onto the market and to construct robust beliefs that these products are needed for the good life" (p. 159). The lucrative marketing of Viagra provides a unique context for exploring these newly "robust beliefs" about aging and male sexuality.

The first part of this chapter looks at the historical shifts in perceptions and practices around male aging and sexuality from negative to positive ageism and the ascendancy of the status of sexual functionality and potency apart from conventional affiliations with procreation.[5] The second part examines erectile dysfunction as a dramatic and recent indication of a population-wide health problem with increasingly refined diagnoses based on "phases," "early warning signs," and preventative regimes, especially as Viagra has became so widely available. Conclusions ponder the consequences that may arise from the pharmacological and scientific technologization of male sexuality and the consumerist "erectile economy" for the redefinition of mid- and late life course identities in the twenty-first century.

Sexual Decline and the Aging Male Body

Before modern medicine fashioned age as a special problem in the nine-teenth century and applied its biological and experimental knowledges to "discovering" and coding it, there was a long and amusing history of writers who praised the arts of living long lives. Their treatises offered a pot-pourri of commonsensical, mystical, scientific, and philosophical advice, most of which counselled moderation in diet, drink, exercise, and sexual activity itself (see Cole, 1992b; Gruman, 1966; Troyansky, 1989). For exam-ple, Renaissance Italian writers warned that male sexual virility could be affected by diet, behaviour, herbal remedies, heat, and humidity condi-tions, stimulants, excessive sexual activity, and diabolical influences (Bell, 1999). Girolamo Menghi, a well-known sixteenth-century Franciscan exorcist, wrote in his *Compendium of the Arts of Exorcism* (1580) that:

> ... evil spirits may directly attack the penis, rendering it flaccid, or alternatively they may close the seminal canals. Externally, they accomplish the same results by working on a man's imagination, especially by having him eat herbs and other things that are not efficacious in themselves but that lead him to think he is impotent. (in Bell, 1999, p. 52)

Further, Menghi reported that male impotence could be caused by the devil mischievously imposing himself between a man and woman during sexual intercourse, a situation only remedied by the couple turning to rit-ual, pilgrimage, and prayer. Thus, sexual function can wane due to a uni-verse of forces aside from aging—behavioural, dietary, climatic, natural and supernatural, real and imaginary.[6]

One of the earliest scientific reports on the human life span and life expectancy was Francis Bacon's *The Historie of Life and Death* (1638). Bacon advises, "the desire of Venery often stirred up and excited, but seldom satisfied in Act, doth strengthen the heate of the Spirits, and so doe some of the affections. So much of the heate of the spirits, being a cause of long life" (1977 [1638], p. 166). For Bacon, it is sexual desire that benefits the aging process and not the "Act" itself, which is "seldom satisfied." Bacon inspired other inventive medical writers in the eighteenth and early nine-teenth centuries, such as Sir John Floyer (1724), Benjamin Rush (1789), Christopher W. Hufeland (1797), Sir John Sinclair (1807), and Sir Anthony Carlisle (1817), who continued to link the loss of vitality in an aging per-son to a diversity of factors: illness, imbalance in vital fluids, improper diet, poor environmental conditions, moral improprieties, emotional dilemmas, and disharmony between physical and spiritual forces. Aging itself was not necessarily a pathological process, nor was sexual decline precisely identified with it.

While sexual functionality was associated with procreation, in pre-modern thinking the relation between sexual desire and physical health in the aging male body was indeterminate. This relation would become reordered in the nineteenth century, however, as modern geriatric medicine, aging studies, sexological morality, and population politics drew closer together to biologize human development and the life course as precarious and crisis-ridden. One of the clearest indicators of this change was the invention and popular usage of the ideas of "the climacteric" and "the climacteric disease."

The Climacteric

Sir Henry Halford, once physician to King George III of England, is credited with producing the first medical treatise on the male climacteric, "On the Climacteric Disease" (1813). Carole Haber notes that Halford's influential notion of the climacteric as a disease marked by the *abrupt* onset of symptoms, only became popular some decades later when aging began to attract wider medical attention (1983, pp. 69-70). In his repub-lished paper, Halford states:

> The period of the occurrence of this change in men, in general, is so very irregular, that it may be occasionally remarked at any time between fifty and seventy-five years of age; and I will venture to question, whether it be not, in truth, a disease, rather than a mere declension of strength and decay of the natural powers. (1831, p. 4)

As a disease, the symptoms involved a "falling away of the flesh in the decline of life, without any obvious source of exhaustion" (p. 5). Added to this vague diagnosis was the problem of exact determination, since the climacteric was assumed to disguise itself within other diseases and com-plaints. In the end Halford admits that there is no cure: "I have nothing to offer with confidence in that view beyond a caution that the symptoms of the disease be not met by too active a treatment" (p. 13). Nevertheless, the climacteric disease marked the onset of old age and became a widening reference point for behavioural, emotional, and physiological changes associated with it. It also legitimized medical intervention into the lives of aging individuals by problematizing male, midlife aging.

Later George Day, a foremost translator of French and German litera-ture on old age (Haber, 1983, p. 64), supported Halford's contentions about the overwhelming yet mysterious power of the climacteric, noting that it is less common in women because men lead more exhausting and active lives (Day, 1849, pp. 62-63). It is also untreatable, but manageable through diet, rest, and the avoidance of excitement (p. 63). Other geriatric research followed (e.g., MacLachlan, 1863; Skae, 1865), expanding the symptomatol-ogy of the climacteric to include sexual decline, not as a physical prob-lem of functionality but as a moral problem requiring adjustment to the passage of time in the body. After all, in the nineteenth century male sex-ual potency was linked to the idea of semen supply and its procreative power (Gullette, 1994). Reserving one's semen was advisable in order to ensure better sexual capabilities, and for those who lived intensively and lasciviously, the consequences could only be negative—dissipation and pathology. "Doctors did not believe that age in itself was a cause of impo-tence; if there was a problem, excess was the cause" (Gullette, 1994, p. 70). Behaviour, especially restraint, and not biology, was key to sexual health across the life course.

Several experts also noted that the climacteric was beneficial to both women and men because it forced their sexual "natures" to converge (see Hepworth and Featherstone, 1998, pp. 295-99; Von Kondratowitz, 1991, pp. 149-50). For women, menopause and the end of reproductive sexuality were seen as potentially restorative developments.[7] As George Day claimed:

> Women, after they have got through the critical period following the cessation of menstruation, their systems have again attained, as it were, a state of equilibrium, generally find themselves better than in the earlier periods of their adult and middle age. ... In the male sex, the opposite is true. (1849, pp. 54-55)

Furthermore, menopausal women, masculinized and sexually neuter, could expect their "sexual feeling" to decline. Dr. J. Braxton Hicks, in "The Croonian Lectures on the Difference between the Sexes in Regard to the Aspect and Treatment of Disease" (1877), asserts that menopause re-establishes women's health because: "when the change is complete, the woman passes much into the state of one who has had her ovaries removed, having a tendency to revert to the neutral man-woman state" (in Jalland and Hooper, 1986, p. 293). At the same time, for men, the passing into a gentler more "feminine" time of less excitation was seen to be a boon to their overall health. Thus, the challenge for men was acceptance of their diminished sexual capacities. Alfred Scott Warthin, author of *Old Age: The Major Involution* (1929) settles these points about men and women:

> Much of the abnormal psychologic manifestations attending senescence and senility have their well-spring in the failure or maladjustment of the individual to his declining virility. On the other hand, the average senescent female meets the loss of sexual function on her part with equanimity, even with relief, and turns to new activities with zest and pleasure, so that the early years of senescence are often for her a period of revivification. (pp. 109-10)

The main argument here about the climacteric is that it problematized a precipitous transitional life course space, in which the individual was caught between middle age and old age and faced the pathological consequences of senility. As such, the climacteric was the prototype for other scientific models of human development about distinct stages of life that fed into industrial concerns with productivity and retirement and contributed to political debates about pensions and social security. As the forerunner to the male midlife crisis or "viropause" in the later twentieth century, the climacteric also made it possible for the aging process to be shaped by modern expertise in ways that articulated it with the moral and technical ideologies of the time. Above all, the idea of the climacteric was a popular crisis furnishing the public with a decline schematic of male life based on age, useful not only for registering a host of new "age-based" problems, including sexual ones, but also for promoting a culture of rejuvenation and anti-aging technology.

Rejuvenation and Positive Gerontologic Aging

In the early twentieth century the widespread hostility towards aging and old age, fostered by climacteric science, new hormonal research, pension reform debates, the idealization of youthfulness, and the industrial era's expectations of machinic bodies renewed the imaginative appeal of life-extending possibilities. Unlike past ideas about life extension, however, modern rejuvenation and prolongevity therapies had a strongly biological focus that bridged coexistent discourses on eugenics, sexology, and reproductive technology (Squier, 1999). Thomas R. Cole divides rejuvenation therapies, informed by these discourses, into three categories of medical and professional, fringe (quackery), and hygienic reform (1992b, p. 179), although the boundaries between them are blurred. The most famous example in the late nineteenth century was French-American neurologist, Dr. Charles E. Brown-Séquard, who experimented with animal gland extracts and promoted the idea that sex-glandular injections especially had remarkable revitalizing powers. In 1889, at age 72 and citing his own rejuvenation as proof, Brown-Séquard inspired a public sensation about his "method" and "formula," which a drug company marketed in an elixir called "Pohl's Spermine Preparations."

In the early twentieth century, doctors such as French-Russian Serge Veronoff, Austrian Eugen Steinach, and American Harry Benjamin (1959), stepped up research into animal gland grafts and surgical rejuvenation in the battle against aging. Surgical rejuvenation most famously involved the "Steinach operation"—cutting and tying off the vas deferens to redirect the testicular ejaculation of sperm into the body. Another Austrian physician, Arnold Lorand, in his popular book *Old Age Deferred* (1912), corroborated the theory that sexual glands, sexual activity, and longevity are related. To Lorand, degeneration follows from damaged or removed sexual glands in both men and women, so that "degenerated conditions of the sexual glands, by producing alterations in important organs, diminish vitality and the chances of an advanced old age" (1912, p. 47). As Hirshbein (2000) has recently argued, however, the rejuvenators were far more ambivalent about the benefits for women, given that "femininity" was still closely tied to reproductive function, and surgical rejuvenation could not restore this. For men, on the other hand, masculinity could be more firmly grounded in the ability to perform sexually, and age-related decline became, literally, a process of demasculinization:

> By reasoning that the sex glands contained the essence of masculinity and that old age was a state of depletion of these glands, the rejuvenators promised to restore manhood itself to aging men who feared that they had lost the ability to function as men within the modern world. (Hirshbein, 2000, p. 293)

While inevitably failing to comprehend the aging process in any lasting way, the advocates above and many others in the rejuvenation movement created a vast archive of sensationalistic, pseudo-scientific experimentation in the first half of the twentieth century. As Susan Squier comments: "They generated controversy in the popular press, became the focus of best sellers, canonical novels, and science fiction short stories, provided the theme for a smash Hollywood movie, and exercised a shaping impact on our attitudes toward aging that persists to the present day" (1999, p. 89). The "attitudes" to which she refers are those that claimed that science could make a miraculous contribution to the plight of the aging body and even transform later life into a enlightened aging experience. These attitudes also made their way into the budding sciences of geriatrics and gerontology in the early twentieth century (see Achenbaum, 1995).

As mentioned earlier in Chapter 6, the term *gerontology* was coined by Elie Metchnikoff (1845-1916), the celebrated Nobel Prize winning scientist who worked at the Pasteur Institute in Paris from 1888 until his death in 1916. He wrote two influential books on the subject of aging: *The Nature of Man* (1903) and *The Prolongation of Life* (1907), respectively subtitled *Studies in Optimistic Philosophy* and *Optimistic Studies*. In *The Nature of Man* Metchnikoff muses: "I think it extremely probable that the scientific study of old age and of death, two branches of science that may be called gerontology and thanatology, will bring about great modifications in the course of the last period of life" (1903, p. 298). While Metchnikoff saw aging as a process of cellular involution, where cell decay outbalances cell growth, he speculated that defense against senile decay could be mustered with the use of animal organ injections and a diet rich in sterilized or sour milk to control harmful bacterial flora.[8] Thus Metchnikoff helped to launch gerontology not only as a science of aging, but one inspired by a discourse of optimism, in particular, an optimism that the pathological ravages of the aging process could be contested and even eliminated once the body was understood as a site of ongoing struggle between vital forces within tissues and cells. Among the chapters that delineate the diseases of senility in *The Prolongation of Life* are others on philosophy and morality, with a section devoted to Goethe and Faust. But something new and important emerges in Metchnikoff's last chapter on *orthobiosis*, which proposes an idealized partnership between individual aging and scientific progress. He says that "bacteriology has placed hygiene on a scientific foundation, so that the latter is now one of the exact sciences. It has now become necessary to give it the chief place in applied morality as it is the branch of knowledge that teaches how men ought to live" (1907, p. 331). Science as morality is thus a theme that becomes apparent when Metchnikoff discusses Goethe's profligate sexual reputation: "The truth is that artistic genius and perhaps all kinds of genius are closely associated with sexual activity" (p. 272), and "from the point of view of a naturalist, I cannot agree with the moralists who have blamed Goethe for his sexuality" (p. 273). Metchnikoff, in the name of science, was making a prophetic claim that would eventually run throughout modern gerontological culture: sexual activity is connected to long life, if not poetic genius.

By the early to mid-twentieth century we have three predominant ideas about men, sexual function, aging, and the life course. First, a pathological, climacteric-induced process, whose crisis points emerge not only in old-old age but in young-old age or middle age as well, characterized aging. In fact the medical and cultural anxieties about male decline moved down into middle age as rejuvenation therapies and early gerontology alighted on this time of life as an opportunity for effective intervention (see Gullette, 1994). Sylvanus Stall's guide to midlife hygiene, *What a Man of Forty-Five Ought to Know* (1901) is a perfect example of the middle aging of decline, linking sexual loss to middle age and suggesting that it is nature's course to diminish sexual power in men once their peak reproductive fitness has passed.

Second, there was the emergent status and problematization of sexual function as an indicator of successful aging. Since impotence and related sexual dysfunctions were seen as biologically derived, the choice was either to accept and adjust to them—although deferral and management could be achieved through a prudent lifestyle—or indulge in the increasingly discredited rejuvenating nostrums of Steinach or Brown-Séquard in an attempt to restore sexual function. Stall reminded his male reader of the benefits of the former approach: "the stress of passion will be past, the imagination will become more chastened, the heart more refined, the lines of intellectual and spiritual vision lengthened, the sphere of usefulness enlarged" (1901, p. 59). Instead, he should,

> fix his thoughts upon those philanthropic and unselfish projects which add beauty to age, and are the crown to gray hairs. What more nauseous and repulsive object than a libidinous and worn-out old man, heating his diseased imagination with dreams and images which his chilled and impotent body can no longer carry into effect? (p. 83)

Later, Dr. R. Reynell, in a presentation to the Royal Society of Medicine in 1931, noted that while impotence is frequently the cause of "intense mental distress," he found it difficult to understand "why this should be the case in say, a man of 50, married with a family" (1931, p. 28).

Edward J. Stieglitz, a leader in the gerontological field, confirmed this perspective on adjustment in the postwar years. In his text, *The Second Forty Years* (1949), and in a vocabulary on sexuality that reflected a growing emphasis on libido and hormones, Stieglitz advises both men and women:

> The personal importance of diminishing libido will depend upon how important the sexual aspect of life has been before the climacteric. It is significant chiefly to those whose interests and pleasures are largely limited to sex. It is calmly welcomed by many as a release from turmoil, permitting greater and deeper enjoyment of other beauties of living. (p. 197)

For men in particular, however, "the only definite evidence of the masculine climacteric is the gradual diminution of sexual potency and libido" (p. 203). "Depression is significant only in those who take intense pride in their virility and to whom the exercise of sexual functions is unduly important" (p. 204). If the masculine climacteric stimulates sexual desire, especially as subjects acknowledge their declining virility, "this may lead to wild extravagances" (p. 204); hence, aging subjects must fatefully acknowledge, along with the author, that "sex, after all, is an activity for youth" (p. 205).

Third, there was the powerful allure of science. Despite its codifying the aging body within an expansive pathologizing discourse of senescence, science was also seen as the solution to the worst manifestations of aging. Beginning with Metchnikoff and continuing in the present, professional gerontologists embraced the *positive* as an ethical and intellectual resource with which to sustain the optimistic promise of their field. As such, gerontological practices have been saturated with positive agendas around ideals of vitality, activity, autonomy, mobility, choice, and wellbeing. In a time of recent changes in demographic patterns, the possibilities of extending the life span, and the rise and empowerment of grey political movements, such agendas are also viewed as essential to the promotion of a buoyant perspective on later life and an antidote to traditionally negative stereotypes of decline, dependency, and decrepitude.[9]

However, in the middle of the twentieth century, this positive development was stymied when confronted with sexual decline, especially since scientific gerontology and sexology had made sexual decline an element of a climactericized middle aging. Metchnikoff may have proclaimed that biological science rather than morality "teaches how men ought to live," but a legitimately positive discourse on sexual decline could only come about as a result of a shift from an organic understanding of impotence to one based on the psychology of aging and its relation to sexuality.

The Psychology of Impotence

While remnants of nineteenth-century conceptions of the "spermatic economy" (Haller, 1989) persisted into the new century,[10] new configurations of physiological and psychological factors were beginning to form in understanding impotence, and psychological explanations rapidly became favoured. Psychological factors behind impotence are not new; Freud's colleague William Stekel wrote about them in the 1920s in *Impotence in the Male* (1927).[11] J. Lombard Kelly summed up the prevailing wisdom by mid-century in the title of his book: *So You THINK You're Impotent!* (1957). Even within this shift in aetiology, impotence was still largely regarded as a disease of the young and a condition of the old. Hirsch (1947), for example, clearly distinguished between the primarily psychic impotence of those aged between 20 and 45 and the more physically derived impotence of those older than 45. While the prognosis for psychotherapy to successfully treat the former was good, so-called normal sexual aging was still viewed as an adjustment to physical decline. However, the psychological paradigm quickly expanded to include aging men as well, who were increasingly told that it was their anxiety over their supposedly inevitable loss of sexual function, their *fear* of loss of potency that was causing their *premature* sexual decline. Edmund Bergler went so far as to identify particular specific crisis points at which the aging man might succumb to psychic impotence:

> There are two especially critical psychological danger spots, both of neurotic origin: the time of the middle and late forties, and the middle sixties. In the former, neurotic expectation of "old age" creeps in making the man believe that he is "definitely through." In the latter, fear of death contributes its share to neurotic impotence. Both types of impotence can be psychiatrically remedied. (1951, p. 10)

Overall, two axioms characterized the advice given to men from the 1960s through the 1980s: first, psychological factors were primarily responsible for loss of sexual function; and second, to cease having sex would hasten aging in itself. As an entry in the 1972 *Encyclopedia of Love and Sex* put it:

> The most common cause of the loss of sexual ability in the older man is mental negativism and fear, rather than physical degeneration. ... Medical opinion is unanimous that, provided a man is generally healthy and has a positive mental attitude, he can continue to lead an active sexual life at least until he is eighty and possibly beyond. By far the most effective way of ensuring that he continues to be sexually active is never to stop. (Fletcher, 1972, p. 164)

These axioms had certainly been underlined in the influential sexological reports of Kinsey (1948, 1953), Masters and Johnson (1966, 1970), and Hite (1976). As part of their demystification of sexuality, these reports mention that sexual activity is enjoyed throughout the life course and often more so later in life than earlier (see Neugebauer-Visano, 1995). Gerontology and sexology shared common ground in asserting that both physiological and psychological factors were fundamental in making sexual activity, particularly sexual intercourse, a healthy and necessary component of successful aging. Indeed, the passive acceptance of age-related changes in sexual capacity that had characterized the professional advice of the past, now became viewed as a pathological adaptive response rooted in ignorance or fear.

In their book *Love and Sex after 60*, gerontologists Robert Butler and Myrna Lewis very clearly encapsulate the new perspective, citing a popular fact in the literature: "It has long been established that at least 90 per cent of impotence in men over sixty was psychologically based, with only about 10 per cent physiologically caused" (1988, p. 45). For these authors, the problem of impotence should be attributed to a number of lifestyle factors including drug interactions and side effects, overwork, poor diet, lack of exercise, physical disability, and stress. Sometimes "the fear of impotence can cause impotence" (p. 99). Hence, psychological and couple counselling are as important as remedies as are the more tricky (and unreliable) hormone therapies, penile prostheses, and vitamin-mineral supplements. Social factors can also contribute to impotence, such as the lack of privacy in homes and care facilities, the prevalence of sexually oppressive attitudes about aging, and the loss of lifelong partners. For modern gerontology, men may still have to adjust to the consequences of lowered testosterone levels, but this adjustment should be directed toward learning to enjoy sex more as they mature, while focussing more on intimacy and less on performance (Adelman, 1995; Hodson and Skeen, 1994; Schlesinger, 1996; Tallmer, 1996; Whitbourne, 1995).

From *Impotence* to *Erectile Dysfunction*

While sex therapy (for both young and old) seemed confident in its assumption of a primarily psychological basis for impotence, a different turn was being taken in urological research. In 1983, Dr. Giles Brindley astounded an audience of his colleagues at a conference by injecting his penis with phenoxybenzamine and displaying, for all to see, an erection obtained by purely chemical means.[12] While this led to the development of new therapies for impotence, such as intracavernosal injection and transurethral therapies, the more revolutionary import was to visibly sever the mechanism of penile erection from any sort of psychological or emotional arousal, or even tactile stimulation, and to reconceptualize it as a primarily physiological event. That "impotence is now recognised to be primarily a disorder of organic causes rather than a psychological problem" convinced many scientists that "a new sexual revolution" was under way (Morgentaler, 1999, p. 1713). Disease models were constructed which de-linked physical sexual decline from bodily aging, evidenced both by erectile difficulties and hormonal changes. McKinlay, Longcope, and Gray (1989), for example, suggested that there was no evidence for a male climacteric syndrome, and that "age per se may be a relatively unimportant contributor to endocrine variability and that anthropometrics and lifestyle phenomena may be at least as important" (p. 103). In a wide-ranging review of the research, Metz and Miner (1995) concluded, "loss of sexual function is due more to comorbid disease processes, side-effect of medication or physical disability than due to the normal aging process" (p. 299). This, then, became the starting point for subsequent research; that it was not age *per se*, but "modifiable para-aging phenomena" (Feldman *et al.*, 1994) that were largely responsible for sexual dysfunction in the aging male.

Significant as well was a reversal of the assumption that fear, depression, anxiety, or other psychological factors could act on the body to produce impotence. Instead, "as the physical causes of impotence have become better appreciated, emphasis has shifted to the potentially very serious emotional consequences of impotence" (Morganstern and Abrahams, 1988, p. 6). This has been a pivotal move in the construction of impotence, now reconceptualized as *erectile dysfunction*, as a threat to both the physical and psychological well-being of an aging population, and hence as a matter for public concern.

Thus, through the 1980s and 1990s, a decisive shift was made from impotence to erectile dysfunction, a shift stabilized by the National Institute of Health's "consensus development conference" on impotence convened in 1992.[13] Made up of a number of leading medical scientists, the panel included among its conclusions and recommendations that "the term erectile dysfunction should replace the term impotence to characterize the inability to attain and/or maintain penile erection sufficient for satisfactory sexual performance" (NIH, 1993, p. 89). Among its other conclusions the panel stressed that, while the likelihood of erectile dysfunction increases with age, it is more related to "age related conditions" than age itself, that erectile dysfunction is a treatable organic disease, and that it is an important public health problem. The consensus panel thus codified assertions about aging and male sexuality that would quickly become doctrine in medical research, therapeutic practices, and health promotion discourses.

The new focus on erectile dysfunction epitomizes the manner in which truth claims about the sexual body have become increasingly medicalized. Such truth claims rest on the privileged access of science to the natural body and increasingly on the ability to visualize and objectively record both the "normal" and "pathological" operations of the sexual body. As one of the scientists later puts it:

> Few fields in medicine can match the rapid progress that has been made in our understanding of male erectile function. These changes have been profound, and fundamental. Baseless speculation about the essential vascular mechanisms of erection and the belief in a predominantly emotional etiology have given way to the identification of the molecular events resulting in an erection and to effective pharmacological treatment of their alterations. The current state of the art is a pre-eminent example of what is achievable by systematic and conscientious application of basic research and clinical observation. (Morales, 1998, p. xv)

This neatly encapsulates the story told by the scientists: it is a narrative of progressive discovery, assisted by new techniques of visualization, which has allowed them to get at "the molecular events resulting in an erection." Erectile dysfunction (ED) becomes a simple mechanical problem. As another scientist later summarizes it, "The man needs a sufficient axial rigidity so his penis can penetrate through labia, and he has to sustain that in order to have sex. This is a mechanical structure, and mechanical structures follow scientific principles" (Dr. Irwin Goldstein, cited in Hitt, 2000, p. 36). At the same time, however, erectile dysfunction is far more than a simple mechanical problem because it is framed as a social problem of supposedly epidemic proportions. It is this framing that illuminates the extent to which anxieties about penile erectility both crystallize broader social anxieties about masculinity, sexuality, and aging and foster a particular mobilization of social resources.

Constructing the Epidemic

While Kinsey's 1948 report on male sexuality took a "glass half full" approach, stressing that impotence was a "relatively rare phenomenon" with only 27 per cent of men becoming impotent by 70 years of age, it has been widely criticized for its non-representative, small sample of older men who were surveyed. Most widely cited is the Massachusetts Male Aging Survey (MMAS), which was a probability sample of 1,700 men aged 40 to 70 conducted in the Boston area between 1987 and 1989 (Feldman *et al.*, 1994; McKinlay and Feldman, 1994).[14] The MMAS found consistent age-related decline in erectile function (defined here as the ability to "get and keep an erection good enough for sexual intercourse") but this decline was extrapolated from cross-sectional, rather than longitudinal data, and was thus unable to account for cohort effects.[15] Significant in the MMAS was the *grading* of degrees of erectile dysfunction by age (mild, moderate, complete), but emphasized in subsequent reporting of the data were overall prevalence rates of "some degree of erectile dysfunction" at 52 per cent. Here, the glass is half empty: "Once a man enters the [40–70] age group his odds of developing erectile dysfunction are at least as high as his odds of avoiding it. If this doesn't constitute an epidemic, I don't know what would!" (Melchiode and Sloan, 1999, p. 9).

Reported prevalence rates in articles citing the MMAS tend to adopt the broadest definition of erectile dysfunction. Not surprisingly, given the advantages of defining the largest market possible for potential treatment, the tendency in both scientific and popular reports is to include all of those suffering from "some degree" of difficulty. This puts reported rates from the United States at 39 per cent of 40-year-olds, and 67 per cent of 70-year-olds. These prevalence rates are then applied against demographic projections of age changes in the population to predict incidence rates, future increases, and policy consequences (see Aytac, McKinlay, and Krane, 1999; Keith, 2000). While Bahr could claim, in 1992, that impotence was the "least publicized epidemic," by the end of the twentieth century, surely it was one of the most publicized. This could only occur in the context of new truths about the relationship between aging and male sexuality. Of course aging itself could not be construed as an epidemic, but erectile dysfunction could be framed as a result of pathological *para-aging* phenomena amenable to both preventative and rehabilitative intervention.

Despite the cross-sectional nature of the data, secondary interpretations routinely imply that degrees of erectile dysfunction can be directly mapped onto phases of erectile dysfunction. Once phases are identified, then erectile dysfunction becomes a progressive disease. Consider one of the clinical case studies reported by Lamm and Couzens: Ron, a 41-year-old electrician, reports on his first visit: "I felt the sex I was having was just okay…. I also knew it should be a lot better…. Getting an erection isn't the problem—it's that I'm not as firm and full as I used to be. Amy, my wife, says it doesn't bother her. But I'm very aware of it and it upsets me." Dr. Lamm's response: "I told Ron that his primary symptoms, which included slower arousal time, the need for increased stimulation to achieve an erection and the inability to maintain an erection, were *early signs* of ED" (1998, pp. 75-76; emphasis added). Thus, erectile dysfunction is rendered a potentially epidemic progressive disease, from which all men are "at risk." As Linda Singer has argued, "in order to represent a phenomenon as socially undesirable … one need only call it an epidemic," a strategy which "mobilizes a certain apparatus and logic, a particular way of producing and organizing bodies politically" (1993, p. 27). The onus on the individual now is no longer to carefully husband their sexual resources as they age, but to take responsibility for managing risk through new regimes of bodily discipline that must start long before the onset of old age.

Risky Business

A large and growing body of literature has suggested that the project of the self in late modernity is largely a body-project (Featherstone, 1991; Shilling, 1993; Williams and Bendelow, 1998). It is characterized, on the one hand, by an increasing individualization of risk, but on the other, an increasing reliance on expert advice and consumer goods (Giddens, 1991; Rose, 1996; Slater, 1997). Both commercial and public health promotion discourses about "positive aging" (Hepworth, 1995) have actively incorporated the fear of erectile failure into more general models of "healthy living." *Men's Health*, a popular men's magazine which emphasizes health, fitness, and sexual performance, has a regular feature called "the game show," where profiles of three men are presented and the reader is invited to discern, from the information given, which one will first manifest the phenomenon of the month (Who will go bald first? Who will look old first?). The October 2000 issue focussed on "Who will be impotent first?" (McDonald, 2000). Each of the three men profiled presented a different set of "risk factors." George is 31, overweight, with a family history of high blood pressure and diabetes. Joe, while only 25, is a competitive cyclist. Carlos is 63; age is his sole risk factor. Each profile also included what they're doing right: George has sex nearly every day, Joe is in excellent physical shape and has sex four times a week, Carlos leads a "health-obsessed" lifestyle and has sex three to five times per week. When we turn the page to find out who wins (loses?), a detailed "scorecard" is provided which assigns a point value to an array of 12 "impotence factors" (age, health, stress, diet, exercise, alcohol, smoking, temper, depression, sexual activity, performance anxiety, saddle sports). Scores could range from a low of −23 to a maximum of +10. George came in at the low score (and hence highest risk) of −4; Carlos, despite his age, got a positive 5; and Joe a very positive 7. Of course, the reader is invited to fill out the scorecard for himself, and if a score of −3 or less is obtained, they are exhorted that "You are high-risk and need to change your lifestyle immediately." Those with a score of −2 to +2 are warned "you've still got it but maybe not for long." Those with a score of +3 are obviously doing something right, but still there is the warning to continue doing it ("Continue what you're doing and enjoy a long, hard life").

That the high-risk individual identified in this feature (George) is only 31 years old and currently reports having sex every day is significant, as is the fact that the "point values" available for scoring are, with the exception of a total of 4 negative points for age and family history factors, all related to matters that are seen to be changeable by lifestyle. George, for example, is told that while he doesn't have problems yet, "his poor diet, sedentary lifestyle, and family history will eventually catch up with him," but that "fortunately, his fate isn't inevitable." He needs to exercise and eat right, which will cause him to "lose weight, control his blood pressure, and increase his sex life expectancy." If not, the experts predict he has "about 10 years left."

The message here is not only one of constant vigilance, even in the absence of any perceptible sense of bodily decline, but also one of equating the loss of erection with the end of life itself. Age, then, is a risk factor among many. While there is an acknowledged link between age and the prevalence of erectile dysfunction, a simple causal link is now severed. As one review article put it: "This prevalence does not represent normal aging … any more than hypertension is considered to be normal in an older adult, and erectile dysfunction is not an inevitable effect of aging" (Kaiser, 1999, p. 1267). Like hypertension, it is a disease that is preventable and manageable through appropriate bodily discipline. Just as Slater notes for obesity or slovenliness, erectile dysfunction can now be understood as a "moral disorder," a reflection on one's inadequacy and one's consumption, or lack thereof, of appropriate or inappropriate goods and knowledge (1997, p. 92).

While medical practitioners have long prescribed various regimes of bodily hygiene as a means of prolonging or restoring one's vital powers, the intensified medicalization of sexuality mandates compulsory tumescence. George Ridley Scott, reviewing the literature on rejuvenation therapies in 1953, suggested that "much of the hostility towards rejuvenation has been engendered through its association with sex," and countered that "there is no way of extending the physical and mental powers of the individual into advancing years without coincidentally keeping the sexual and endocrinal glands functioning" (1953, pp. 9-10). By contrast, there is nothing coincidental at all about the emphasis on sexual function in contemporary health promotion discourses. The image of the erect penis, long the most vulgar of indecent "exposures," is now elevated to

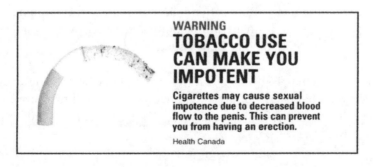

WARNING
TOBACCO USE CAN MAKE YOU IMPOTENT
Cigarettes may cause sexual impotence due to decreased blood flow to the penis. This can prevent you from having an erection.
Health Canada

the status of a vital organ symbolizing the healthfulness of midlife successful aging. When Health Canada introduced new, graphic warnings on cigarette packages in 2001, among them was a picture of a drooping cigarette, with the warning that "Tobacco use can make you impotent."[16]

This thought is echoed by Melchiode and Sloan (1999) who suggest that "no malfunction of the human apparatus—not even cancer or heart disease—can be more painful to the male ego or catastrophic to the male psyche than sexual impotence" (p. 17). Men are thus exhorted to eat a healthy diet, get lots of rest, stop smoking, drink in moderation, and engage in a regular exercise program in order to minimize the likelihood of "problems that impede blood flow to his penis" (Whitehead and Malloy, 1999, p. 169) or to ensure "penile health" within a broader "virility program" which includes a number of dietary supplements (Lamm and Couzens, 1998) or penis-conditioning exercises (Drew, 1998).

Maintaining penile erectility is not just a benefit of a healthy lifestyle; it is a compelling reason for that lifestyle and stands as a signal indicator of successful, ageless aging. The erect penis becomes a visible index (almost in a Durkheimian sense) of masculinity, emotional health, and physical health, and one that is no longer tied to bodily age. Whether through preventative bodily discipline or remedial therapy, the onus is on the responsibly aging individual to remain *forever functional*. If one event can be singled out as securing this view of male sexual fitness, then it would have to be the introduction of Viagra, which hit the North American market in the spring of 1998.

The Pharmaceutical Fix

> To come in to a doctor and say: I am losing (or I have lost) my sexual power, I wish you would give me some prescription for it …which so many poor patients do, shows only the unsophisticatedness of the layman and his boundless belief in the miraculous power of medicine. (Robinson, 1930, p. 159)

> For the generation that refuses to grow old, Viagra is the drug everyone has been waiting and praying for. The pill that promises a lifetime of great sex — for just about everyone. (Whitehead and Malloy, 1999, p. 2)

Within months of its release, Viagra attained iconic status. Not only were millions of prescriptions written, but a slew of mass-market paperbacks hit the stands; extensive coverage appeared in every mainstream media outlet; it was the subject of countless comedy monologues, cartoons, and jokes; and hundreds of Internet sites emerged which offered on-line prescriptions and home delivery. Both the popular media and the medical therapeutic community heralded Viagra as revolutionary. Far more than a pharmaceutical product, the little blue diamond-shaped pill has become a cultural signifier of virility, bio-perfection, potentially unlimited sexual performance, and a new era in sexuality (Marshall, 2002). Viagra, sildenafil citrate, is a pharmacological compound that suppresses an enzyme that allows blood to flow out of the penis, thus facilitating the achievement and maintenance of an erection. While biotechnical remedies for rehabilitating erections have been common practice for many years,[17] what sets Viagra apart is its relationship to the development of a molecular science of sexuality, its location by the medical and therapeutic communities within the "natural" sexual response cycle, and its cultural acceptance as the magic bullet that will usher in a whole new era of both sexual medicine and sexual relations (Marshall, 2002).

While the initial justification for the disease model of erectile dysfunction was clearly framed in terms of a discernible physiological basis and its relationship to potentially serious health problems such as diabetes, hypertension, and arterial sclerosis, the efficacy of Viagra in producing erections regardless of the etiology, not to mention the huge profitability of expanding the market, has considerably broadened the clinical framing of erectile dysfunction.[18] In fact, it is asserted that the existence of a highly successful and well-tolerated treatment reveals the "true incidence of erectile dysfunction" (Broderick, 1998, p. 205), which has hitherto been clearly "underdiagnosed" (Seiden, 1998, p. 3). The user is now configured not just as the man who, for whatever reason, is unable to get or keep an erection much of the time, but includes all those whose erections could be "improved." Both the popular literature and recent advertising suggest that you might have ED and not even know it![19] One doctor sums it up well: "Should a man take the pill to improve erections if he doesn't think he has ED? The issue can be side-stepped by saying that if a man takes the pill and his erections improve, then he had ED after all" (Lamm and Couzens, 1998, p. 82).

Originally marketed to a mature audience as a treatment for an identifiably age-related condition within the context of stable heterosexual relationships (with Bob Dole as its most memorable spokesman), Viagra is now being pitched to an ever younger, and potentially single, market. The original print and television advertisements featured white-haired couples dancing. Subsequent ads featured younger and younger looking couples in happy embraces. The most recent campaigns eliminate the partner altogether with a recent television ad showing a man in his late thirties or early forties getting dressed and groomed to go out, with a blistering blues soundtrack ("I'm ready for you, I hope you're ready for me ..."). The pill becomes one more tool in the project of constructing the sexually functional male body, with both its maleness and its functionality defined by penile erectility, as an ageless body, a project that now must begin earlier and earlier in the life course.

Along with the lifestyle discipline required to maintain erectile function, pharmaceutical and other biotechnical advances figure prominently in the expanding horizon of sexual fitness, with its emphasis on prevention and the refusal of bodily limits.[20]

> In sports, what were once considered insurmountable barriers—the four-minute mile, the seven-foot high jump, and so forth—are now accomplished routinely. Furthermore, the peak years of an athlete have been dramatically extended by conditioning procedures, nutritional knowledge, and medical breakthroughs. I can see no reason why the years of active sexuality cannot be expanded, and with it the penis power of aging men. (Danoff, 1993, p. 158)

Viagra (or Viagra-like drugs) may also have prophylactic potential, similar to that of aspirin in warding off heart disease: "Some experts are predicting that, in the near future, the drug will be taken two or three times a week, even when the man is not engaging in sex, to ensure erectile health" (Lamm and Couzens, 1998, p. 137). However, it is the possibility of prevention through advances in molecular biology that seems to have captured the scientific imagination, and "the future of the genetic therapy of human erectile dysfunction seems bright indeed" (Christ, 1998, p. 193). As one scientist confidently predicts, "It is clear that early in the new millennium, ED will not only be effectively treated but also potentially prevented" (Padma-Nathan, 1998, p. 216).

Conclusions: The Sexually Dysfunctional

Viagra has already shed more light on the once forbidden area of sexual function than any medical discovery since the dawn of time ...[it] has thrown open the door to frank discussion and enlightened study of human sexuality in a way that no scientific development has ever done before. (Melchiode and Sloan, 1999, pp. 230-31)

If the advent of Viagra has brought about a new discursive explosion on sexuality, it has been one that Foucault might have characterized as consolidating yet another "strategic unity" which forms "specific mechanisms of knowledge and power centering on sex" (Foucault, 1980a, p. 103): the "sexually dysfunctional."[21] But, as we noted at the outset, the sexual body here is also a gendered body and an aging body, and it is in this convergence that we wish to locate our discussion. Evident is a new bodily configuration in the making, one arising, on the one hand, from the pharmacological and scientific technologization of male sexuality and, on the other, from a contemporary politics of life that fosters an ageless aging while creating, paradoxically, an anxiety-ridden and somatized middle age. Even after the late twentieth-century reassertion of an overwhelmingly physiological basis for impotence, the assumption that to remain sexually active is to remain young seems unquestioned: "The strenuous use of your penis will sharpen your mind, exalt your soul and keep you feeling vigorous. In short, you don't stop having sex because you get old, *you get old because you stop having sex*" (Danoff, 1993, pp. 155-156; emphasis in the original).

On the one hand, the entwining of the climacteric panic of midlife decline with the positive and expansive purview of the gerontological and sexological sciences in the latter twentieth century has attracted attention to a new series of health risks and concerns about how to live properly, responsibly, and sexually. Further, the configuration of successful midlife lifestyles has meant that anxiety over midlife decline is culturally fostered at increasingly younger ages. As Gullette notes, "as the century has progressed, everyone has been getting older younger" (1998, p. 17). On the other hand, positive aging has created a bind: by loosening sexual decline from the aging body in order to address ageist conventions of sexual oppression, it has also reassigned it to a broad range of factors considered vital to identity in midlife and successful aging thereafter. And the broadening of sexual decline to include psychological, emotional, and social factors has meant that the older tension between the body and age has become libidinously internalized. Masculinity remains anchored in the erect penis across the life course, and that functional penis remains the visible indicator of interior character and successful living. The aging male is now a sexualized subject within a modern life course regime, who, like Foucault's nineteenth-century sexually strategic figures (1980a, pp. 104-05), finds himself in a struggle against the very orders of power and truth that shape him.

Notes

Barbara L. Marshall and I are fellow members of the Sociology Department at Trent University. When we discovered that our work around sexuality and aging intersected in many interesting ways, we decided to write a paper together, which we submitted to and published in the British journal *Body and Society* 8 (4), 2002, pp. 43-70. This paper has given each of us special opportunities to present conference papers in our respective fields. We would also like to acknowledge the financial support of a research grant from Trent University's SSHRC Committee on Research, as well as the assistance afforded by superb archives staff at the libraries of the Wellcome Institute, the Kinsey Institute, and Cornell University, and the interlibrary loans staff at Trent's Bata Library. I thank Barbara and Sage Publications for permission to reprint the essay here. The authors would also like to thank Health Canada for permission to use and reproduce the health warning image on p. 179.

1. This point is elaborated elsewhere (Katz, 1996, 1997; Tulle-Winton, 2000).
2. An exception to the almost exclusive focus on women is the important work of Mike Featherstone and Mike Hepworth in the 1980s on male menopause and sexuality, consumer lifestyles, and midlife crises (1982a, 1982b, 1985a, 1985b, 1986).
3. That sex equals penile penetration of a vagina is an assumption that runs through the literature on sexual dysfunction. The heterosexuality of the body is assumed and inscribed in the most basic of scientific research (Marshall, 2001a). That masculinity is largely measured by the possession of a penis, which is capable of penetrating a vagina, is also evident in other contexts, such as the degree to which this is used as a diagnostic criterion in pediatric intersexuality (Fausto-Sterling, 1997).
4. However, no magic bullet such as Viagra has yet been developed for women, although several drugs and mechanical therapies are in clinical trials.

5. A number of historical investigations of impotence have demonstrated that, while intertwined with shifting conceptions of masculinity and changing assumptions about male bodies, impotence has remained a significant concern and source of anxiety for men. See, for example, Hall (1991, 1995), Haller (1989), McLaren (1997), Mumford (1992), and Nye (1989). The relationship between aging and sexual decline does not figure prominently in these investigations. It does, however, emerge as a significant theme in the large body of popular sexological literature aimed at men; for example, see Caprio (1952), Chesser (1947), Fere (1932), Kelly (1957), Peterson (1968), Saxe and Gerson (1964), Stall (1901), and Stone (1938).

6. One of the most popular Renaissance treatises on prolongevity was *How to Live for a Hundred Years and Avoid Disease* (1558), written by Louis Cornaro, a sixteenth-century Venetian nobleman. While Cornaro explains the success of his health regimes for living into his centenarian years, which focus obsessively on diet, hygiene and temperance, he hardly considers sexual function, desire, or decline as part of them.

7. The idea of sexual convergence did not compensate for the prevailing sexist and ageist attitudes about female menopause and older women (e.g., Colombat, 1845; Napier, 1897; Tilt, 1882). As Hepworth and Featherstone note about Victorian ideas, "Ironically, the menopause signalled the end of one disruptive bodily leakage only to replace it with another 'obscenity'" (1998, p. 283). For critical treatments see Formanek (1990), Shaw (1995), and Smith-Rosenberg (1985).

8. Throughout his career Metchnikoff maintained that lactic bacteria in soured milk and fermented foods were essential to balancing and detoxifying the effects of harmful intestinal phagocytes, an idea that also inspired a sour milk craze in Paris in 1902 (Cole, 1992b, p. 189).

9. Several critical gerontologists are less sanguine about their profession's positive turn, castigating it for imposing unrealistic expectations on elderly persons and neglecting their material difficulties, especially in deep old age (Cohen, 1998, p. 71; Cole, 1992b, pp. 227-33; Ekerdt, 1986; Hepworth, 1995; Holstein, 1999; Katz, 2000a; Moody, 1988a).

10. Bernard McFadden, for example, warned men of the danger of oversexed women who would sap their "vital economy":

    If your wife is abnormally sexed and seems to enjoy these relations at all times, then you have a problem before you which is not by any means easy to solve. A very plain talk is absolutely essential under such circumstances, if you wish to avoid serious inroads upon your vital economy. (1923, p. 54)

11. Stekel (1927) differed from many of his contemporaries in suggesting that the generally accepted relationship between sexual excess and premature sexual

decline was "a widely prevalent falsehood." Instead, he countered: "Whoever shows strong sexuality at an early age, in spite of masturbation and so-called excesses, will preserve it to advanced age" (p. 10).

12. This incident is widely recounted in both the scientific and popular literatures as a watershed in the shift from psychological to physiological aetiologies of impotence. See Broderick (1998), and Whitehead and Malloy (1999).

13. The shift in terminology has been uneven, despite the rather decisive shift in paradigms of understanding. *Impotence* continues to be used in a range of contexts (including some of the major scientific journals), but it now refers more precisely to the condition of erectile dysfunction.

14. The other major study cited is the National Health and Social Life Survey of 1992, which was a probability sample of men and women, aged 18 to 59. Rates of erectile dysfunction were determined by a yes/no answer to the question: "During the last 12 months, has there ever been a period of several months or more when you ... had trouble achieving or maintaining an erection?" The NHSLS researchers suggest that a "yes" answer to this question would be comparable to the MMAS definition of moderate to complete impotence, but their results show only a 13.9 per cent prevalence for 40- to 59-year-olds, with the highest prevalence (22 per cent) in the 50- to 55-year-old-group, declining to 10 per cent in the 55- to 59-year-old group (Laumann, Paik, and Rosen, 1999).

15. *Cohort effect* refers to the possibility that differences between age groups may result from different historically linked experiences or practices common to each group rather than differences related to the aging process. Another finding of the MMAS which does not get reported in the ubiquitous citations to this study is that: "Despite the marked declines in actual events and behavior and in subjective aspects of sexuality, men in their sixties reported levels of satisfaction with their sex life and partners at about the same level as younger men in their forties" (McKinlay and Feldman, 1994, p. 272). The researchers attribute this to differing normative expectations associated with specific age groups. Part of the construction of the ED epidemic then, is a reorientation of these normative expectations.

16. Canada is not alone in using the threat of impotence in campaigns against smoking. The state of Oregon introduced both television and print advertising in 2000 which showed men "striking out" with women as their cigarettes went limp.

17. These run the gamut from early forms of splints and supports, hormonal and glandular therapies, rejuvenation "tonics," herbal remedies, and penile exercises, to more recently standardized treatments including penile implants and prostheses, vacuum cylinders, penile injections, urethral suppositories, and oral medications. Historically, this is an arena of treatment in which struggles for legitimacy

and authority over diagnosis and prescription have figured prominently.

18. Numerous clinical trials have demonstrated that Viagra is most effective in cases of erectile dysfunction for which no organic origin has been identified (classified as *psychogenic*) (Shabsigh, 1999; Steers, 1999). That it so effectively works in these cases acts to reinforce the conviction that the dysfunction must have been a physiological matter after all.

19. Nor, indeed, might your partner: "Erectile dysfunction can range widely in severity from men who are completely 'impotent' in every negative and absolute sense of the word to men whose problems are so slight that not even their partners are aware they have it" (Katzenstein, 1998, p. 5).

20. Zygmunt Bauman (1998) has usefully distinguished between "health" and "fitness" by arguing that although the former term has some criteria of fulfillment, the latter term has no boundaries.

21. For a more general discussion of both male and female dysfunction, and how conceptions of these have shifted in post-Viagra science, see Marshall (2002).

ten

Growing Older Without Aging? Postmodern Time and Senior Markets

I would like to begin this chapter with a diaper story. When Proctor and Gamble introduced a new, extra-large size six *Pampers* diaper, called "Huggies," to handle the untrained toiletry habits of three-year-old children weighing over 35 pounds, the company claimed it was responding to evidence that increasingly fewer children in the United States are out of diapers by the age of three. It seems that both career-weary parents, who are continually advised by experts to reduce the pressure they put on children to "train," and their appreciative children, who apparently enjoy the freedom not to master one of the fundamental functions of life until they feel prepared to do so, are embracing the new product.[1] At a local level, this is just another story about another leakproof, disposable technological wonder-diaper that frees parents and children from facing anxious-making decisions. On a larger level, however, this is a story about technological expertise in a postindustrial society carving out of the life course yet another commercial opportunity and, in so doing, fostering in children those attributes germane to their future lives as consuming, self-fashioning subjects. In particular, the move from with-diaper to without-diaper stages of maturation depends, in part, on the child's ability to speak about and *choose* the lifestyle commodities that best suit his or her personal development. Needless to say, early reports indicate that the diapers are a huge success, and we can anticipate the consequences for future generations who were prematurely market-niched and comfort-zoned into consumer independence by being able to negotiate their own toilet training at the age of three. The irony is that by getting their children out of diapers later, parents may be pushing their children into adulthood earlier.

However, the diaper story suggests two interesting questions to be explored in this chapter. First, how is consumerism and its associated marketing vocabularies and technologies shaping new notions of maturity, fitness, human development, and sexuality around the central concept of *lifestyle*? Secondly, how has the rise of positive images of growing older and the celebration of an anti-aging culture configured a new postmodern life course, moored to standards of timelessness and bodily perfection?

The Course of Life in Postmodern Time

Traditionally, gerontologists and life course researchers, despite their different approaches, have faced a common problem, which is how to produce comprehensive models or narratives of life when the aging process has no single developmental logic. At whatever biological, cognitive, or social register one studies the life course, one finds more diversity than unity, more paradox than consistency, more ambiguity than certainty. The multifarious realities of aging have been illustrated in cross-cultural studies of aging that tackle the plurality of life course models across the world's societies (Amoss and Harrell, 1981; Cohen, 1998; Lock, 1993; Shweder, 1998) and in historical investigations of the rich and varied representations of the ages and stages of human existence through time (Cole, 1992b; Pelling and Smith, 1991; Shenk and Achenbaum, 1994). Social critics of Western modernity have also underscored the connection between the bureaucratic standardization of age-graded behaviours and identities and the industrial segmentation of the life course into distinct age differences (Chudacoff, 1989; Hockey and James, 1993). Indeed, what is accepted as the modern life course is closer to what Martin Kohli calls a "life course regime" (1986a, 1987), that is, an administrative rationality that politicizes the temporalization of everyday life. Furthermore, the life course regimes typical of modern Western societies have been shaped according to white, masculine, heterosexual, middle-class values and cultural patterns. Hence, the critics point out as well that life course politics constitute a critical arena of struggle whereby race, gender, sexual, and class divisions intersect with those based on age (see Dannefer, 2003; Fry, 2003).

Thus, it would appear that while aging is a universal phenomenon, its configuration in life courses is not, despite customary attempts by gerontologists to identify one with the other. On a macro-scale, life courses are aggregations of knowledges, structures, ethics, and hierarchies through which the complexities of aging are refracted and socially organized. On a micro-scale, they are lived-out embodiments of time from which people distill a rich and versatile archive of meaning, memory, passion, and identity. Life courses span rather than separate macro and micro dimensions of aging, even where they emerge in tandem with bureaucratic or administrative authorities. As such they can be thought of as a "folding" in the sense of the term used by late French philosopher Gilles Deleuze, that is, a dynamic shaping and pleating of subjective worlds as they interact with the external imperatives for living in time. In short, as foldings, life courses are "the inside *of* the outside"; hence, they are both uniquely individual and collectively sustained according to the cultural priorities of historical societies (Deleuze, 1988, p. 97; see also Deleuze, 1993).

Thinking of life courses in the plural and as coexisting regimes and macro-micro foldings returns our thinking to the connection between life course, the postindustrial landscape, and consumer society, a connection around which an interdisciplinary literature has recently blossomed in the humanities (Basting, 1998; Gullette, 1997; Featherstone and Wernick, 1995), social sciences (Biggs, 1999; Blaikie, 1999; Gilleard and Higgs, 2000), and feminism (Ray, 1999; Woodward, 1999). Focussing their critique on the temporal, bodily, and spatial manifestations of the postindustrial landscape, this literature examines how, in the late twentieth and early twenty-first centuries, modern chronological and generational boundaries, which had set apart childhood, middle age, and old age, became blurred and indeterminate because of new labour and retirement structures; the importance of leisure and consumerism on a global scale; the medical, pharmacological, and commercial stretching of middle age into later life; and the improved health and increasing size of aging populations in Western society.[2]

On the one hand this movement has inspired real estate, financial, cosmetic, and leisure enterprises to target a growing and so-called "ageless" seniors market (usually pegged at 55+) and to fashion a range of positive "uni-age" bodily styles and identities that recast later life as an active, youthful, commercial experience (Meyrowitz, 1984). On the other hand, the postmodern life course has created new avenues of self-definition that inspire seniors' groups to innovate imaginative arts of life for themselves and those who will follow. In both cases, the mobilization of new retiree segments by the private sector, in anticipation of extracting the "gold in grey" (Minkler, 1991), has expanded the significance of senior citizenry from professional and policy realms to include symbolic and cultural meanings. This transformation is accompanied by an explosion of popular demographic terms such as "boomers," "empty-nesters," and "third agers" that gloss over the negative realities of poverty and inequality in old age. The advertising industry has chimed in with its portrayals of the new anti-ageist, positive senior as an independent, healthy, sexy, flexi-retired "citizen," who bridges middle age and old age without suffering the time-bound constraints of either (Ekerdt and Clark, 2001; Hepworth, 1995; Katz, 1999, 2000a). Thus, the overall characterization of this period, as Gilleard and Higgs remark, is that "post-traditional culture extends equally to life after retirement as well as before" (2000, p. 25).[3]

Most importantly, within this culture the postmodern treatment of traditional age categories has fostered new experiments with time and timelessness, or what Bryan Turner refers to as the proliferation of "contingent life strategies" (1994, p. 110). Historians have demonstrated that industrial society operated within a calendrical world, where the values of mechanical factory time and historical progress were intrinsically linked to the family and generational practices of everyday life (see Chudacoff, 1989; Daly, 1996; Gillis, 1996). Here the clock face became the figurative face of modernity itself and its preoccupation with uniformity and permanence. The economies associated with postmodern time, however, emphasize replication, speed, impermanence, simultaneity, and immortality, as all activities from leisure to education to health, including ironically death and dying (Wernick, 1995), have become personal, consumerist, and lifelong experiences. Zygmunt Bauman characterizes postmodern timelessness, as it confronts the linear continuity and ordered fullness of modern time, in the following way:

> In a life composed of equal moments, speaking of directions, projects and fulfilments makes no sense. Every present counts as much, or as little, as any other. Every state is as momentary and passing as any other, and each one is—potentially—the gate opening into eternity. Thus the distinction between the mundane and the eternal, transient and durable, mortal and immortal, is all but effaced. Daily life is a constant rehearsal of both mortality and immortality—and of the futility of setting one against the other.
>
> *Simultaneity* replaced history as the location of meaning.

What counts—what has the power to define and shape—is what is around here and now. "Older" and "younger" objects are all on the same plane, that of the present. (1992b, pp. 168-69)

A good example of the expression of postmodern time is the development of retirement communities and Sun Cities. These spaces are akin to the touristic theme parks and fast-food restaurants that are so pervasive in North America whereby "every place can be anyplace in an essentially placeless world" (Rowles, 1994, p. 122). The retirement communities are often publicized as "escapes," "villages," "havens," and "parks" and constitute what Andrew Blaikie calls the "landscapes of later life" (1999, pp. 169-96). In reality they tend to isolate aging groups and potentially mask the aging process itself by naturalizing retirement living as continuously active and problem-free (Laws, 1995b, 1996; McHugh, 2000). Hence, new retirement developments can have the ironic effect of presenting agehood as an ageless and timeless experience, while separating it from the life course at the same time. This leads Robert Kastenbaum to observe that in an Arizona Sun City, "time is the time of busy and robust adults in their prime years ... it's a funny kind of time, though" (1993, pp. 177-78).

Another example is the reconceptualization of sexuality that has accompanied the popularity of sexual dysfunction medications such as Viagra and related health promotion campaigns that link sexual "fitness" to healthy aging. This postindustrial version of sexual vigour glosses over those cases where sexual dysfunction or impotence might actually be an effect of aging, disease, or psychological or personal problems that require specialized care or long-term counselling, as argued in Chapter 9. Thus, eternal (hetero)sexual functionality is yet another ageless, lifelong ambition seemingly attainable through the technological, consumerist, and lifestyle resources of postindustrial society (Hepworth and Featherstone, 1998; Katz and Marshall, 2003). The widespread uses of cosmetic surgery, rejuvenation, and life-extension therapies, as well as "boomer" fashion and recreation industries, are other areas that similarly reduce to a singular historical existence the opportunities for living in time within a global diversity of life courses.

It is important to note that the scientific community itself is divided about the possibilities of anti-aging. A recent *Scientific American* article on "The Truth about Human Aging" (13 May 2002) cites 51 leading research scientists who debate and critique anti-aging and enhancement technologies: specifically, antioxidant supplements, genetic therapy, telomere cellular shortening, caloric restrictive diets, hormonal enhancements, and

cloning and embryonic stem cell technology. At the end of their survey
the scientists all agree on three seemingly obvious points. First, aging is
not a disease, but even if all age-related causes of death were eliminated,
humans would still suffer from the biological processes of aging. We cannot live forever; we cannot grow younger; and only very few people can
survive to the current edge of the human life span projection of 122 years.
Secondly, anti-aging medicine, despite its popularity, can only address
some of the manifestations and consequences of aging by attempting to
mask or retard them, but it has no influence on the aging process itself. (It
is estimated that even if a cure were found for Alzheimer's Disease, only
19 days would be added to the average life expectation). Thirdly, optimum
lifestyles, exercise, and dietary regimes may contribute to life expectancy
and prevent age-related diseases, but in themselves do not increase
longevity or alter the processes of age. So, while future research on anti-
aging may be very promising, presently the scientists conclude with a
warning urging "the general public to avoid buying or using products or
other interventions from anyone claiming that they will slow, stop or
reverse aging."

However, the cultural responses to aging that derive from popular
gerontological, commercial, marketing, media, and even governmental
spheres appear to contradict these obvious points, preferring instead to
project images of aging that foster a more timeless and ageless experience
of growing older. They point to the expectation that we can become successful members of a new and bold senior citizenry if we could just grow
older unburdened by the limitations of aging. But how can we grow older
without aging, and why is this desirable? Why is this happening now, and
what cultural conditions support it? Is the problem that we struggle
against morbidity and decline, or that we refuse to give morbidity and
decline any meaningful place in our society? And most importantly, who
benefits and who suffers from a culture that idealizes growing older while
denying aging?

Positive Aging or Positive Ageism?

While few would complain that images of activity, independence, and
mobility are replacing past negative stereotypes of aging decline, poverty,
and obsolescence, our culture's positive turn has also tended to overlook
the hardships experienced by many senior and older persons, which are
also the consequence of postmodern living. As Kastenbaum (1993) and

other critical gerontologists point out, popular images and professional programs that connect positive aging to anti-aging can lead to the very marginalization they profess to eradicate (Ekerdt, 1986; Hepworth, 1995; Moody, 1988a). For instance, in Canada, although child poverty is promoted as the most prominent social issue, 20.8 per cent of seniors aged 65 and older have relatively low incomes (with single women leading the group), which is only slightly less than the child poverty rate (Prince, 2000, p. 109). As Western welfare states continue to (neo)liberalize and privatize social services, diminish their budgets for universal social security programs, and relay the responsibilities of public support onto local communities and families, older people who lack the middle-class financial and cultural capital to secure successful, self-financed, and self-caring lifestyles will face even greater struggles to meet social expectations. Another Canadian study of senior working people aged 55 to 64 argues that, although the number of mostly male seniors who left the labour market in Canada in the past decade has ballooned (due to early retirement programs, job loss, and poor health), their chances of being poor and dependent are high compared to middle-aged people. The benefits of being a senior in Canada can also be a liability, a problem the authors conclude will have serious repercussions for future aging cohorts who must "first go through the senior years before reaching old age" (Cheal and Kampen, 1998, p. 164). The critics also point out the sexist implications of related models of *productive aging* that reinforce structures of gender inequality (Holstein, 1999).

These and other critical arguments remind us that the *positive* is not necessarily the successor to or the opposite of the *negative*, but rather part of a continuum of images and forces that configures old age and the life course. Many older people are not the exemplars of senior citizenry idealized by the current imagery and do face tremendous emotional and health problems that require sustainable social support, effective care solutions, and informed public sympathy. As Mike Hepworth comments,

> Positive and negative styles of ageing into old age are not objectively distinctive physical conditions waiting to be discovered, but are socially constructed moral categories reflecting the prevailing social preference for individualised consumerism, voluntarism and decentralisation.
>
> [These] foster an accelerating age-consciousness where the fear of ageing into old age tends to predominate, and old age is

consequently perceived as a "social problem" which can only be
resolved by normalising styles of ageing prescriptively designated
"positive" ... and discouraging or even punishing styles of ageing defined as deviant. (1995, p. 177)

In equating the virtues of positive aging with successful aging, and anti-
ageism with timeless anti-aging, both professional and commercial fields
share common ground in their struggle to represent the new aging. At the
same time, positive agendas based on activity and mobility can downplay
traditionally crucial values such as wisdom and disengagement by translating them into (negative) problems of *inactivity* and *dependency*. Thus,
this internal critique of the positive construction of aging not only draws
our attention to the vacuity of popular anti-aging imagery, but also to the
deeper tension that exists between seniors cultures as empowering political and social forces and seniors cultures as commercially "imagineered"
(to use a suggestive term by Glenda Laws, 1995b, p. 276) communities of
marketing demographics, an area to which this essay now turns.

Marketing Maturity

Seniors marketing literature is a prime example of how the postmodern
agenda for timeless, positive aging is aligned to new frameworks for
growing older based on consumerism. Some of the leading texts in this
field have been Jeff Ostroff's *Successful Marketing to the 50+ Consumer: How to
Capture One of the Biggest and Fastest-Growing Markets in America* (1989),
Stephan Buck's *The 55+ Market: Exploring a Golden Opportunity* (1990),
Rosemary Breckler's *If You're Over 50, You are the Target* (1991), George
Moschis's *Gerontographics: Life-Stage Segmentation for Marketing Strategy
Development* (1996), Barrie Gunter's *Understanding the Older Consumer* (1998),
and Ken Dychtwald's *Age Power: How the 21st Century Will Be Ruled by the New
Old* (1999). These texts are accompanied by hundreds of papers and stud-
ies in journals such as *American Demographics*, *Psychology and Marketing*, and
Journal of Consumer Research, and in the reports, brochures, and websites of
new American consulting and marketing organizations such as AgeWave,
Primelife, Lifespan Communications, and Lifestage Matrix Marketing.

In order to convince the corporate world that marketing to seniors is a
booming industry, this literature has developed sophisticated technical
vocabularies that transfigure the life course into market segments and

consumer profiles. As a result, aging, as a chronological process, is masked or disappears entirely. This is necessary, as marketing professors Dale A. Lunsford and Melissa S. Burnett report in a paper on "self image," because the "new age elderly" have a "cognitive age younger than their chronological age" (1992, p. 56); hence the appeal to a younger self-image can increase the purchase of new products or the switching of brands. In other words, new age elderly consumers are not attracted to products specifically marketed to "older people," even though marketing surveys have shown that traditional values based on thrift, honesty, and hard work overdetermine the attraction to "the new" or "the latest" (see also Carrigan, 1999). The authors conclude "the challenge for marketers is to develop products that meet the unique needs of the elderly without becoming a visible emblem of age that others can see" (Lunsford and Burnett, 1992, p. 58). This observation has also been extended to rehabilitation products, according to a recent marketing study, which claims that "the traditional view of older people needing a rehabilitation product as being 'desperate' needs to be abated, and the messages used to communicate need to concentrate more heavily upon humour and wit" (Lancaster and Williams, 2002, p. 409).

Thus masking age becomes a key strategy in developing what has become the "mature market," with maturity being used with increasing frequency because it is a chronologically neutral term endlessly available as a sign for positive images and lifestyles. Yet, choosing what kinds of images and lifestyles should be used in the media for mature advertising, if age is to be masked, is also a challenge (see Carrigan and Szmigin, 2001; Sawchuk, 1995). So is differentiating the mature market from older and younger markets. For example, a study of American insurance trends announces that insurers are starting to use the term "longevity market" and are creating "longevity products" to signal that they "now consider America's oldest citizens to be an insurance niche, worthy of its own nomenclature and product development activity (and dollars)" (Coco, 1995, p. 27). In this case, the longevity market differs from the senior market (aged 50 to 75) in that the former are people aged 75 and over who are at risk of outliving their assets.

Such research can also alter or transform traditional images and realities of later life. Grandparenting is a case in point. Marketers are now increasingly interested not only in the consumer activities of grandparents, but also in how grandparentage itself can be enlarged beyond its generational definitions to include marketing criteria (Fisher, 1996, p. 13).

Indeed, another study is concerned with the lack of databases on "grand-parent lists," because, as one advertising director notes, "grandparents are very hard to find" (Markets, 1996, p. 22). Hence, Lifestyle Change Communications of Atlanta and Caring Grandparents of America (Washington, DC), among others, are today busy expanding and design-ing new grandparent lists.

Marketing language is a component of the strategy to depict maturity and consumerism as intrinsic to the development of each other, even as the life course itself in marketing literature seems to have no particular timelines, goals, or boundaries except to enter into transient networks of spending, owning, and investing. Subjectivity in later life is reduced to a spurious cluster of consumer identities. In short, as the title of Patrick Flanagan's report in *Management Review* recommends: "Don't call 'Em Old, Call 'Em Consumers" (1994). But in order to call them consumers, marketers require more than just new vocabularies and imagery; they also need to reconstruct the determinants and contours of population aging in terms of demographic targets and segments.

To establish the art of market segmentation in later life, George Moschis has invented the term *gerontographics*. Moschis is a professor of marketing and Director of Georgia State University's Center for Mature Consumer Studies, a member of the university's Gerontology Program Faculty, and the instructor of a first-of-its-kind course on "Marketing to Older Adults." His text, *Gerontographics: Life-Stage Segmentation for Marketing Strategy Development* (1996), is a sophisticated compendium of research in social gerontology, life course studies, and consumer behav-iour. In the author's words, gerontographics "is a life-stage model" devel-oped "to help marketers better understand the heterogeneous older con-sumer market" (p. xiii). It consists of a quartet of segmented subgroups, the schematic results of a comprehensive survey of biophysical, behav-ioural, health, and contextual factors. Each subgroup aged 55 and over, is differentiated on the basis of their product preferences and lifestyle profiles. Other studies look to different factors such as restaurant use pat-terns (Morgan and Levy in Stephenson, 1996) or household credit and financial indices (Morgan and Levy, 1996). Overall, gerontographics is part of the larger trend to define, segment, and empower a new con-sumer-oriented senior citizenry. Yet, the discussion of such a citizenry rarely mentions gender or ethnic differences, class and poverty, or rising health care and housing costs. Not only does the "gold in grey" financial marketing strategy assume that middle and older ages are periods in which wealth naturally and easily accumulates for everyone, but also that the life course has an unvarying gravitational pull towards consumer lifestyles and identities premised on the expanding exercise of choice.

On the one hand, while the new marketing literature uniformly criticizes negative images of aging, decries the invisibility of later life in promotional culture and advertising, and advises marketers, according to the theme of one report, "to love the older consumer" (Carrigan and Szmigin, 2001), much of its so-called "maturity" segmentation typologies is patronizing and simplistic. The supposedly positive characterizations of social types and roles can be as stereotyping as the more conventional images, which the marketers denounce (e.g., Gabriel, 1990). On the other hand, there may be more bridges connecting the marketing and gerontological camps than walls separating them, for three reasons.

First, increasingly more marketing research is utilizing gerontological thinking and proclaims an alliance with it. For example, in a paper called "Grey Marketing," the authors cite the work of Carroll Estes and Meredith Minkler on the commercialization of aging (Coleman and Militello, 1995). David Wolfe, (author of *Serving the Ageless Market*, 1990), backs up his views in a commentary on the role of values in older consumer behaviour with the work of Carl Jung, Abraham Maslow, and James Birren (1992, 1994). Again in *Gerontographics*, George Moschis provides lengthy discussions on gerontological theory that would not be out of place in a university-level gerontology course. Other texts link ethnicity to geographical location (Campanelli, 1994, p. 69) and utilize classical sociological distinctions between individual/society and traditional/modern to model the mature Canadian population (Adams, 1997, p. 62). In fact, most literature provided to managers and marketers today contains substantial gerontological, psychological, and sociological data. Andrew Blaikie makes the insightful point that, "market researchers sometimes appear to know more about what goes on in the minds of today's elders and mid-lifers than social scientists" (1999, p. 74).

Second, the legacy of gerontological thinking is already steeped in individualist, activity-type theories of the life course. Thus, the critique of the marketing literature throws much-needed reflective light on gerontological academic traditions. This is too large a point to expand upon here, but one case to consider might be the proliferation of professional activity checklists and social service assessments for older people.[4]

Thirdly, if the critics of postmodernity and neoliberalism are right in concluding that timelines, life-scripts, and life courses are being reordered through the dislocating effects of consumer society as new aging identities are loosened from past conventions, then gerontologists are challenged to extend their multidisciplinary scrutiny to new areas, however prosaic and commercial they may be. We might also learn a great deal from these areas about the kinds of aged identities, bodies, populations, and social spaces upon which competing discourses on the life course are converging in order to recreate it. Chris Gilleard puts it very well when he says: "Exploration of the cultural means by which older people develop their identities should become the central task for a re-fashioned social gerontology; central to that task is the place of consumer culture in the lives of the newly retired population" (1996, p. 496). If gerontologists, professionals, and scholars in the aging field leave it up to the corporate world to frame our understanding of contemporary later life, however, then a great opportunity would have been missed for them to provide genuine anti-ageist leadership in an era of growing anti-aging gerontographical enterprises.

Indeed, futuristic writers are already pursuing critiques of aging in consumer society. For example, science fiction writer Bruce Sterling's *Holy Fire* (1996) is a compelling cyber-fable about a spooky gerontocracy that comes to dominate social life in the twenty-first century, where growing older without aging is the norm. Sterling takes us into a future where the "scope of gerontological research alone was bigger than agriculture" (p. 57) and where much of this research goes into the preservation of older posthuman bodies. His cautionary perspective is neatly encapsulated in one scene where the novel's central female character, who is over 90, enters a virtual architect's office.

> The chairs were puffy, overstuffed, and swaddling comfortable. Old people's chairs. They were the kind of chairs the top-flight furniture designers had begun making back in the 2070s, when furniture designers suddenly realized that very old people possessed all the money in the world, and that from now on very old people were going to have all the money until the end of time. (p. 29)

While appearing at first to have little in common, perhaps Bruce Sterling's fantasies and the prognostications of George Moschis and his marketeers have similarly mapped out a contested ground, intersected by the forces of positive aging, anti-ageism, and anti-aging, where the realities of aging and dreams of timelessness are inevitably destined to clash and transform each other.

As for that other end of life with which this essay began, we can also conclude by asking how the children of today will age, as the twenty-first century's first, fully postindustrial generation? What kinds of environments and technologies, desires and lifestyles, and intergenerational relations will they seek? How will they, as consumers, confront the dreams of their consumer society with the realities of aging, which have been folded into their lives from the earliest ages along with those extra-size diapers?

Notes

This essay is an expanded and altered version of "Growing Older Without Aging? Positive Aging, Anti-Aging and Anti-Ageism," which appeared in the special issue on "Anti-Aging" in the journal *Generations* 25(4), 2001, pp. 27-32. I thank Thomas R. Cole for encouraging and inviting me to write the original essay and the Publication Division of the American Society on Aging for permission to use parts of it here. I also thank the journal *Gerontechnology* and editor-in-chief Johanna E.M.H. van Bronswijk for allowing me to voice some of my ideas on the "postmodern landscape" as a "Shorty," in *Gerontechnology* 2(3), 2003, pp. 255-59.

1. This story comes from Kim Boatman, *Englewood Sun Herald* (Florida), 31 December 1998.

2. Gerontologists who champion positive images of aging have also contributed to this chronological blurring. For example, the late Bernice Neugarten, a pioneer in social and psychological gerontology, espoused the idea of an "age-irrelevant" society in her work that addresses American social policy in the early 1980s (Neugarten, 1982) and was criticized by fellow gerontologists and gero-advocacy groups for doing so. For Neugarten's own views on this controversy and her influential conceptualizations of "young-old" and "old-old" demographic segments, see Neugarten in Riley (1988).

3. Although I deal only with later life here, similar conditions apply to younger consumer categories as well. Children and teenagers, locked into the amorphous category of "youth," are certainly the target of marketing strategies because of the opportunity to build lifelong brand loyalties (even though younger people typically have less income than their elders). For example, *Chips and Pop: Decoding the Nexus Generation* (Barnard, Cosgrave, and Welsh, 1998) is a fascinating corporate survey of the newly minted nexus generation, an offshoot of Generation X. For more caustic treatments on how consumerism has redefined youth and robbed it of political and generational meaning, see the collection of "salvos"

from *The Baffler* magazine, *Commodify Your Dissent* (Frank and Weiland, 1997), and *Kinterculture: The Corporate Construction of Childhood* (Steinberg and Kincheloe, 1997).

4. For instance, one of the first checklists developed by Neugarten, Havighurst, and Tobin (1961) constructed categorical types who fit between behavioural qualities of "zest" and "apathy." In many ways their types prefigure some of the marketing typologies used today.

eleven

Spaces of Age, Snowbirds, and the Gerontology of Mobility: The *Elderscapes* of Charlotte County, Florida

Gerontology is a field befittingly fixed on the problems of aging-in-time and the temporal conditions of growing older. Consequently, researchers focus on *when* people retire and the social roles, economic challenges, and cohort experiences associated with such a momentous life course passage. At the same time the place of retirement has become an increasingly vital dimension of later life because, as more people retire, issues of mobility, residence, and community are linked to gerontologic ideals of independence and successful aging. Thus, this chapter is oriented to the questions of *where* people retire and how they create cultural spaces for retirement. Specifically, the research examines several sites or *elderscapes* unique to Charlotte County in the Gulf coastal area of southwestern Florida as evidence of the growth of new retirement and aging communities. My objective is not to produce a conventional ethnographic analysis but to sketch a social topography of spaces of age. As such, the data combine documents, photographs, personal reflections, and interviews collected during a field research project conducted in Florida during 1998-99. The resulting experimental methodological weave is an attempt to represent the complexity of migrational retirement culture and the spatial dynamics that shape its regions, flows, and environments.

In this chapter I use photographic materials and diary entries as the personal means by which I can include my identity and journey as a researcher within the montage of places I visited. In addition, the photographic and visual materials enrich the depiction of physical and built spaces and their relevance to cultural gerontology. Indeed, visual gerontology is a highly valuable yet surprisingly underdeveloped resource within the field. Where it has been central to the research, as in Dena Shenk and Ronald M. Schmid's work (2002) on the *Rural Older Women's Project in Minnesota* in the 1980s and 1990s, the results are innovative and edifying. As these authors note about their gerontology, "the benefits of using photography as a research tool include providing evidence that is difficult to put into words. Photography can also be viewed as a way to portray the context within which other kinds of data can be analyzed and understood" (p. 260). In another fascinating study British cultural sociologist Andrew Blaikie demonstrates the historical influence of photographic imagery on cultural constructions of retirement, aging, and old age in the United Kingdom (Blaikie, 1999). In these cases visual gerontology has an inherent reflexive dimension because it not only looks to images as valuable sources of data, but it also considers the conditions under which images are used to create data. As visual ethnographer Sarah Pink reminds us, the import of photographic representations is contingent upon how they are situated and interpreted; hence, photographic research is also a reflexive exercise whereby the researchers, in part, construct the cultural environments they analyze (Pink, 2001, pp. 19-21). This means that multiple narratives, ambiguous meanings, and the researcher's subjective experiences can coexist in photographic imagery along with the objective goals of the research itself (p. 126). This is certainly the case with photographic research on aging, challenged as it is by our society's dominant negative images of aging and old age and the restriction of their meanings to demeaning stereotypes that prefigure other kinds of reception and interpretation.

With these methodological considerations in view, the first part of this chapter surveys gerontology's spatial inquiries and postmodern critiques of commercial retirement communities, drawing upon recent cultural theories of global processes whereby technologies, networks, and populations are identified by their movements across geo-social spaces rather than by their locations within them. The second part of the essay portrays the selected *elderscapes* of Charlotte County, Florida with a concentration on *snowbird culture*, a migrational intercultural world where northern Americans and Canadians spend their winter months living in warm southern states.

Towards a Gerontology of Mobility

The Inquiries of Spatial Gerontology

If one could summarize gerontology's primary professional goal, it would be to determine the conditions and contexts in which an individual's adaptation to aging is either facilitated or limited. These include spatial and residential arrangements as key adaptational resources, which academic gerontologists investigate at three levels of inquiry: (1) institutional ethnographies, (2) "aging-in-place" debates, and (3) community networks. In their combination, as the survey below indicates, these inquiries have constituted a significant literature on elder environments and their impact on an individual's health care, quality of life, independent living, and functional capabilities.

Institutional ethnographies are produced by sociological researchers who have been inspired by Erving Goffman's *Asylums* and related social interactionist and ethnomethodological frameworks to tackle the internal environmental relationships and subjective conditions within institutional, residential, and community-care spaces (e.g., Diamond, 1992). Jaber F. Gubrium's social constructivist research is the most well-known for building this level of inquiry into a leading contribution to social gerontology (1997 [1975], 1993). For Gubrium and his associates a nursing home is not simply a building or residence; rather, it is a micro-complex of architectural, administrative, financial, clinical, familial, symbolic, and emotional interactions and power relations.[1] Institutional ethnographers show how everyday existence is organized both formally, according to the structured roles, statuses, and authorities of nursing home administrators, staff, residents, and visitors, and informally, according to the residents' subjective experiences with meals, toileting, sleeping, bathing, activities, family visits, and medical treatment. Everyday existence, as Gubrium notes, is a whole "social world" whereby "worlds are the operating frameworks that make what participants do immediately reasonable in their everyday lives" (Gubrium and Holstein, 1999, p. 295). In such worlds, within and outside institutions, even the most mundane and routine activities in the most microcosmic of spaces, such as residents meeting in the lobby of an old-age home or friends meeting in a fast-food restaurant, take on special social meaning and shape age-identities in elaborate ways (Gamliel, 2000; Cheang, 2002). In *Facing the Mirror* (1997), author Frida Furman discovers an entire social world of older women and their wider community of self-care and sisterhood within the confines of their local hair salon.

The second type of inquiry within spatial gerontology revolves around "aging-in-place" debates. These tend to concentrate on two issues: first, the benefits and disadvantages of people living at home or in familiar surroundings as they age; and second, the transformation of homes or familiar surroundings as people suffer physical disabilities and/or cognitive limitations. Obviously a powerful component of a person's aging is their attachment over time to their homes, neighbourhoods, parks, shopping areas, schools, religious centres, restaurants, and local points of community history. Personal identity is constantly spatialized because people narrate the things and places around them as part of their biographical development. A walk through a neighbourhood or a room-to-room tour of a house and its cherished objects are also poignant narrative experiences full of memories and stories. Therefore, the possibility of not being able to live (or die) at home can be one of the most terrifying aspects of growing older, even where home life creates its own disadvantages. Most aging-in-place research addresses this problem by measuring an individual or family's level of subjective well-being at home against the physical, accidental, and financial risks home residence can generate (*Generations*, 1992; Heumann and Boldy, 1993). As Graham Rowles, a pioneer in spatial gerontology points out, aging-in-place thinking must neither romanticize nor exaggerate "familiarity and emotional affiliation with place" nor "overstate the negative consequences of relocation for the elderly" (Rowles, 1994, p. 122). Rather we must take into account all the pragmatic, intergenerational, income-related, situational and technical realities that go into residential decision-making (see also Rowles, 1978; Rowles and Ravdal, 2002; Heywood, Oldman, and Means, 2002).

If the first issue elucidated by aging-in-place debates is the relation between residence and the continuity of successful aging, the second issue has to do with home environment design modifications and social services that allow people to live in their homes (Lanspery and Hyde, 1997; Taira and Carlson, 1999). For example, simple yet effective home aids such as the installation of hand rails, non-slip floors, easy-to-reach cupboards, or volume-enhanced telephones and doorbells can make home life so much easier for older individuals who experience physical decline.

In homes where stairs are a major impediment to a resident's mobility, sleeping, bathroom, and kitchen areas can be relocated on the same floor. More complicated, however, are those cases where residents, despite their lifelong competencies around cleaning, gardening, cooking, travel, and personal care, require professional home visits or special assisted living services in order to remain at home. Such interventions can upset the delicate domestic balance between private and public spaces, as Julia Twigg (2000) outlines in her research on home residents and visiting careworkers in Britain. In addition to cases of theft and elder-abuse (p. 85), Twigg observes that, "care, in coming into this territory [home], brings its own rationalities, and these are in many ways in conflict within those of home and domestic life" (p. 105). Another disturbing issue is that homes can become very isolating places for older residents who live alone or in secluded areas, and thus residents become house-bound and suffer further physical and psychological problems. Hence, aging-in-place debates correlate the personal circumstances surrounding privacy, identity, bodily, and subjective well-being with the social, spatial, and residential features of homes, homecare, and home-like environments in public settings (Kontos, 1998). The idea of home as a place and a resource, with its own set of risks and rewards, is also an important element of community network research, the third general inquiry within spatial gerontology.

Community network research is a more technical level of inquiry than ethnographic or aging-in-place investigations because here researchers set out to map the gerontological networks by which homes, community facilities, senior centres, geriatric clinics, hospitals, and related areas are linked to the movements, visits, and stays of the older individuals, caregivers, friends, and families who travel between them. Of primary importance is the question of how people cope with spatial transitions, uprooting, displacement, and relocations. Journals such as *Journal of Housing for the Elderly* (Haworth Press) and the social environmental research inspired by M. Powell Lawton and others (Lawton, Windley, and Byerts, 1982; Altman, Lawton, and Wohlwill, 1984; Newcomer, Lawton, and Byerts, 1986) examine the constant interaction between competency, adaptation, context, and environment in the lives of older persons. Such interaction has also been termed the "person-environment fit" whereby "competence does not reside solely in the individual nor in the environment" but occurs "when the capabilities of the individual match the environmental demands and resources" (Schaie and Willis, 1999, p. 183). The information generated by community network and person-environment studies is vital to future health care policy because it helps to determine the conditions under which people can live *autonomously*, that is, in ways by which they negotiate control over both dependent and independent features of their aging. For example, Susan Garrett's report on poor rural communities in Virginia, *Miles To Go* (1998) illustrates how location, identity, and spatial relations configure the experience of aging and determine the efficacy of professional intervention. There is still much research to do in this area, however, as Laura Strain demonstrates in her survey of Manitoba senior centres (2001). Strain found that senior centre rates of participation are unpredictable, often low, or variable with very little information available as to why this is the case. This situation lead her to conclude that "our research knowledge regarding senior centres, their participants, and their activities must be considered in its infancy" (p. 488).

Contemporary social policy has also contributed a different set of political meanings to "community" that profoundly affect person-environment relations. Today the institutional supports that had been built into modern Western welfare states are eroding in favour of greater political reliance upon, and often burdening of, local and community resources. One result is that social program policies coalesce around the transfer of financial state responsibilities to non-state and community social spaces and services (Aronson, 2002; Broad and Antony, 1999; Rose, 1999; Schofield, 2002). Where such spaces and services become enfolded within privatized and community-state partnerships, significant consequences for aging groups have arisen because of the fiscal limitations such partnerships entail and because their articulation within public discourses takes on a crisis-oriented tone, such as those that attempt to "oversell" the problems of population aging (Gee and Gutman, 2000). Community living for aging groups is a neoliberal dilemma. On the one hand, the enhancement of familiar, local, and community spaces which support older persons is desirable, especially given the largely negative and "medicalized" connotations associated with care institutions, nursing, and retirement homes and other specialized environments. Good examples are where local community banks and businesses offer senior homeowners helpful reverse mortgage arrangements, tax incentives, home-sharing options, mixed-age co-op housing, reduced transportation expenses, or low-cost landscaping services. There is also evidence that "naturally occurring retirement communities" (NORCs) are on the rise, whereby sizable groups of retired senior residents happen to find themselves living in a selected area by chance. As such they independently and inventively initiate community mutual aid and other supportive networks, which, in turn, evolve into new community assets (Callahan and Lansperry, 1997; Pine and Pine, 2002). On the other hand, the idealized sense of the "local community" and its assumed beneficence for older persons is promoted in Canada and elsewhere as a political and economic panacea to problems of dependency with little regard to the gender, ethnic, class, and regional inequalities that exist in communities. In other words, as we learn from gerontological community and network research about the *local* as a genuinely creative and resourceful gerontological system of support, we must also consider its increasing role in being made to subsidize governmental fiscal policy, consumer-based health care models, and market-driven retirement planning. Thus, a key challenge of this kind of research is to advance a critical analysis of both the ideals and the practices that make up gerontological communities and spatial networks.

The three areas of inquiry within spatial gerontology outlined here—institutional ethnographies, aging-in-place debates, and community network mapping—create a fascinating subfield that underscores the point that any social space can be the inspiration for important commentary on the state of contemporary later life and gerontological research itself. There are many other examples than the ones offered above. However, one of the most interesting and unique spatial developments has been retirement communities. Unlike other elder spaces and networks, retirement communities call for a somewhat different kind of analysis because lifestyle and leisure values, rather than historical community and social relationships, frame their spatial characteristics and affiliated retiree identities. In particular the American "Sunbelt" or "Sun City" type of communities exemplify the new cultural connection between lifestyle and residence in retirement. As such, these communities have been accused of promoting an overly commercialized and idealized image of successful aging to the disregard of the disadvantaged living conditions faced by many older persons and their families who require sustainable support. Taking this criticism into account, the next section discusses how Sun City retirement communities, lifestyles, and identities might offer spatial gerontology a fresh approach, beyond traditional and local analyses, to the larger cultural forces at work redefining age in an anti-aging culture.

Sun Cities and the Mobility of Retirement

In previous chapters I have discussed how contemporary images of time-less, ageless, and "positive" cultures of aging feed into the postindustrial and postmodern blurring of conventional life course roles and transitions. Within these cultures, and despite current and popular expectations that older people will devise active, independent, self-caring, and mobile lifestyles, those who lack the middle-class financial and cultural capital to do so face an even greater struggle to gain social support and recognition. In the midst of these contradictions Sun City retirement communities, built mostly in Florida, Arizona, Texas, and California since the 1960s, are spatial expressions of the new social aging and its idealistic imagery. In reality, their "gated" exclusivity and predominantly white and owner-res-ident features tend to isolate aging groups and potentially mask the aging process itself by naturalizing retirement living as continuously active and problem-free (Kastenbaum, 1993; Laws 1995b, 1996; McHugh, 2000). Hence, new retirement developments that celebrate active, healthy aging can also separate it from how aging is experienced in real communities. As McHugh comments, "Sun Belt retirement communities are defined as much by the absent image—old poor folks in deteriorating neighbour-hoods in cold, grey northern cities and towns—as by the image presented: handsome, healthy, comfortably middle-class 'seniors,' busily filling sun-filled days" (2000, p. 113). From this critical perspective Sun Cities can appear as simulated lifestyle enclaves, marketed as the just rewards for a life of hard work, and where even the harsh Arizona desert can become a retirement-friendly *elderscape*. In this sense Sun Cities are little more than massive real estate ventures beckoning to well-to-do mid-lifers who are already anxious about their retirement-fit futures.

However, Sun Cities and associated retirement communities also encompass wider and non-commercial issues significant to spatial and cultural gerontological inquiries, such as mobility, migration, and *tran-sculturality*. Indeed, for those sociologists who study spatial processes at the global level the concept of *society* itself is no longer an adequate theo-retical base from which to understand the contemporary movements of peoples and cultures.[2] In this regard British sociologist John Urry pro-vides a new set of ideas stemming from his instructive examination of "mobilities for the twenty-first century" (2000). For Urry, social relations and forces now operate beyond societies due to the impact of global social and populational *flows* (including diasporas), transcultural lifestyles, transnational economic networks, virtual connectivity webs, and borderless transportation systems. Within these mobile forms, "*Scapes* are the networks of machines, technologies, organisations, texts, and actors that constitute various interconnected nodes along which the flows can be relayed" (p. 35). For example, local rapid transportation systems, informational channels, and communication satellites all compete to become connected or plugged into dominant scapes via their own "nodes." Some scapes create incredible power and prestige while others are globally ignored or bypassed altogether. "By contrast with the structured scapes, the *flows* consist of peoples, images, information, money and waste, that move within and especially across national borders and which individual societies are often unable or unwilling to control directly or indirectly" (p. 36). Inequalities in "flows" are based on the degree of their accessibility and the extent to which flows create health or environmental risks in some areas but not in others. Flows can also facilitate mobility and new nomadic lifestyles because of inexpensive travel, cheapened global consumer goods, and electronic connectivity. According to Urry, therefore, places are "a set of spaces where ranges of relational networks and flows coalesce, interconnect and fragment" across distances (p. 140).

Taken together, global *scapes*, flows, and places create the conditions under which global citizenries can emerge, whereby people can "migrate from one society to another," "stay at least temporarily with comparable rights as the indigenous population," and "return not as stateless and with no significant loss of rights" (Urry, 2000, p. 174). Global citizens can also expect to encounter hybrid cultures that contain some of the elements of their own culture. Most importantly, such citizens are,

> ... able to inhabit environments which are relatively free of risks to health and safety produced by both local and distant causes; to sense the quality of each environment directly rather than to have to rely on expert systems which are often untrustworthy; and to be provided with the means by which to know about those environments through multi-media sources of information, understanding and reflection. (Urry, 2000, p. 174)

The overall cultural effect of these historic global processes, as Welsch (1999) reminds us, is that cultural differences "no longer come about through a juxtaposition of clearly delineated cultures (like in a mosaic), but result between transcultural networks, which have some things in common while differing in others, showing overlaps and distinctions at the same time" (p. 201). If typical theories of globalization assume that cultures around the world are becoming homogenized or the "same," transculturality combines local and global cultures anew by merging particular cultural details with universalistic processes. In short, "transcultural identities comprehend a cosmopolitan side, but also a side of local affiliation. Transcultural people combine both" (p. 205).

Unfortunately Urry, Welsch, and other global theorists neglect to include retirement as a key contemporary "mobility" whose migrational patterns are set to become even more extensive in the years ahead. Nevertheless, their characterizations of global citizenry are appropriate to the inhabitants of retirement areas and communities framed by Sunbelt and Snowbird cultures. If we extend their ideas about social spaces (scapes, flows, places) and global transcultural citizens to migrational and mobile retirement cultures, then these, along with related spatial gerontological inquiries and postmodern Sun City critiques, can be considered part of a larger subfield we can call the *gerontology of mobility*. The gerontology of mobility would include the transculturality of both people and places as they age and change while adding a dynamic sense of retirement "flow" to the more static tradition of retirement "time." In line with these proposed defining features of the gerontology of mobility, the second part of this chapter offers a medley of sociological, visual, spatial, and reflexive materials based on three elderscapes in Charlotte County, Florida: Warm Mineral Springs, the Port Charlotte Cultural Center, and Maple Leaf Estates. At the same time the study considers Canadian snowbird culture as an exemplary case of life course "flow" from which to explore the opportunities and contradictions of global life in an era of unprecedented population aging.

Spaces of Age in Charlotte County, Florida

Diary, December 12, 1998: *9 am. Pearson International Airport, Toronto, waiting to depart on Canadian Airways Flight 242 to Miami. Filling the large waiting area are mostly middle-aged and older people, couples, some already with a pre-tanned skin, putting their feet up on matching "his" and "hers" luggage, migrational souls relaxed, travel-tuned and waiting for take-off. The pre-boarding announcement for people with small children immediately inspires the elder crowd to ready themselves. Once on the plane, among*

the seats behind me I see a sprouting of books, bottles of water, crossword puz-
zles, and headphones; hear the quick snapping of seat-belts, closing of over-
head hand luggage doors, zipping up of seat tables, and the stripping off of
parkas, sweaters, and other wintry wear to reveal sensible summer wear, polo
shirts and short-sleeved cotton blouses. Rockport shoelaces are everywhere
loosened and cell phones tucked away, grey heads that line the rows of seats
lay back and smile. These folks know what they're doing. Once airborne, an
elderly male cabin attendant makes his way forward with a trolley for drinks.
As we descend towards the Miami Airport, I wonder if aircraft passenger
cabins have become micro elderscapes and how they might change in the
future accordingly.

Charlotte County, Florida was established in 1921. The story behind the
county's name is that it is an Anglicized corruption of the Spanish
"Carlos" which came from the original native Calusa word "Calos." What
the Spanish called Carlos Bay in 1565 the English called Charlotte
Harbour in 1775 in honour of Queen Charlotte Sophia, wife of King
George III (*Charlotte County Statistical Prospectus* 1998-99, p. 1). The lovely
waterfront and semi-tropical area lies 50 miles south of Sarasota, 24 miles
north of Fort Myers, and 160 miles northwest of Miami. The county
includes the towns of Englewood, Punta Gorda, and Port Charlotte. Port
Charlotte, located north of the Peace River along US Highway 41, is one
of the country's fastest growing areas. However, most of the growth in the
county is tied to the fact that the median age of the residents is 52.1 with
32.9 per cent of them aged 65 and older (*Florida Statistical Abstract*, 1998).
Future projections are for increased immigration and a rising median age.
Put another way, 40 per cent of Charlotte County is 55 or older, and in
some areas 50 per cent or more are 65 years or older.[3] A recent ten-year
health study of Charlotte County's senior residents, according to the
local newspaper, found that "they are healthier and happier than their
peers across the nation" (*Charlotte Sun Herald*, 25 February 1999). The
Senior Community Service and Employment Program affiliated with the
regional AARP (American Association of Retired Persons) Foundation
office in Port Charlotte reported a 73 per cent job placement success rate
in 1998, making the office's success rate second in the country and winning it a bronze award. Charlotte County also hosts the popular weeklong
Senior Fit for Life Games.

Hence, it is little wonder that the social landscape of the county is
dominated by a large number of resident-owned retirement communities, financial, and recreational organizations and health care facilities and

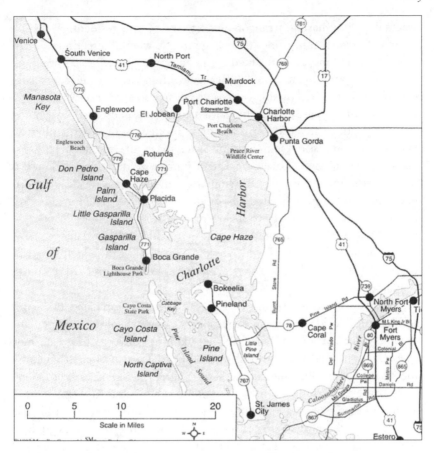

Gulf Coast map showing Charlotte County. Source: *The Gulf Coast of Florida: A Complete Guide.* **Chelle Koster Walton. Stockbridge, MA.: Berkshire House Publishers, 1993, p. 42**

volunteer societies. In brief, there is a five-fold grid of residential options, depending on income level, health status, and individual autonomy: Home Health Care, Retirement communities, Continuing Care Retirement Communities (CCRCs), Assisted Living Facilities (ALFs), and Nursing Homes (*Senior Living Guide of South Florida*, 1998, pp. 27-28). Home Health Care provides visiting professional services for residents who live at home. Retirement communities are mostly private and available to those who live independently but desire a range of leisure activities and resident conveniences. CCRCs are self-contained resident communities that also offer nursing and other care services such as housekeeping and personal assistance in one location, depending on the contractual or purchasing arrangement set out by the resident. ALFs are catered, personal care homes that range in size where recreational activities, meals, bathing, and routine daily needs are provided. ALFs are more of a care environment than CCRCs and often include residents with Alzheimer's disease. Nursing homes are designed for those who require full-time nursing care and facilities for a complete spectrum of assistance. All these options are costly or require the resident to meet strict physical and income admission standards in order to qualify for financial assistance (where it exists). Given the size of Florida's elderly population, it is not surprising that the state's nursing home industry has recently experienced insurance, financial, and labour crises which have combined to create what some critics call "a long-term-care storm" (Polivka-West *et al.*, 2001). Meanwhile, researchers have also found that affordable government-subsidized housing for low-income residents is unequally distributed in Florida, with many people living in underserved counties (Golant, 2002).

However, Charlotte County, as an area heavily populated by senior residents in Florida, is also an experimental zone where the aging demographic forces of North American populations converge to create new spatial, mobile, and transcultural ways of life. This is particularly true in the case of Canadian snowbirds, semi-migrational retirees who spend their winters in Florida while maintaining their homes in Canada. It is estimated that 500,000 Canadians spend three months or more in Florida each year with another 350,000 people heading to other states such as Arizona, California, and Texas. Snowbirds who come to the Gulf coastal areas of southwestern Florida are mostly Anglo-Canadians and live in a variety of residences, the most notable being retirement communities or parks.[4] While snowbird culture is elaborated later in the essay, the point stressed here is that Charlotte County's elderscapes illustrate something of how retirement and later life are shaped both by the material struggles over health and security and by the innovative networks and flows of a unique social topography.

Warm Mineral Springs

Diary, December 16, 1998: *I had been shopping in Sarasota, where most shops cater to elderly customers looking for good deals, restaurants advertise "early bird" special meals, and clothing stores sell the same leisure wear and comfort clothing without extending their imagination to those shoppers who*

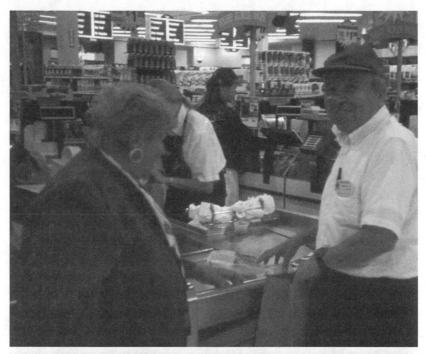

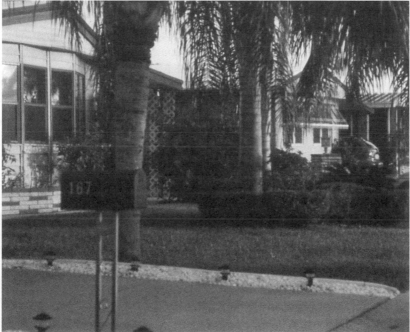

Port Charlotte

maintain a lifelong interest in fashion, elegance, sexiness, and creative expressions of self. Driving back to my place in Englewood, a dark feeling surfaces as I pass identical malls, gated residences and condos, seafood "palaces," video rentals, and gigantic drug-marts. The feeling is one of loneliness and desperation, a secret, fearful retirement culture that exposes the real illusion of an American Dream that not only doesn't last but may never have really existed. Along the roads connecting the towns, new buildings and communities seem to have been burned right out of the environment, in asphalted areas that separate the resorts and golf courses from the original residences that have come to appear as "quaint" or "historic" in comparison. Sometimes the alligators make an appearance as a reminder of what once was. This is a largely white world, cared for and serviced by a world of mostly non-white black or Hispanic labourers, cleaners, drivers, and landscapers. But then all this is thrown into relief when I came to visit Warm Mineral Springs, Charlotte County's fountain of youth.

Warm Mineral Springs is just south of Venice and near the town of North Port in Florida. The spa opened in 1940 and is famous for its highly mineral and sulphurous 2.5-acre lake, whose waters are maintained at a luxuriously warm 87°F year-round. The lake is believed to have youth-giving and healing powers; the water is also drunk as a curative and mild laxative. The area and buildings that once housed rooms for massage, hydrotherapy, hotpacks, whirlpool, and sauna now show their age, and what services are on offer look like they have had better days, although new vacation villas at the Springs are being planned along with a town centre (www.warmmineralsprings.com). There are also apartments to rent or resorts nearby to accommodate people who visit the springs. Despite appearances, Warm Mineral Springs is a unique and fascinating facility that joins the world's great international spas and adds to their mythical accounts about the restorative miracles of drinking and bathing in vital waters. At Warm Mineral Springs, stories and testimonials abound of people tossing away canes and walkers, even wheelchairs, after weeks of bathing or sitting on chairs in the rejuvenating lake. At the lake, mostly elderly bathers swim slowly around the perimeter of the swimming area, enjoying the mineral-rich, steamy water, and soothing their aches and pains. There is a large Eastern European clientele, and visitors to Warm Mineral Springs lean towards traditional health-management techniques involving baths, muds, minerals, massages, open air, calming views, stretching, and water therapy; they appear wary of the current cultural obsession with anti-aging chemicals, surgery, diets, and antioxidants.

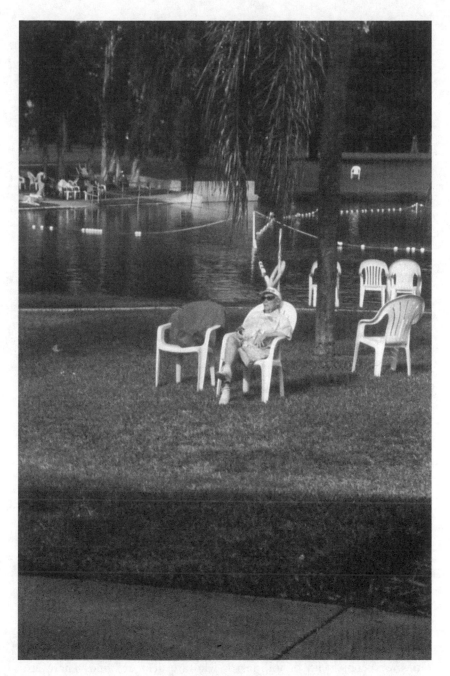

Warm Mineral Springs

Appropriately, Warm Mineral Springs was declared a historic site in 1977. When Ponce de Leon colonized Florida in 1513 (at the age of 53), he was intent on finding the legendary Fountain of Youth but unfortunately he never made it to Warm Mineral Springs.

The Port Charlotte Cultural Center

> Diary, December 17, 1998: *While doing a run to the local grocery store, I discover that many of the part-time workers in drugstores and grocery stores are older and retired, but still working. Indeed older workers are everywhere: behind the counters, the cash registers, carrying out bags, and stacking shelves. At the nearby Publix I talk with Joe, a retiree from the American airforce who now flies around the store aisles gathering shopping carts. He tells me how great it is that younger and older people work in the same place, since the young have so much to learn from the old. In other words, sharing a "job niche" is a great opportunity despite the different values that are placed on life at different points of the life course. Joe and the others know about the Port Charlotte Cultural Center, which they consider "their" center not because it is* for *seniors but because it was built* by *seniors for everybody in Charlotte County.*

When I visited the Port Charlotte Cultural Center on December 24, 1998, I was greeted by volunteers who immediately offered me a cool drink, gave me a tour of the rooms and buildings, and left me with a sense that I had entered a special place: a temple, a micro-world operating on a different basis than the larger society. I was reminded that this was one of the largest, most successful centres of its kind and, as its brochure boasts, "There's nothing like it anywhere else in America." I can believe it. I talked with Judy Ventrella, Director of the Volunteers Office, who showed me several crowded schedules listing the hundreds of hours each month worked by volunteers and the ongoing projects that self-fund the Center. "Miracles happen all the time here," says Judy, because people come in and offer all kinds of skills and talents creating a volunteer pool that is unrivalled elsewhere. The Center also reaches out to provide for those with special needs, such as a course for older drivers, free eye screening, legal support for those working on wills and power-of-attorney arrangements, support groups for widows and widowers, and volunteer opportunities for people with disabilities or who are deaf or blind. There are intergenerational programs being developed to include younger groups so that the Center remains a broadly appealing "cultural" rather than

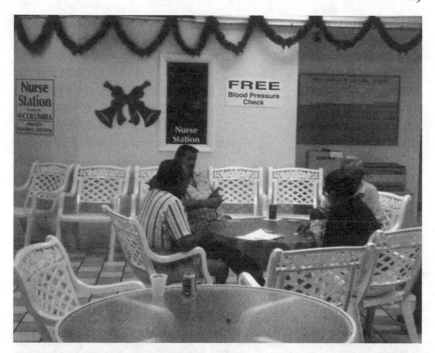

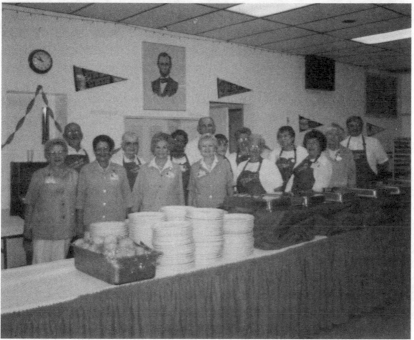

Port Charlotte Cultural Center

strictly "seniors" facility.

Indeed the Port Charlotte Cultural Center is really a complex of spaces and activities, consisting of meeting and music rooms, clothing boutique, school and classrooms, library, woodworking shop, art gallery, travel agency, President's Room Museum, kitchen and cafeteria, the Trash and Treasure Shop, nurses' station, Administrative and Volunteer Offices, and a 418-seat theatre, all housed in four buildings covering five acres of land. Amazingly, along with about 30 paid employees, over 1,000 mostly retired and older volunteers, including its Board of Trustees, run the Center almost entirely. The original buildings were built in 1960 by the General Development Corporation (now called Atlantic Gulf Communities), which constructed housing estates in the area. Retired residents who moved to Port Charlotte organized an adult education school with grants from the county library and school board to build a library, theatre, and classrooms. Hence, the group was referred to as PCU or "Port Charlotte University." In the 1960s PCU and the Center grew through new additions, vigorous lobbying, and sizable donations until it was officially dedicated as the Cultural Center in January 1968. As local histories, such as Jim Robertson's *At The Cultural Center* (1996) demonstrate,[5] it is a case of senior power, senior resources, and senior culture. Robertson's book is based on his radio series on the Cultural Center in the 1990s, and he devotes several chapters to volunteer profiles to celebrate and commemorate their ingenuity and hard work. On a deeper level, Robertson and others who write about the Center are sociologically describing a unique elderscape, one that is constantly in transition as it attracts and coordinates an expansive mutual aid society. The number of social recreation and learning opportunities is stunning; The Activities Center and The Theatre offer a host of theatrical, musical, travel, health, and lifestyle programs, and at The Learning Place over 140 volunteer-taught classes are available across a range of academic, lifestyle, professional, and language subjects. The Cultural Center is also a social magnet that attracts regular public and media attention, public and private funding, renovation projects, partnerships, and community support to Port Charlotte itself; thus, the Center extends its importance within the vibrant elder network throughout the county.

Concluding my visit to the Center I join some of the men playing cards in the club room. As we talk, most of the players tell me that they are from the northeastern part of the country where they spent most of their working lives. And while they came to Florida to retire and escape the grueling winters of the north, they found they still needed to work at something in order to maintain a rich social life and stimulate their intellectual interests. So they are fortunate to be exactly where they want to be. As I leave the Cultural Center and drive around Port Charlotte, I realize the important role the Center plays as a counter space to the commercial sites surrounding it, which announce atop their flashing billboards the seemingly endless places and services catering to eyes, muscles, hearing, rehabilitation, exercise, hair loss, and teeth. Because medicine and consumerism are made to meet and mingle so well here, drugstores articulate the many malls and mini-malls around their clinical glow, absorbing into their commercial authority other opportunities for sociality, activity, and collective meaning. Invisible or non-existent are computer, hardware, music, book, and kitchen shops—places of doing, learning, and growing. This is why the Cultural Center's members, volunteers, and participants, wise in establishing themselves as an autonomous, enterprising, and inclusive community, can walk outside their special elderscape and squint skeptically in the Florida sun at the age-resistant culture around them.

Snowbird Culture

"The Life of the Retired in a Trailer Park," is a short paper written by G.C. Hoyt in the *American Journal of Sociology* in 1954, but it is generally credited as one of the first sociological treatments of migrational or seasonal retirement culture. Hoyt, in his study of the historical Bradenton Trailer Park in Florida, founded in 1936, asks why the residents, whose median age is 69, "leave relatives, friends, and other associations in the home community?" (p. 361). He reasons that the climate is obviously an important factor, but more so is the idea that a new kind of community is possible and desirable, one built on a sociality dedicated to retirement living and a "different code of conduct" (p. 369). Since Hoyt's study and despite the growth of migrational or snowbird retirees living in Florida during the winter months, there has been relatively little research on these retirees or the communities and spatial relations that have developed around them. In other words, we are still asking Hoyt's questions.

Charles Longino Jr., professor at Wake Forest University in North Carolina, is one of the few gerontologists who has made a career of concentrating on migrational retirement (Longino Jr. 1984, 1989, 1995, 1998, 2001; Longino Jr., Perzynski, and Stoller, 2002). During the late 1980s and early 1990s Longino Jr. teamed up with Richard D. Tucker, Larry Mullins, and Victor W. Marshall to write an important series of research papers on the first large-scale survey of Canadian snowbirds, whose members today form the largest group of Canadians to be in one place outside the country since the Canadian armed forces were in Europe during World War II (Tucker *et al.*, 1988; Longino Jr. *et al.*, 1991; Tucker *et al.*, 1992; see also Mullins and Tucker, 1988; Marshall and Tucker, 1990). The team discovered three central socio-spatial components of Canadian snowbird culture. First, the relation between migration and permanence is a matter of degree or gradient rather than a binary distinction between a "here" and a "there," with seasonal migrants forming the "middleground of the continuum" between permanent migrants and vacationers (Longino Jr. and Marshall, 1990). Thus, snowbirds are a kind of migrational flow in the sense of the term used by Urry above; their movements give new meaning to traditional definitions of residence, territory, distance, and portability of resources. Sometimes this flow works in a reverse or "counterstream" direction whereby snowbirds move back home because of financial decline, health problems, or changing family relationships, which leads Stoller and Longino Jr. to question whether in such cases people are "going home" or "leaving home"? (2001).⁶ Second, since most Canadian snowbirds are middle class and financially independent, they bring to their Florida communities and host economies an intercultural prosperity through their taxes, real estate, and consumer purchasing. Despite concerns from American hosts that wealthier snowbirds in central, less urban areas would draw away medical resources from local needs, it has been shown that this is not the case and that snowbird medical demands on Florida geriatric services are minimal (Longino Jr. *et al.*, 1991; Marshall and Tucker, 1990). Similar findings have been reported for snowbird groups in Arizona (McHugh and Mings, 1994). Third, snowbirds form their own mobile networks that attract other snowbirds. Mullins and Tucker found that Canadian snowbirds "were nomadic in the sense that their social ties were primarily with the same migrants in the communities they shared at both ends of the move. Their ties were not to places but to the migrating community itself" (Longino Jr. and Marshall, 1990, p. 234). Such networks are also symbolically fortified through the availability of Canadian TV and newspapers such as *Canada News*, *The Sun Times of Canada*, *Le Soleil de la Floride*, and *RV Times*.

   This networking component of Canadian snowbird culture has been augmented by the Canadian Snowbird Association, whose clubs, activities, and snowbird "extravaganza" trade show and exhibitions in Florida, California, Arizona, Texas, and Toronto, contribute to the social expression of a migrational citizenry.[7] Specifically, the Canadian Snowbird Association (CSA) is an advocacy organization that lobbies the government on behalf of senior travellers, provides accessible travel and health insurance packages (Medipac), and acts as a travel information service. The CSA began in March 1992 to challenge budget-slashing governmental attacks on out-of-province health care insurance and limits on travellers' prescription pharmaceutical allowances. The CSA has also inspired other businesses and agencies to focus on snowbirds and their cross-national circumstances; for example, American-Canadian banks now offer special "snowbird services" and favourable currency exchange deals. The 100,000 members to whom the CSA caters, with its images of active, healthy, independent, mobile, and financially secure lifestyles, are mostly a privileged group. However, the CSA also represents the spatial dimensions of an expansive and accomplished snowbird world, a continent of *Snowbirdia*, ranging across great distances in Canada and the United States and mobilized through extensive transportation, internet, and social networks.

Outside of Canada the CSA sponsors the organization of regional snowbird clubs and retiree groups that hold special events, dinners, and golf tournaments and act to provide snowbird groups with support and community. In the Port Charlotte area when I did my fieldwork in 1998, Hazan Walters was President of the Canadian Club of Charlotte County and a very active member of the CSA. The club has been meeting since the mid-1960s and has grown in tandem with the migrational population. Like other clubs, the Port Charlotte group is more of a social network than a structured organization requiring a centre or an office. When I spoke with Hazan at his condo complex near Port Charlotte on December 18, 1998, he explained that while the area has always been marketed as a kind of "dream land" for retirees, older Canadians are challenged by the fluctuating and often declining Canadian dollar, the escalating out-of-province health insurance, and American inflationary costs in health and other services. "The average Canadian is squeezed from both ends," although Charlotte Club members are mostly homeowners (85-90 per cent) and therefore increases in rentals do not greatly affect them. Culturally, Hazan noted that snowbirds are quite comfortable with their bi-national identities and that travelling in both directions feels like "going home." For those who own and live in recreational vehicles, there is even the added sense of being "without an address" and living in the culturally in-between (which can also cause border-crossing problems).[8]

When I asked Hazan if his work with the club and many other activities as a snowbird citizen has made him as busy as when he was working full time back in his native Newfoundland, he replied "more so." Organizing the interplay between snowbird elderscapes and migrational flows obviously takes ingenuity and work; characteristics not lost on the residents of the last place I visited, Maple Leaf Estates.

Maple Leaf Estates

> Diary, December 28, 1998: *When I first drove around Maple Leaf Estates, my attention was drawn to the energetic seniors on bikes or golf-carts, wearing crisp polo shirts and sensible sun hats, zooming around residential streets or trotting across the surrealistic greens of the golf course. It really had the feel of an early and eerie 1960s science fiction movie set, an elder-island inhabited by invading senior aliens. It is so interesting to observe the centrality of golf here, not only as an activity but also as a crystallizing force that bonds the social with the environmental into an accessible, international symbol of retirement life. Of course as I stopped to talk with people, I soon heard about their very real lives. These are people who raise money, help each other, mourn losses, develop networks of friendship and trust; they have fought in wars, worked hard throughout their lives, and survived the upheavals and challenges of the twentieth century. Now, in the twenty-first century, they want to live well, or as best they can.*

Maple Leaf Estates, also called The Maple Leaf Golf and Country Club, is a Port Charlotte resident-owned snowbird community. Sitting on 285 acres of land, the park consists of over 1,000 homes, three clubhouses, four swimming pools, five tennis courts, a library, fitness centre, greenhouse, golf course, and a lake stocked with fish. There are dozens of amenities, services, and activities, including an internal newsletter and a CATV station that broadcasts the park's many events throughout the day. Since at least 60 per cent of the residents are Canadian, the eight miles of streets boast Canadian names such as Maple Lane, McKenzie Lane, Iroquois Trail, Huron Crescent, and Nanaimo Circle. Canadian newspapers are available, and near the entrance security gates the American and Canadian flags fly side by side, emblematizing how the two nations are also cultural allies in the retirement state of Florida, far from the 49th parallel. Indeed Maple Leaf Estates is a place dedicated to Canadian snowbirds, whose numbers swell the park's population to nearly 2,000 residents during the winter months when the mainly Canadian Board of

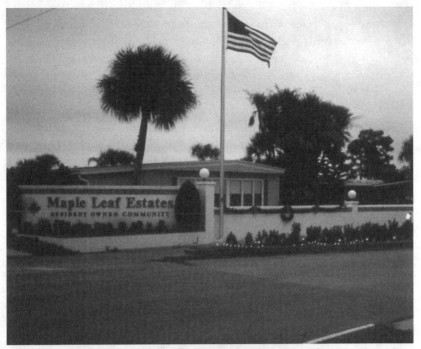

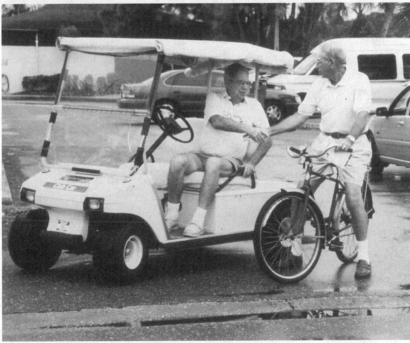

Maple Leaf Estates

Directors organizes the main business and managerial meetings. And when the snowbirds pack up to return to Canada during the summer, the park shrinks to 500 or less with about 250 permanent residents. The park was established in the late 1970s, and the residents purchased it in 1990. They have developed their own governance and social management according to the rights and privileges associated with several intersecting layers of rental, leasing, purchasing, membership, and ownership arrangements. There are also strict regulations around driving, parking, and cycling; use of pools and golf facilities; and treatment of property and design of residences. The most important rule, however, is that the park exists for and is dedicated to people 55 years and older. Children and younger people are allowed to visit, but not to stay. For example, a note in the December 1998 issue of *Accents*, a Maple Leaf Estates Homeowners' newsletter, tries to establish generational guidelines for Christmas visitors:

> We believe that as homeowners and residents of MLE we have an opportunity to deal both creatively and proactively with the projected influx of children into our Park during the coming Christmas Season. We are referring primarily to teenagers who are betwixt and between adults and the young children. Younger children are constantly under the supervision of parents or family members, and their use of Park facilities is largely limited to the kiddies swimming pool. Our challenge is to develop some creative recreational opportunities for teenagers during their stay in MLE. (*Accents*, 1998, p. 10)

On the one hand, Maple Leaf Estates appears to conform to some of the characteristics of Sun City retirement communities described by the postmodern critics above: privileged, leisure-oriented, lifestyle enclaves built by property developers who profit by fostering fantastical and protective age-segregated communities. Dominated by promotional images that embellish healthy aging (and anti-aging) with exhaustive regimes of activity, classes, and clubs, such elderscapes create a bond between new aging identities and the consumer environments and products of postmodern capitalism. In this sense Maple Leaf Estates may have an affinity with other Sun Cities as "a landscape to be consumed" (Laws, 1997, p. 96), where even the children who visit must submit to sunny retirement activities as elders-in-training. On the other hand and despite its emphasis on security and selectivity, Maple Leaf Estates is also an example of a micro-society of migrational processes where the imagery of leisured land-scapes and lifestyles is crosscut by the movements of people across different cultures and various places. The resulting complex of interpersonal, interactional, and intercultural relations is dense and delicately networked to the wider snowbird topography of Charlotte County. The earthbound features of what appears to be just another modular park of seasonal mobile bungalows built on the health/profit/lifestyle corner-stones of the Floridian economy are transcended by the communal energies and creative strategies of its inhabitants. One resident told me that when a new piano was needed for the choir, it took only a "day or less" to raise the money for it. Another resident explained how lifts were built for people in wheelchairs to get in and out of the swimming pool with money raised, again, virtually "on the spot." Flea markets, bake sales, casino days, and auctions are just the edge of a mutual aid society where volunteer labour is everywhere and part of everything. Akin to the Port Charlotte Cultural Center and other spaces of age in the area, Maple Leaf Estates is an interesting world where artless bingo coincides with the arts of sociali-ty to create meaningful cultural resources, similar to the "definitional ceremonies" described by Barbara Myerhoff in her seminal gerontologi-cal ethnographies of aging communities in California (1978, 1986): "Definitional ceremonies deal with problems of invisibility and marginal-ity; they are strategies that provide opportunities for being seen and in one's own terms, garnering witnesses to one's worth, vitality and being" (Myerhoff, cited in Kaminsky, 1993, p. 261).

On December 28-29, 1998, I interviewed several of the Canadian resi-dents at Maple Leaf Estates, including Joan and Bill Charles (fictional names), both in their mid-70s, who have been staying at their park home an average of five to six months since they first bought it in 1982. Indeed, they purchased their property before they retired in 1985. Joan and Bill enjoy their time at MLE because of the social network, the volunteer opportunities for people to help each other, and the freedom to feel one's age apart from the expectations of the younger society that exists back in Canada. They are also pleased to let younger members of their family "take charge" and allow the couple the time and space to withdraw on their own. To Joan and Bill their life in Canada is more constrained than it is in Florida. Besides the colder weather, work and family configure their social relations in Canada, while in Florida the mobile sense of a retirement community allows them the freedom to do things they could not do otherwise. They admit that the long-distance travel, international communications, and moving between places require careful planning, organizing, and fortitude. Upset with the image that snowbirds are a drain on both Canadian and American health care services, the couple is especially keen to see to their health care needs and insurance arrangements in Canada "so that they [insurance providers] will hear from us less." The decline of the Canadian dollar at that time had also required greater attention to financial resources, although since then a rising Canadian dollar has eased snowbird financial pressures somewhat.

One of the most poignant realizations for Joan and Bill Charles is that "eighty percent of the people that were here when we first came are no longer here," and so "it is always sad when we come back." Given the age and cohort identities of the park's population it is not surprising that the number of people who are dying is growing and the question of their replacements troubling. This issue was also raised by others whom I met, such as Ted Smith, the President at the time of the Maple Leaf Estate Homeowners Corporation. Ted, a Canadian from Ontario, patiently explained to me the economics of the park's management and the complexities of the transcultural real estate market, taxes, and rules of ownership. The park is "in transition" because, as original owners may not be physically able to continue their snowbird lifestyles, approaches to the next "coming-of-age group" are still being worked out. There is no doubt that the Port Charlotte area is experiencing tremendous retirement development, but how this will affect Maple Leaf Estates is not completely clear. Will the park become more Americanized, as was the case with neighbouring Victorian Estates, while it waits for younger cohorts to mature into retirement? Will younger cohorts make new demands on the park, look for alternative activities, and seek different residency arrangements? Will rules disallowing children to live in the park have to change? Will selectivity criteria have to become more flexible and accommodating to a future retirement culture loosened from industrial and patriarchal models of the life course?

As I left Maple Leaf Estates with these questions in mind and trying to reconcile its replication of a restrictive suburban utopia with its lively elder village atmosphere, I too wondered what will happen here. Will the next retiring generation care about such a place or care about getting old at all? Maybe retirement communities will become completely different cultural sites and re-network the spaces of age in Port Charlotte and other areas into remarkable new patterns. Future speculations aside, my visit to Maple Leaf Estates and other elderscapes gave me pause to reflect upon how a gerontology of mobility might begin with the proposition that the paradoxes of aging in time might be best understood within the contexts in which they are lived out and journeys through which they flow.

Conclusions: The Uncharted Territory in a Nation of Age

According to Andrew Blaikie, "much of the sociology of later life remains uncharted territory ... sociology may have clarified how 'being elderly' is a learned social role, but is not particularly good at explaining what it is like to become and be old" (1999, p. 169). Blaikie's criticism that sociologists pay scant attention to the lived experience of older individuals in favour of traditional ideas about social "role" is also relevant to the pervasive sociological portrayals of retirement and life course identities as static and bounded phenomena. Accordingly, the goal of this chapter's reviews of spatial gerontological inquiries, Sun City cultural critiques, and theories of global societies has been to illuminate that part of the "uncharted territory" of the sociology of later life related to socio-spatial dynamics. At the same time the study's excursions into the Charlotte County migrational worlds of snowbirds and other retirees have been directed to the question of lived experience as new experimental and mobile cultures challenge the definitions of what it means to grow older today. Arguably the sites selected here are shaped in part by the privileged and mobile demographic status of their occupants and participants. Nevertheless, such sites have become inventive social spaces where experiential and biographical resources culled from diverse backgrounds are summoned to counter the dominant culture's marginalization of older persons and denigration of late life transitions. Our consumer culture is one that openly subdues human values associated with continuity, memory, and tradition and their means of expression despite its rhetorical promotion of "positive aging." This makes identity maintenance in time and place an arduous task of negotiation between postmodern scripts of individualistic choice and structural demands for independent lifestyles, even in the face of suffering, illness, and loss. Thus, the collective strategy to redevelop roots in multiple contexts across intercultural spaces is a critical response and an indication of where the future of aging, and social gerontology, might be heading. I certainly sensed this possibility as I left Florida on January 7, 1999 from the Tampa airport where younger people were heading north and older people were arriving in the south. On the ground the terminal seemed to be a teeming traffic node where ages converged and aspirations were exchanged. And from the air, within my own mobility, I looked down at Florida and wondered how it would grow, provide leadership, and resolve its contractions as it takes shape as a nation of age.

Notes

This chapter appears for the first time here. I would like to thank Trent University's Committee on Research for its financial support of this project and the staff at the Canadian Snowbird Association in Toronto for their help and materials. I owe much appreciation to Patricia Stamp for her photographic assistance. I am deeply grateful to the people in Florida with whom I spoke, snowbirds and others, who offered me their time and patience. I also wish to express my sympathies to all those contacts and friends who lost their homes, properties, and communities due to the destruction wrought by Hurricane Charley in August, 2004.

1. Although physical design problems of institutional settings invite their own critical scrutiny (see Rule, Milke, and Dobbs, 1994).
2. The use of concepts and metaphors of space in sociology, due largely to the influence of Michel Foucault and Pierre Bourdieu, is generally considered a distinguishing mark of contemporary sociological theory (see Silber, 1995).
3. While Charlotte County is certainly one of the "oldest" areas in the United States, the entire population of the recently created City of Laguna Woods, Orange County, California, is over 55 and the median age is 78! Dominated by the private retirement community called Leisure World, the city's residents successfully challenged the building of a nearby airport (see Ross and Liebig, 2002). The city is a unique opportunity to observe what can happen when a retirement community becomes an independent polity.
4. Francophone Canadians also live in this part of Florida but have their main snowbird and holiday hubs on Florida's east coast, such as Hollywood Beach located between Fort Lauderdale and Miami. Much of this area's commerce, banks, real estate, and health care facilities are geared to an estimated 100,000 Canadians that visit each year. Here restaurants offer Québec fare, stores sell Québec newspapers, Québec satellite TV is available, and a seasonally transplanted Québec community lacks few of the amenities of home (Stephanie Nolan, *The Globe and Mail*, 15 March 1999).
5. Also see the Center's website for extensive information on programs, volunteers, and facilities, www.theculturalcenter.com.
6. In the United States, retirees who escape southern heat by heading north are

called "sunbirds." In a study by Hogan and Steinnes (1996) of Arizona sunbirds, patterns emerged whereby snowbirds became eventual sunbirds, thus migrating in both directions.

7. These three socio-spatial elements also apply to other cases, such as Swedish snowbirds who retire in Spain (Gustafson, 2001) and whose trans- and multi-local experiences of mobility and expatriate culture not only invite "further investigation of retirement migration and other forms of later life mobility" but also new knowledge "about globalisation and transnationalism" (p. 392).

8. Dorothy and David Counts capture the fascinating culture of senior recreational vehicle (RV) groups and lifestyles in their book, *Over the Next Hill: An Ethnography of RVing Seniors in North America* (2001).

afterword

Aging Together

The essays in this book have reminded me how much our ideas, metaphors, and meanings of aging are materially inscribed, yet how so little account we take of the material life of aging around us and outside of our particular human experience of it. That fact that we are surrounded by fascinating and divergent temporal conditions, from the deep time of the earth's geological eras to the micro life spans of cellular species, should inspire us to think of aging as encompassing biological, geological, historical, and cosmic spheres. For example, one of the oldest forms of life is the giant California sequoia, with the General Sherman Tree in California's Sequoia National Park estimated to be between 3,000 to 4,000 years old. This alone tells a story of how time is governed by different and wider movements, tempos, environments, and cycles than the ones determining the span and development of our human lives.

This reflective exercise prompted me to look around the home I share with my wife, Patricia Stamp, to see what kinds of aging, outside of myself, exist. There is our African drum; its outer skin, slowly being worn through my years of playing it, is beginning to reveal another skin underneath, a drum-skin that will wear as well and constantly produce different looks and textures that resound to the changing rhythms of its aging. There are the cast-iron frying pans in our kitchen that, with use, oiling, and care, become better cooking utensils. Aging and wear augment their beauty and utility.

In the yard, garden composting bins are reminders that it takes time for compost to age and become the organically powerful and historically vital material that it is. Looking at firewood curing and weathering beside the fireplace and our "old" rocking chair nearby encourages thinking about the place of wood in our everyday products and environments and how we respect its aging and celebrate its endurance.

Even a Chicago peace rose in the flowerbed, so-named for the ending of World War II but whose original stock dates from before that war, signals that rose stock has a history that is understood by gardeners. A rose is not just a rose, but, like other material objects, it is a living gateway to the dynamics between material culture, the contingencies of time, and the spirit of renewal that confront the new paradoxes of cultural aging and its postmodern timelessness with an eternity of other possibilities.

References

Achenbaum, W.A. (1978). *Old Age in the New Land: The American Experience since 1790.* Baltimore, MD: The Johns Hopkins University Press.

Achenbaum, W.A. (1983). *Shades of Gray: Old Age, American Values, and Federal Policies Since 1920.* Boston, MA: Little, Brown and Company.

Achenbaum, W.A. (1991). The State of the Handbooks on Aging in 1990. *The Gerontologist* 31: 132-34.

Achenbaum, W.A. (1993). One Way to Bridge the Two Cultures: Advancing Qualitative Gerontology through Professional Autobiographies. *Canadian Journal on Aging* 12: 143-56.

Achenbaum, W.A. (1995). *Crossing Frontiers: Gerontology Emerges as a Science.* New York, NY: Cambridge University Press.

Achenbaum, W.A. (1996). Handbooks as Gerontologic Maps. *The Gerontologist* 36: 825-26.

Achenbaum, W.A. (1997). Critical Gerontology. In A. Jamieson, S. Harper, and C. Victor (Eds.), *Critical Approaches to Ageing and Later Life* (pp. 16-26). Buckingham, UK: Open University Press.

Adams, M. (1997). *Sex in the Snow: Canadian Social Values at the End of the Millennium.* Toronto, ON: Penguin Books.

Adelman, D.S. (1995). The Biological Facts: Myth vs. Reality. In R. Neugebauer-Visano (Ed.), *Seniors and Sexuality: Experiencing Intimacy in Later Life* (pp. 35-72). Toronto, ON: Canadian Scholars Press.

Adkins, L. (1999). Community and Economy: A Retraditionalization of Gender? *Theory, Culture and Society* 16: 119-39.

Adkins, L. (2001). Risk Culture, Self-Reflexivity, and the Making of Sexual Hierarchies. *Body and Society* 7: 35-55.

Allen Memorial Art Museum Bulletin. (1977-78): 35.

Altman, I., Lawton, M.P., and Wohlwill, J.F. (Eds.). (1984). *Elderly People and The Environment.* New York, NY: Plenum Press.

Amoss, P.T., and Harrell, S. (Eds.). (1981). *Other Ways of Growing Old: Anthropological Perspectives.* Stanford, CA: Stanford University Press.

Andel, R., and Liebig, P.S. (2002). City of Laguna Woods: A Case of Senior Power in Local Politics. *Research on Aging* 24: 87-105.

Andrews, M. (1991). *Lifetimes of Commitment: Aging, Politics, Psychology.* Cambridge, UK: Cambridge University Press.

Andrews, M. (1999). The Seductiveness of Agelessness. *Ageing and Society* 19: 301-18.

Arber, S., and Ginn, J. (Eds.). (1991). The Invisibility of Age: Gender and Class in Later Life. *Sociological Review* 39: 260-91.

Arber, S., and Ginn, J. (1995). "Only Connect": Gender Relations and Ageing. In S. Arber and J. Ginn (Eds.), *Connecting Gender and Ageing: A Sociological Approach* (pp. 1-14). Buckingham, UK: Open University Press.

Arbuckle, T.Y., Gold, D.P., Chaikelson, J.S., and Lapidus, S. (1994). Measurement of Activity in the Elderly: The Activities Checklist. *Canadian Journal on Aging* 13: 550-65.

Ariès, P. (1981). *The Hour of Our Death.* Trans. H. Weaver. New York, NY: Alfred A. Knopf.

Armenini, G.B. (1988 [1587]). *De' veri precetti della pittura.* Turin: G. Einaudi.

Aronson, J. (2002). Frail and Disable Users of Home Care: Confident Consumers of Disentitled Citizens? *Canadian Journal on Aging* 21: 11-25.

Atchley, R.C. (1989). A Continuity Theory of Normal Aging. *The Gerontologist* 29: 183-90.

Atchley, R.C. (1991). The Influence of Aging or Frailty on Perceptions and Expression of the Self: Theoretical and Methodological Issues. In J.E. Birren, J.E. Lubben, J.C. Rowe, and D.E. Deutchman (Eds.), *The Concept and Measurement of Quality of Life in the Frail Elderly* (pp. 207-25). New York, NY: Academic Press.

Auster, C.J. (1985). Manuals for Socialization: Examples from Girl Scout Handbooks 1913-1984. *Qualitative Sociology* 8: 359-67

Aytac, I.A., McKinlay, J.B., and Krane, R.J. (1999). The Likely Worldwide Increase in Erectile Dysfunction Between 1995 and 2025 and Some Possible Policy Consequences. *British Journal of Urology International* 84: 50-56.

Baars, J. (1991). The Challenge of Critical Gerontology: The Problem of Social Constitution. *Journal of Aging Studies* 5: 219-43.

Baber, Z. (1991). Beyond the Structure/Agency Dualism: An Evaluation of Giddens' Theory of Structuration. *Sociological Inquiry* 2: 219-30.

Bacon, Sir Francis. (1977 [1638]). *The Historie of Life and Death with Observations Naturall and Experimentall for the Prolonging of Life*. New York, NY: Arno Press.

Bahr, R. (1992). *The Virility Factor: Masculinity Through Testosterone, the Male Sex Hormone*. Mobile, AL: Factor Press.

Bailey, T. (1857). *Records of Longevity*. London, UK: Darton and Company.

Baines, C., Evans, P., and Neysmith, S. (Eds.). (1991). *Women's Caring: Feminist Perspectives on Social Welfare*. Toronto, ON: McClelland and Stewart.

Baker, G.T., and Achenbaum, W.A. (1992). A Historical Perspective on Research on the Biology of Aging from Nathan W. Shock. *Experimental Gerontology* 27: 261-73.

Barnard, R., Cosgrave, D., and Welsh, J. (1998). *Chips and Pop: Decoding the Nexus Generation*. Toronto, ON: Malcolm Lester Books.

Barry, A., Osborne, T., and Rose, N. (Eds.). (1996). *Foucault and Political Reason: Liberalism, Neo-Liberalism and Rationalities of Government*. London, UK: UCL Press.

Barthes, R. (1974). *Mythologies*. St. Albans, UK: Granada Publishing.

Basting, A.D. (1998). *The Stages of Age: Performing Age in Contemporary American Culture*. Ann Arbor, MI: University of Michigan Press.

Basting, A.D. (2001). "God Is a Talking Horse": Dementia and the Performance of Self. *The Drama Review* 45: 78-94.

Battle, K. (1997). Pension Reform in Canada. *Canadian Journal on Aging* 16: 519-52.

Bauman, Z. (1992a). Survival as a Social Construct. *Theory, Culture and Society* 9: 1-36.

Bauman, Z. (1992b). *Mortality, Immortality and Other Life Strategies*. Oxford, UK: Polity Press.

Bauman, Z. (1998). On Postmodern Uses of Sex. *Theory, Culture and Society* 15: 19-33.

Baxandall, M. (1988). *Painting and Experience in Fifteenth Century Italy: A Primer in the Social History of Pictorial Style*. 2nd ed. Oxford and New York: Oxford University Press.

Bazerman, C., and Paradis, J. (1991). Introduction. In C. Bazerman and J. Paradis (Eds.), *Textual Dynamics of the Professions* (pp. 3-10). Madison, WI: University of Wisconsin Press.

Beard, G.M. (1874). *Legal Responsibility in Old Age*. New York, NY: Russells' American Steam Printing House.

Beauvoir, Simone de. (1972). *Old Age*. Trans. P. O'Brian. Middlesex, UK: Penguin.

Beeson, D. (1975). Women in Studies of Aging: A Critique and Suggestion. *Social Problems* 23: 52-59.

Beizer, J. (1994). *Ventriloquized Bodies: Narratives of Hysteria in Nineteenth-Century France*. Ithaca, NY: Cornell University Press.

Bell, S. (1987). Changing Ideas: The Medicalization of Menopause. *Social Science and Medicine* 24: 535-43.

Bell, R.M. (1999). *How to Do It: Guides to Good Living for Renaissance Italians*. Chicago, IL: University of Chicago Press.

Bellah, R.N. (1985). Social Science as Public Philosophy. In R.N. Bellah, R. Madsen, W. M. Sullivan, A. Swidler, and S. M. Tipton, *Habits of the Heart: Individualism and Commitment in American Life* (pp. 297-307). Berkeley, CA: University of California Press.

Bengtson, V.L., Parrott, T.M., and Burgess, E.O. (1996). Progress and Pitfalls in Gerontological Theorizing. *The Gerontologist* 36: 768-22.

Bengtson, V.L., Burgess, E.O, and Parrott, T.M. (1997). Theory, Explanation, and A Third Generation of Theoretical Development in Social Gerontology. *Journal of Gerontology* 52B: S72-S88.

Bengtson, V.L., and Schaie, K.W. (Eds.). (1999). *Handbook of Theories of Aging*. New York, NY: Springer.

Benjamin, H. (1959). Impotence and Aging. *Sexology* (November): 238-43.

Bennett, A. (1988). A Book Designed for a Noblewoman: An Illustrated *Manuel des Péchés* of the Thirteenth Century. In L.L. Brownrigg (Ed.), *Medieval Book Production: Assessing the Evidence*, (pp. 163-81). Los Altos Hills, CA: Anderson-Lovelace and Red Gull Press.

Bergler, E. (1951). *Neurotic Counterfeit Sex: Impotence, Frigidity, Mechanical and Pseudosexuality, Homosexuality*. New York, NY: Grune and Stratton.

Best, D.L., and Ruther, N.M. (1994). Cross-Cultural Themes in Developmental Psychology: An Examination of Texts, Handbooks, and Reviews. *Journal of Cross-Cultural Psychology* 25: 54-77.

Biggs, S. (1997). Choosing Not to be Old? Masks, Bodies, and Identity Management in Later life. *Ageing and Society* 17: 553-70.

Biggs, S. (1999). *The Mature Imagination: Dynamics of Identity in Midlife and Beyond*. Buckingham, UK: Open University Press.

Biggs, S. (2001). Toward Critical Narrativity. Stories of Aging in Contemporary Social Policy. *Journal of Aging Studies* 15: 303-16.

Birren, J.E., and Clayton, V. (1975). History of Gerontology. In D.S. Wooduff and J.E. Birren (Eds.), *Aging: Scientific Perspectives and Social Issues* (pp. 15-27). New York, NY: D. Van Nostrand Company.

Birren, J.E., and Bengtson, V.L. (Eds.). (1988). *Emergent Theories of Aging*. New York, NY: Springer.

Birren, J.E. (1995). New Models of Aging: Comment on Need and Creative Efforts. *Canadian Journal on Aging* 14: 1-7.

Blaikie, A. (1999). *Ageing and Popular Culture*. Cambridge, UK: Cambridge University Press.

Bogue, R. (1989). *Deleuze and Guattari*. London and New York: Routledge.

Bois, J-P. (1989) *Les Vieux de Montaigne aux premières retraites*. Paris, FR: Librairie Arthème Fayard.

Bond, J., Briggs, R., and Coleman, P. (1990). The Study of Aging. In J. Bond and P. Coleman (Eds.), *Aging in Society: An Introduction to Social Gerontology* (pp. 17-47). London, UK: Sage.

Bookstein, F.L., and Achenbaum, W.A. (1993). Aging as Explanation: How Scientific Measurement Can Advance Critical Gerontology. In T.R. Cole, W.A. Achenbaum, P.L. Jakobi, and R. Kastenbaum (Eds.), *Voices and Visions of Aging: Toward a Critical Gerontology* (pp. 20-45). New York, NY: Springer.

Bourdieu, P. (1990a). Fieldwork in Philosophy (Interview). In *In Other Words: Towards a Reflexive Sociology* (pp. 3-33). Stanford, CA: Stanford University Press.

Bourdieu, P. (1990b). Landmarks. In *In Other Words: Essays Towards a Reflexive Sociology* (pp. 34-55). Stanford, CA: Stanford University Press.

Bourdieu, P. (1993). The Historical Genesis of a Pure Aesthetic. In R. Johnson (Ed.), *The Field of Cultural Production: Essays on Art and Literature* (pp. 254-66). Cambridge: Polity Press.

Boyle, J.M., and Morriss, J.E. (1987). *The Mirror of Time: Images of Aging and Dying*. Westport, CT: Greenwood Press.

Bradley J.F., and Specht, D.K. (1999). Successful Aging and Creativity in Later Life. *Journal of Aging Studies* 13: 457-72.

Breytspraak, L.M. (1984). *The Development of Self in Later Life*. Boston, MA: Little, Brown and Company.

Brinckmann, A.E. (1925). *Spätwerke grosser Meister*. Frankfurt am Main: Frankfurt Verlags-Anstalt A.G.

Broad, D., and Antony, W. (Eds.). (1999). *Citizens or Consumers? Social Policy in a Market Society*. Halifax, NS: Fernwood Press.

Broderick, G.A. (1998). Impotence and Penile Vascular Testing: Who Are These Men and How Do We Evaluate the Etiology and Severity of their Complaints? *Journal of Sex Education and Therapy* 23: 197-206.

Brooks, M.L. (1992). *Retirement Communities in Florida*. Sarasota, FL: Pineapple Press.

Brown, C.V. (Ed.). (1998). *Women, Feminism, and Aging*. New York, NY: Springer.

Brown, R.H. (Ed.). (1992). *Writing the Social Text: Poetics and Politics in Social Science Discourse*. New York, NY: Walter de Gruyter.

Buck, S. (Ed.). (1990). *The 55+ Market: Exploring a Golden Opportunity*. Maidenhead, UK: McGraw-Hill Book Company.

Bunton, R., Nettleton, S., and Burrows, R. (Eds.). (1995). *The Sociology of Health Promotion: Critical Analysis of Consumption, Lifestyle and Risk*. London and New York, NY: Routledge.

Burchell, G. (1993). Liberal Government and Techniques of the Self. *Economy and Society* 22: 267-82.

Burchell, G., Gordon, C., and Miller, P. (Eds.). (1991). *The Foucault Effect: Studies in Governmentality*. Chicago, IL: University of Chicago Press.

Burrow, J.A. (1986). *The Ages of Man: A Study in Medieval Writing and Thought*. Oxford, UK: Clarendon Press.

Bury, M. (1995). Ageing, Gender, and Sociological Theory. In. S. Arber, and J. Ginn (Eds.), *Connecting Gender and Ageing: A Sociological Approach* (pp. 15-29). Buckingham, UK: Open University Press.

Butler, R.N. (1969). Age-Ism: Another Form of Bigotry. *The Gerontologist* 9: 143-46.

Butler, R.N. (1990). A Disease Called Ageism. *Journal of the American Geriatrics Society* 38: 178-80.

Butler, R.N., and Lewis, M.L. (1988). *Love and Sex After 60*. Rev. Ed. New York, NY: Harper and Row.

Buxton, W., and Turner, S. (1992). From Education to Expertise: Sociology as a "Profession." In T.C. Halliday and M. Janowitz (Eds.), *Sociology and Its Publics* (pp. 373-407). Chicago, IL: University of Chicago Press.

Callahan, J.J., and Lansperry, S. (1997). Can We Tap the Power of Naturally Occurring Retirement Communities (NORCs)? *Perspectives on Aging* 26: 13-15.

Campanelli, M. (1994). Selling to Seniors: A Waiting Game. *Sales and Marketing Management* (June): 69.

Campbell, E.J. (2003). Old Age and the Politics of Judgment in Titian's Allegory of Prudence. *Word & Image* 19: 261-70.

Campbell, E.J. (2002). The Art of Aging Gracefully: The Elderly Artist as Courtier in Early Modern Art Theory and Criticism. *Sixteenth Century Studies Journal* XXXIII: 321-31.

Canada News/The Sun Times of Canada (1997-1999). Auburndale, FL: Canadian Media Enterprises.

Caprio, F. (1952). *The Sexually Adequate Male*. New York, NY: Citadel Press.

Carlisle, Sir Anthony. (1817). *An Essay on the Disorders of Old Age*. London, UK: Longman, Hurst, Rees, Orme, and Brown.

Carpenter, B. (1998-99). *Charlotte County "Statistical Prospectus."* Port Charlotte, FL: Charlotte County Chamber of Commerce, Inc.

Carrigan, M. (1999). "Old Spice"—Developing Successful Relationships with the Grey Market. *Long Range Planning* 32: 253-62.

Carrigan, M., and Szmigin, I. (2001). Learning to Love the Older Consumer. *Journal of Consumer Behaviour* 1: 22-34.

Castel, R. (1991). From Dangerousness to Risk. In G. Burchell, C. Gordon, and P. Miller (Eds.), *The Foucault Effect: Studies in Governmentality* (pp. 281-98). Chicago, IL: University of Chicago Press.

Cavan, R.S., Burgess, E.W., Havighurst, R.J., and Goldhamer, H. (1949). *Personal Adjustment in Old Age.* Chicago, IL: Science Research Associates.

Chambon, A., Irving, A., and Epstein, L. (Eds.). (1999). *Reading Foucault for Social Work.* New York, NY: Columbia University Press.

Charcot, J-M., and Loomis, A.L. (1881). *Clinical Lectures on the Diseases of Old Age.* Trans. L.H. Hunt. New York, NY: William Wood.

Cheal, D., and Kampen, K. (1998). Poor and Dependent Seniors in Canada. *Ageing and Society* 18: 147-66.

Cheang, M. (2002). Older Adults' Frequent Visits to a Fast-Food Restaurant: Nonobligatory Social Interaction and the Significance of Play in a "Third Space." *Journal of Aging Studies* 16: 302-21.

Chesser, E. (1947). *Love Without Fear: How to Achieve Sex Happiness in Marriage.* New York, NY: Roy Publishers.

Chopra, D. (1993). *Ageless Body, Timeless Mind: The Quantum Alternative to Growing Old.* Toronto, ON: Harmony Books.

Christ, G.J., and Melman, A. (1998). The Application of Gene Therapy to the Treatment of Erectile Dysfunction. *International Journal of Impotence Research* 10: 111-12.

Christ, G.J. (1998). The Control of Corporal Smooth Muscle Tone, the Coordination of Penile Erection, and the Etiology of Erectile Dysfunction: The Devil is in the Details. *Journal of Sex Education and Therapy* 23: 187-93.

Chudacoff, H.P. (1989). *How Old Are You? Age Consciousness in American Culture.* Princeton, NJ: Princeton University Press.

Clark, K. (1972). *The Artist Grows Old.* Cambridge: Cambridge University Press.

Clifford, C.G. (1990). *Canada's Fighting Seniors.* Toronto, ON: James Lorimer.

Cloet, A. (1993). *University of the Third Age (U3A): The Rank Fellowship Report.* London, UK: The Third Age Trust.

Cockerham, W.C., Rutten, A., and Abel. T. (1997). Conceptualizing Contemporary Health Lifestyles: Moving beyond Weber. *The Sociological Quarterly* 38: 321-342.

Coco, L. (1995). Longevity Products Aren't for the Faint of Heart. *National Underwriter* (26 June): 27.

Cohen, G.D. (2001). *The Creative Age: Awakening Human Potential in the Second Half of Life.* New York:, NY Harper Collins Publishers.

Cohen, L. (1994). Old Age: Cultural and Critical Perspectives. *Annual Review of Anthropology* 23: 137-58.

Cohen, L. (1998). *No Aging in India: Alzheimer's, The Bad Family, and Other Modern Things.* Berkeley, CA: University of California Press.

Cohen-Shalev, A. (1989). Old Age Style: Developmental Changes in Creative Production from a Life-Span Perspective. *Journal of Aging Studies* 3: 21-37.

Cohen-Shalev, A. (1993). The Development in Artistic Style: Transformations of a Creator's Core Dilemma. *Human Development* 36: 106-16.

Cohen-Shalev, A. (2002). *Both Worlds at Once: Art in Old Age.* Lanham, MD: University Press of America.

Cole, T.R. (1986). The "Enlightened" View of Aging: Victorian Morality in a New Key. In T.R. Cole and S.A. Gadow (Eds.), *What Does it Mean to Grow Old? Reflections from the Humanities* (pp. 115-30). Durham, NC: Duke University Press.

Cole, T.R. (1992a). The Humanities and Aging: An Overview. In T.R. Cole, D.D. Van Tassel, and R. Kastenbaum (Eds.), *Handbook of the Humanities and Aging* (pp. xi-xxiv). New York, NY: Springer.

Cole, T.R. (1992b). *The Journey of Life: A Cultural History of Aging in America.* Cambridge, UK: Cambridge University Press.

Cole, T.R. (1993). The Prophecy of *Senescence*: G. Stanley Hall and the Reconstruction of Old Age in Twentieth-Century America. In W.K. Schaie and W.A. Achenbaum (Eds.), *Societal Impact on Aging: Historical Perspectives* (pp. 165-81). New York, NY: Springer.

Cole, T.R., Achenbaum, W.A., Jakobi, P.L., and Kastenbaum, R. (Eds.). (1993). *Voices and Visions of Aging: Toward a Critical Gerontology*. New York, NY: Springer.

Cole, T.R., and Ray, R.E. (Eds.). (2000). *Handbook of the Humanities and Aging*. 2nd ed. New York, NY: Springer.

Coleman, L.J., and Militello, J. (1995). Gray Marketing. *Health Marketing Quarterly* 12: 27-35.

Colombat, M. (1845). *A Treatise on the Diseases and Special Hygiene of Females*. Trans. C. Meigs. Philadelphia, PA: Lea and Blanchard.

Conrad, C. (1992). Old Age in the Modern and Postmodern Western World. In T.R. Cole, D. D. Van Tassel, and R. Kastenbaum (Eds.), *Handbook of the Humanities and Aging* (pp. 62-95). New York, NY: Springer.

Copper, B. (1988). *Over the Hill: Reflections on Ageism between Women*. Freedom, CA: Crossing Press.

Cornaro, L. (1935 [1558]). *How to Live for a Hundred Years and Avoid Disease*. Trans. G. Herbert. Oxford, UK: The Alden Press.

Counts, D.A., and Counts, D.R. (2001). *Over the Next Hill: An Ethnography of RV-ing Seniors in North America*. 2nd ed. Peterborough, ON: Broadview Press.

Courtright, N. (1996). Origins and Meanings of Rembrandt's Late Drawing Style. *Art Bulletin* 78: 485-510.

Covey, H.C. (1991). *Images of Older People in Western Art and Society*. New York, NY: Praeger.

Cowdry, E.V. (Ed.). (1942 [1939]). *Problems of Ageing: Biological and Medical Aspects*. Baltimore, MD: Williams and Wilkin.

Cropper, E. (1984). *The Ideal of Painting: Pietro Testa's Düsseldorf Notebook*. Princeton, NJ: Princeton University Press.

Cruickshank, B. (1994). The Will to Empower: Technologies of Citizenship and the War on Poverty. *Socialist Review* 23: 29-55.

Cruikshank, B. (1999). *The Will to Empower: Democratic Citizens and Other Subjects*. Ithaca, NY: Cornell University Press.

Cumming, E., and Henry, W.E. (1961). *Growing Old: The Process of Disengagement*. New York, NY: Basic Books.

Daly, K.J. (1996). *Families and Time: Keeping Pace in a Hurried Culture*. Thousand Oaks, CA.: Sage.

Dannefer, D. (1999). Neoteny, Naturalization, and Other Constituents of Human Development. In C. Ryff and V.W. Marshall (Eds.), *Self and Society in Aging Processes* (pp. 67-93). New York, NY: Springer.

Dannefer, D. (2003). Whose Life Course Is It, Anyway? Diversity and "Linked Lives." In R.A. Settersten, Jr. (Ed.), *Invitation to the Life Course: Toward New Understandings of Later Life* (pp. 259-268). Amityville, NY: Baywood Publishing.

Danoff, D.S. (1993). *Superpotency: How to Get It, Use It, and Maintain It for a Lifetime*. New York, NY: Warner Books.

Daston, L. (1988). *Classical Probability in the Enlightenment*. Princeton, NJ: Princeton University Press.

Daston, L. (1991). Marvelous Facts and Miraculous Evidence in Early Modern Europe. *Critical Inquiry* 18: 93-124.

Davies, D. (1975). *The Centenarians of the Andes*. London, UK: Barrie and Jenkins.

Davis, N. D., Cole, E., and Rothblum, E.D. (Eds.). (1993). *Faces of Women and Aging*. New York, NY: Harrington Park.

Day, G.E. (1849). *A Practical Treatise on the Domestic Management of Most Important Diseases of Advanced Life*. Philadelphia, PA: Lea and Blanchard.

Dean, M. (1994). *Critical and Effective Histories: Foucault's Methods and Historical Sociology*. London, UK: Routledge.

Dean, M. (1995). Governing the Unemployed Self in an Active Society. *Economy and Society* 24: 559-83.

Dean, M. (1999). *Governmentality: Power and Rule in Modern Society.* London, UK: Sage.

Deats, S.M., and Lenker, L.T. (Eds.). (1999). *Aging and Identity: A Humanities Perspective.* Westport, CT: Praeger.

Deleuze, G. (1988). *Michel Foucault.* Trans. S. Hand. Minneapolis, MN: University of Minnesota Press.

Deleuze, G. (1993). *The Fold: Leibniz and the Baroque.* Trans. T. Conley. Minneapolis, MN: University of Minnesota Press.

Deleuze, G., and Guattari, F. (1986). *Kafka: For a Minor Literature.* Trans. D. Polan. Minneapolis, MN: University of Minnesota Press.

Deleuze, G., and Guattari, F. (1987). *A Thousand Plateaus.* Trans. B. Massumi. Minneapolis, MN: University of Minnesota Press.

Deleuze, G., and Guattari, F. (1990). What is a Minor Literature? In R. Ferguson, M. Gever, T.T. Minh-ha, and C. West (Eds.), *Out There: Marginalization and Contemporary Cultures* (pp. 59-69). Cambridge, MA.: MIT Press.

Dempsey, C. (1977). *Annibale Carracci and the Beginnings of Baroque Style.* Glückstadt: J.J. Augustin Verlag.

Dennis, W. (1956). Age and Achievement: A Critique. *Journal of Gerontology* 2: 331-33.

Dennis, W. (1966). Creative Productivity Between the Ages of 20 and 80 Years. *Journal of Gerontology* 21: 1-8.

Diamond, T. (1992). *Making Gray Gold: Narratives of Nursing Home Care.* Chicago, IL: University of Chicago Press.

Didi-Huberman, G. (1982) *Invention de l'hystérie: Charcot et l'iconographie de la Salpêtrière.* Paris, FR: Macula.

Donahue, W. (1960). Training in Social Gerontology. *Geriatrics* 15: 801-09.

Dormandy, T. (2000). *Old Masters: Great Artists in Old Age.* London and New York: Hambledon & London.

Dowgibbin, I.R (1991). *Inheriting Madness: Professionalization and Psychiatric Knowledge in Nineteenth-Century France.* Berkeley, CA: University of California Press.

Dowling, J.R. (1995). *Keeping Busy: A Handbook of Activities for Persons with Dementia.* Baltimore, MD: The Johns Hopkins University Press.

Drew, B. (1998). *Viagra and the Quest for Potency.* Sarasota, NY: Health Publishers.

Du Gay, P. (1996). *Consumption and Identity at Work.* London, UK: Sage.

Easton, J. (1799). *Human Longevity.* London, UK: John White.

Einem, H. von (1973). Zur Deutung des Altersstiles in der Kunstgeschichte. In J. Bruyn et al. (Eds.), *Album Amicorum J.G. Van Gelder* (pp. 88-92). The Hague: Martinus Nijhoff.

Ekerdt, D.J. (1986). The Busy Ethic: Moral Continuity Between Work and Retirement. *The Gerontologist* 26: 239-44.

Ekerdt, D.J., and Clark, E. (2001). Selling Retirement in Financial Planning Advertisements. *Journal of Aging Studies* 15: 55-68.

Elder, G.H., Jr. (1974). *Children of the Great Depression: Social Change in Life Experience.* Chicago, IL: University of Chicago Press.

Elias, N. (1985). *The Loneliness of the Dying.* Trans. E. Jephcott. Oxford, UK: Basil Blackwell.

Ernst, K., and Kurz, O. (1979 [1934]). *Legend, Myth and Magic in the Image of the Artist.* Trans. A. Laing. New Haven, CT and London: Yale University Press.

Estes, C.L. (1979). *The Aging Enterprise.* San Francisco, CA: Josey-Bass.

Estes, C.L. (1983). Austerity and Aging in the United States: 1980 and Beyond. In A-M. Guillemard (Ed.), *Old Age and the Welfare State* (pp. 169-85). Beverly Hills, CA: Sage.

Estes, C.L. (1991). The New Political Economy of Aging: Introduction and Critique. In M. Minkler and C.L. Estes (Eds.), *Critical Perspectives on Aging: The Political and Moral Economy of Growing Old* (pp. 19-36). Amityville, NY: Baywood Publishing.

Estes, C.L., Binney, E.A., and Culbertson, R.A. (1992). The Gerontological Imagination:

Social Influences on the Development of Gerontology, 1945-Present. *International Journal of Aging and Human Development* 35: 49-65.

Fausto-Sterling, A. (1997). How to Build a Man. In R.N. Lancaster. and M. di Leonardo (Eds.), *The Gender/Sexuality Reader* (pp. 244-48). London, UK: Routledge.

Featherstone, M. (1991). The Body in Consumer Culture. In M. Featherstone, M. Hepworth, and B.S. Turner (Eds.), *The Body: Social Process and Cultural Theory* (pp. 170-96). London,UK: Sage.

Featherstone, M. (1995). Post-Bodies, Aging and Virtual Reality. In M. Featherstone and A. Wernick (Eds.), *Images of Aging: Cultural Representations of Later Life* (pp. 227-44). London, UK: Routledge.

Featherstone, M., and Hepworth, M. (1982a). Ageing and Inequality: Consumer Culture and the New Middle Age. In D. Robbins, C. Caldwell, G. Day, K. Jones, and H. Rose (Eds.), *Rethinking Social Inequality* (pp. 97-126). Aldershot, UK: Gower.

Featherstone, M., and Hepworth, M. (1982b). *Surviving Middle Age.* Oxford, UK: Basil Blackwell.

Featherstone, M., and Hepworth, M. (1985a). The History of the Male Menopause 1848-1936. *Maturitas* 7: 249-57.

Featherstone, M., and Hepworth, M. (1985b). The Male Menopause: Lifestyle and Sexuality. *Maturitas* 7: 235-46.

Featherstone, M., and Hepworth, M. (1986). New Lifestyles for Old Age. In C. Phillipson, M. Bernard, and P. Strang (Eds.), *Dependency and Interdependency in Old Age* (pp. 85-94). London, UK: Croom Helm.

Featherstone, M., and Hepworth, M. (1991). The Mask of Aging and the Postmodern Lifecourse. In M. Featherstone, M. Hepworth, and B.S. Turner (Eds.), *The Body: Social Process and Cultural Theory* (pp. 371-98). Thousand Oaks, CA: Sage.

Featherstone, M., and Hepworth, M. (1995). Images of Positive Aging: A Case Study of *Retirement Choice* Magazine. In M. Featherstone and A. Wernick (Eds.), *Images of Aging: Cultural Representations of Later Life* (pp. 29-48). London, UK: Routledge.

Featherstone, M., and Wernick, A. (Eds.). (1995). *Images of Aging: Cultural Representations of Later Life.* London, UK: Routledge.

Feinson, M.C. (1985). Where Are the Women in the History of Aging? *Social Science History* 9: 429-52.

Feldman, H.A., Goldstein, I., Hatzichristou, D.G., Krane, R.J., and McKinlay, J.B. (1994). Impotence and its Medical and Psychosocial Correlates: Results of the Massachusetts Male Aging Study. *Journal of Urology* 151: 54-61.

Fere, C.S. (1932). *The Sexual Urge: How it Grows or Wanes.* New York, NY: Falstaff Press.

Field, C.T. (1997). Age and Gender in the US Women's Rights Movement: Elizabeth Cady Stanton's "Development Ideal," 1848-1902. Paper presented at the conference on *Agehood and Childhood.* Odense University, Denmark, April.

Fillenbaum, G.G. (1987). Activities of Daily Living. In G.L. Maddox (Ed.), *The Encyclopedia of Aging* (pp. 3-4). New York, NY: Springer.

Fischer, D.H. (1978). *Growing Old In America.* Exp. ed. New York, NY: Oxford University Press.

Fisher, C. (1996). Grandparents Give of Themselves. *American Demographics Business* Reports (June): 13-14.

Fisher, B.J., and Specht, D.K. (1999). Successful Aging and Creativity in Later Life. *Journal of Aging Studies* 13: 457-72.

Flanagan, P. (1994). Don't Call 'Em Old, Call 'Em Consumers. *Management Review* 83: 17-21.

Fletcher, D. (1972). Does a Man Get Too Old for Sex? *The Encyclopedia of Love and Sex* (pp. 163-65). New York, NY: Crescent Books.

Florida for Canadians: Sarasota and the Gulf Coast. (1996). Toronto, ON: Polar Bear Press.

Florida Statistical Abstract. (1998). Gainesville, FL: Bureau of Economic and Business Research, Warrington College of Business Administration.

Floyer, Sir John (1979 [1724]). *Medicina Gerocomica: Or the Galenic Art of Preserving Old Men's Habits.* New York, NY: Arno Press.

Formanek, R. (Ed.). (1990). *The Meanings of Menopause: Historical and Clinical Perspectives.* Hillsdale, NJ: The Analytic Press.

Foucault, M. (1977). Nietzsche, Genealogy, History. In D.L. Bouchard (Ed.), *Language, Counter-Memory, Practice* (pp. 139-64). Ithaca, NY: Cornell University Press.

Foucault, M. (1979). *Discipline and Punish: The Birth of the Prison.* New York, NY: Pantheon Books.

Foucault, M. (1980a). *The History of Sexuality. Volume I: An Introduction.* New York, NY: Pantheon Books.

Foucault, M. (Ed.). (1980b). *Herculin Barbin: Being the Recently Discovered Memoirs of a Nineteenth-Century French Hermaphrodite.* Trans. R. McDougall. New York, NY: Pantheon.

Foucault, M. (1981). "*Omnes et Singulatim*": Towards a Criticism of "Political Reason." In S. McMurrin (Ed.), *The Tanner Lectures on Human Values, Vol. 2* (pp. 223-54). Salt Lake City, UT: University of Utah Press.

Foucault, M. (1983). The Subject and Power. In H.L. Dreyfus and P. Rabinow (Eds.), *Michel Foucault: Beyond Structuralism and Hermeneutics* (pp. 208-26). Chicago, IL: University of Chicago Press.

Foucault, M. (1984a). What is Enlightenment? In P. Rabinow (Ed.), *The Foucault Reader* (pp. 32-50). New York, NY: Pantheon Books.

Foucault, Michel. (1984b). Polemics, Politics, and Problemizations: An Interview. In P. Rabinow (Ed.), *The Foucault Reader* (pp. 381-90). New York, NY: Pantheon Books.

Foucault, M. (1985). *The Use of Pleasure: The History of Sexuality. Volume Two.* New York, NY: Pantheon Books.

Foucault, M. (1986). Of Other Spaces. Trans. Jay Miskowiec. *Diacritics* 16: 22-27.

Foucault, M. (1988). The Political Technology of Individuals. In L.H. Martin, H. Gutman, and P.H. Hutton (Eds.), *Technologies of the Self: A Seminar with Michel Foucault* (pp. 145-62). London, UK: Tavistock.

Foucault, M. (1991). Governmentality. In G. Burchell, C. Gordon, and P. Miller (Eds.), *The Foucault Effect: Studies in Governmentality* (pp. 87-104). Chicago, IL: University of Chicago Press.

Foucault, M. (1997). The Masked Philosopher. In P. Rabinow (Ed.), *Michel Foucault: Ethics, Subjectivity and Truth* (pp. 321-28). New York, NY: The New Press.

Frank, T., and Weiland, M. (Eds.). (1997). *Commodify Your Dissent.* New York, NY: Norton.

Frankel, B. (1997). Confronting Neoliberal Regimes: The Post-Marxist Embrace of Popularism and Realpolitik. *New Left Review* 226: 57-92.

Freeman, J.T. (1965). Medical Perspectives in Aging (12th-19th Century). *The Gerontologist* 5: 1-24.

Freeman, J.T. (1967). A Centenary Essay: Charcot's Book. *The Gerontologist* 7: 286-90.

Freeman, J.T. (1979). *Aging: Its History and Literature.* New York, NY: Human Sciences Press.

Friedan, B. (1993). *The Fountain of Age.* New York, NY: Simon and Shuster.

Fry, C. L. (2003). The Life Course as a Cultural Construct. In R.A. Settersten, Jr. (Ed.), *Invitation to the Life Course: Toward New Understandings of Later Life* (pp. 269-94). Amityville, NY: Baywood Publishing.

Fuller, S. (1993). Disciplinary Boundaries and the Rhetoric of the Social Sciences. In E. Messer-Davidow, D.R. Shumway, and D.J. Sylvan (Eds.), *Knowledges: Historical and Critical Studies in Disciplinarity* (pp. 125-49). Charlottesville, VA: University Press of Virginia.

Furman, F.K. (1997). *Facing the Mirror: Older Women and Beauty Shop Culture.* New York and London: Routledge.

Gabriel, J. (1990). Portraits of the Over-55s in the United Kingdom. In S. Buck (Ed.), *The 55+ Market* (pp. 21-39). Maidenhead, UK: McGraw-Hill Book Company.

Galenson, D.W. (2001). *Painting Outside the Lines: Patterns of Creativity in Modern Art.* Cambridge, MA: Harvard University Press.

Galton, F. (1869). *Hereditary Genius: An Inquiry into its Laws and Consequences*. London: Henry King.

Gamliel, T. (2000). The Lobby as an Arena in the Confrontation Between Acceptance and Denial of Old Age. *Journal of Aging Studies* 14: 251-71.

Gardiner, J.K. (Ed.). (1995). *Provoking Agents: Gender and Agency in Theory and Practice*. Chicago, IL: University of Chicago Press.

Garland, D. (1997). "Governmentality" and the Problem of Crime: Foucault, Criminology, Sociology. *Theoretical Criminology* 1: 173-214.

Garrett, S. (1998). *Miles to Go: Aging in Rural Virginia*. Charlottesville, VA: The University Press of Virginia.

Gastill, J. (1992). Undemocratic Discourse: A Review of Theory and Research on Political Discourse. *Discourse and Society* 3: 469-500.

Gee, E.M., and Gutman, G.M. (Eds.). (2000). *The Overselling of Population Aging: Apocalyptic Demography, Intergenerational Challenges, and Social Policy*. Don Mills, ON: Oxford University Press.

Generations 16. (1992). Special Issue on "Aging in Place."

Generations 25. (2001). Special Issue on "Images of Aging in Media and Advertising." .

Giddens, A. (1984). *The Constitution of Society: Outline of the Theory of Structuration*. Cambridge, UK: Polity Press.

Giddens, A. (1990). Comments on the Theory of Structuration. *Journal for the Theory of Social Behaviour* 20: 75-80.

Giddens, A. (1991). *Modernity and Self-Identity: Self and Society in the Late Modern Age*. Cambridge, UK: Polity Press.

Giddens, A. (1999). *Runaway World: How Globalization is Reshaping Our Lives*. London, UK: Profile Books.

Gilbert, C. (1967). When Did a Man in the Renaissance Grow Old? *Studies in the Renaissance* 14: 7-32.

Gilleard, C. (1996). Consumption and Identity in Later Life: Toward a Cultural Gerontology. *Ageing and Society* 16: 489-98.

Gilleard, C., and Higgs, P. (1998). Old People as Users and Consumers of Healthcare: A Third Age Rhetoric for a Fourth Age Reality? *Ageing and Society* 18: 233-48.

Gilleard, C., and Higgs, P. (2000). *Cultures of Ageing: Self, Citizen and the Body*. London, UK: Prentice Hall.

Gillis, J. (1996). *A World of Their Own Making: Myth, Ritual, and the Quest for Family Values*. Cambridge, MA.: Harvard University Press.

Gilman, S. (1988). *Disease and Representation: Images of Illness from Madness to AIDS*. Ithaca, NY: Cornell University Press.

Gilman, S. (1991). *The Jew's Body*. New York, NY: Routledge.

Glanz, D., and Neikrug, S. (1997). Seniors as Researchers in the Study of Aging: Learning and Doing. *The Gerontologist* 37: 823-26.

Global Aging Initiative. *Center for Strategic and International Studies*. Washington, DC. www.csis.org/gai.

Goetz, C.G. (Trans. and Ed.). (1987). *Charcot the Clinician: The Tuesday Lessons*. New York, NY: Raven.

Golant, S.M. (2002). Geographic Inequalities in the Availability of Government-Subsidized Rental Housing for Low-Income Older Persons in Florida. *The Gerontologist* 42: 100-08.

Goldstein, I., and Berman, J.R. (1998). Vasculogenic Female Sexual Dysfunction: Vaginal Engorgement and Clitoral Erectile Insufficiency Syndromes. *International Journal of Impotence Research* 12: S152-57.

Goldstein, J. (1987). *Console and Classify: The French Psychiatric Profession in the Nineteenth Century*. New York, NY: Cambridge University Press.

Goodich, M.E. (1989). *From Birth to Old Age: The Human Life Cycle in Medieval Thought, 1250-1350* Lanham, MD: University Press of America.

Gordon, C. (1991). Governmental Rationality: An Introduction. In G. Burchell, C. Gordon, and P. Miller (Eds.), *The Foucault Effect: Studies in Governmentality* (pp. 1-51). Chicago, IL: University of Chicago Press.

Gould, G.M., and Pyle, W.L. (1898). *Anomalies and Curiosities of Medicine.* Philadelphia, PA: W.B. Saunders.

Graebner, W. (1980). *A History of Retirement: The Meaning and Function of an American Institution: 1885-1978.* New Haven and London: Yale University Press.

Gratton, B. (1986). *Urban Elders: Family, Work, and Welfare among Boston's Aged, 1890-1950.* Philadelphia, PA: Temple University Press.

Gratton, B., and Haber, C. (1993). In Search of "Intimacy at a Distance": Family History from the Perspective of Elderly Women. *Journal of Aging Studies* 7: 183-94.

Gray, D.A. (1995). *The Canadian Snowbird Guide: Everything You Need to Know About Living Part-Time in the USA.* Toronto, ON: McGraw-Hill Ryerson Ltd.

Green, B.S. (1993). *Gerontology and the Construction of Old Age: A Study in Discourse Analysis.* New York, NY: Aldine de Gruyter.

Gruman, G.J. (1966). *A History of Ideas About the Prolongation of Life: The Evolution of Prolongevity Hypotheses to 1800.* Transactions of the American Philosophical Society 56. Philadelphia, PA: American Philosophical Society.

Gubrium, J.F. (1992). *Out of Control: Family Therapy and Domestic Disorder.* Thousand Oaks, CA: Sage.

Gubrium, J.F. (1993). *Speaking of Life: Horizons of Meaning For Nursing Home Residents.* Hawthorne, NY: Aldine de Gruyter.

Gubrium, J.F. (1997 [1975]). *Living and Dying at Murray Manor.* Charlottesville, VA: The University Press of Virginia.

Gubrium, J.F., and Holstein, J.A. (1993). Family Discourse, Organizational Embeddedness, and Local Enactment. *Journal of Family Issues* 14: 66-81.

Gubrium, J.F., and Holstein, J.A. (1995). Individual Agency, The Ordinary, and Postmodern Life. *The Sociological Quarterly* 36: 555-70.

Gubrium, J.F., and Holstein, J.A. (1997). *The New Language of Qualitative Method.* New York, NY: Oxford University Press.

Gubrium, J.F., and Holstein, J.A. (1998). Narrative Practice and the Coherence of Personal Stories. *The Sociological Quarterly* 39: 163-87.

Gubrium, J.F. and Holstein, J.A. (1999). Constructionist Perspectives on Aging. In V.L. Bengtson and K.W. Schaie (Eds.), *Handbook of Theories of Aging* (pp. 287-305). New York, NY: Springer.

Gubrium, J.F., and Wallace, J.B. (1990). Who Theorises Age? *Ageing and Society* 10: 131-49.

Gullette, M.M. (1994). Male Midlife Sexuality in a Gerontocratic Economy: The Privileged Stage of the Long Midlife in Nineteenth-Century Age-Ideology. *Journal of the History of Sexuality* 5: 58-89.

Gullette, M.M. (1997). *Declining to Decline: Cultural Combat and the Politics of Midlife.* Charlottesville, VA: University Press of Virginia.

Gullette, M.M. (1998). Midlife Discourses in the Twentieth-Century United States: An Essay on the Sexuality, Ideology, and Politics of "Middle-Ageism." In R.A. Shweder (Ed.), *Welcome to Middle Age! (And Other Cultural Fictions)* (pp. 3-44). Chicago, IL: University of Chicago Press.

Gullette, M.M. (2000). Age Studies as Cultural Studies. In T.R. Cole and R.E. Ray (Eds.), *Handbook of the Humanities and Aging.* 2nd ed. (pp. 214-34). New York, NY: Springer.

Gunter, B. (1998). *Understanding the Older Consumer.* London and New York: Routledge.

Gusfield, J. (1981). *The Culture of Public Problems: Drinking-Driving and the Symbolic Order.* Chicago, IL: University of Chicago Press.

Gustafson, P. (2001). Retirement Migration and Transnational Lifestyles. *Ageing and Society* 21: 371-94.

Haber, C. (1983). *Beyond Sixty-Five: The Dilemma of Old Age in America's Past.* Cambridge, UK: Cambridge University Press.

Haber, C. (1986). Geriatrics: A Specialty in Search of Specialists. In D. Van Tassel and P.N.

Stearns (Eds.), *Old Age in Bureaucratic Society: The Elderly, the Experts, and the State in American History* (pp. 66-84). Westport, CT: Greenwood Press.

Haber, C., and Gratton, B. (1994). *Old Age and the Search for Security: An American Social History.* Bloomington, IN: Indiana University Press.

Habermas, J. (1991). *The Theory of Communicative Action. Volume 2: Lifeworld and System: A Critique of Functionalist Reason.* Cambridge, UK: Polity Press.

Halford, Sir Henry. (1831). *Essays and Orations.* London, UK: John Murray.

Hall, G.S. (1922). *Senescence: The Last Half of Life.* New York, NY: D. Appleton.

Hall, L.A. (1991). *Hidden Anxieties: Male Sexuality, 1900-1950.* Cambridge, UK: Polity.

Hall, L.A. (1995). The Age-Old and Hidden Torments of Impotence. *British Journal of Sexual Medicine* 22: 24-26.

Haller, J.S. (1989). Spermatic Economy: A 19th-Century View of Male Impotence. *Southern Medical Journal* 82: 1010-16.

Hamann, R. (1923). *Der Impressionismus in Leben und Kunst.* 2nd Ed. Marburg: Verlag des Kunstgeschichtlichen Seminars.

Hammond, W.A. (1887). *Sexual Impotence in the Male and Female.* Detroit, MI: George S. Davis.

Harding, J. (1997), Bodies at Risk: Sex, Surveillance, and Hormone Replacement Therapy. In A. Petersen and R. Bunton (Eds.), *Foucault, Health and Medicine* (pp. 134-50). London, UK: Routledge.

Harper, S., and Thane, P. (1989). The Consolidation of "Old Age" as a Phase of Life, 1945-1965. In M. Jeffreys (Ed.), *Growing Old in the Twentieth Century* (pp. 43-61). London, UK: Routledge.

Hauser, R. (1999). Adequacy and Poverty Among Retired People. *International Social Security Review* 52: 107-24.

Havighurst, R.J., and Albrecht, R. (1953). *Older People.* New York, NY: Longmans, Green.

Hazan, H. (1986). Body Image and Temporality among the Aged: A Case Study of an Ambivalent Symbol. *Studies in Symbolic Interaction* 7: 305-29.

Hazan, H. (1994). *Old Age: Constructions and Deconstructions.* Cambridge, UK: Cambridge University Press.

Hazan, H. (1996). *From First Principles: An Experiment in Ageing.* Westport, CT: Bergin and Harvey.

Held, J. S. (1987). Commentary. *Art Journal* (Summer): 127-33.

Held, T. (1986). Institutionalization and Deinstitutionalization of the Life Course. *Human Development* 29: 157-62.

Hendricks, J. (1992). Generations and the Generation of Theory in Social Gerontology. *International Journal of Aging and Human Development* 35: 31-47.

Hendricks, J. (1993). Recognizing the Relativity of Gender in Aging Research. *Journal of Aging Studies* 7: 111-16.

Hendricks, J. (2003). Structure and Identity—Mind the Gap: Toward A Personal Resource Model of Successful Aging. In S. Biggs, J. Hendricks, and A. Lowenstein (Eds.), *The Need for Theory: Critical Approaches to Social Gerontology for the 21st Century* (pp. 63-87). Amityville, NY: Baywood.

Hepworth, M. (1995). Positive Ageing. What is the Message? In R. Bunton, S. Nettleton, and R. Burrows (Eds.), *The Sociology of Health Promotion* (pp. 176-90). London, UK: Routledge.

Hepworth, M. (1999). In Defiance of an Ageing Culture. *Ageing and Society* 19: 139-48.

Hepworth, M. (2000). *Stories of Ageing.* Buckingham, UK: Open University Press.

Hepworth, M., and Featherstone, M. (1998). The Male Menopause: Lay Accounts and the Culture Reconstruction of Midlife. In S. Nettleton and J. Watson (Eds.), *The Body in Everyday Life* (pp. 276-301). London, UK: Routledge.

Hess, Beth B. (1993). "Afterward: A Personal Reflection." *Journal of Aging Studies* 7: 195-96.

Heumann, L.F., and Boldy, D.P. (Eds.). (1993). *Aging in Place with Dignity: International Solutions to the Low-Income and Frail Elderly.* Westport, CT: Praeger.

Heywood, F., Oldman, C., and Robin Means, R. (2002). *Housing and Home in Later Life*. Buckingham, UK: Open University Press.

Hindess, B. (1997). Politics and Governmentality. *Economy and Society* 26: 257-72.

Hirsch, E. (1947). *Sex Power in Marriage*. Chicago, IL: Research Publications.

Hirshbein, L.D. (2000). The Glandular Solution: Sex, Masculinity and Aging in the 1920s. *Journal of the History of Sexuality* 9: 277-304.

Hite, S. (1976). *The Hite Report*. New York, NY: Macmillan.

Hitt, J. (2000). The Second Sexual Revolution. *New York Times Magazine* (20 February): 34-41, 50, 62, 64, 68-69.

Hochschild, A.R. (1994). The Commercial Spirit of Intimate Life and the Abduction of Feminism: Signs from Women's Advice Books. *Theory, Culture and Society* 11: 1-24.

Hockey, J., and James, A. (1993). *Growing Up and Growing Old: Ageing and Dependency in the Life Course*. London, UK: Sage.

Hodson, D.S., and Skeen, P. (1994). Sexuality and Aging: The Hammerlock of Myths. *Journal of Applied Gerontology* 13: 219-35.

Hogan, T.D., and Steinnes, D.N. (1996). Arizona Sunbirds and Minnesota Snowbirds: Two Species of the Elderly Seasonal Migrant Genus. *Journal of Economic and Social Measurement* 22: 129-39.

Holstein, M. (1999). Women and Productive Aging: Troubling Implications. In M. Minkler and C.L. Estes (Eds.), *Critical Gerontology: Perspectives from Political and Moral Economy* (pp. 359-73). Amityville, NY: Baywood Publishing.

Hopflinger, F. (1993). From Ageism to Gerontologism? Emerging Images of Aging in Gerontology. In C. Hummel and C.J. Lalive D'Epinay (Eds.), *Images of Aging in Western Societies: Proceedings of the 2nd "Images of Aging" Conference* (pp. 90-97). Geneva: University of Geneva: Centre for Interdisciplinary Gerontology.

Howell, T.H. (1988). Charcot's Lectures on Senile Diseases. *Age and Ageing* 17: 61-62.

Hoyt, G.C. (1954). The Life of the Retired in a Trailer Park. *American Journal of Sociology* 59 : 361-70.

Hufeland, C.W. (1854 [1797]). *The Art of Prolonging Life*. Boston, MA: Ticknor, Reed and Fields.

Jalland, P., and Hooper, J. (Eds.). (1986). *Women From Birth to Death: The Female Life Cycle in Britain 1830-1914*. Atlantic Highlands, NJ: Humanities Press International.

Jameson, F. (2003). The End of Temporality. *Critical Inquiry* 29: 695-718.

Jamieson, A., Harper, S., and Victor, C. (Eds.). (1997). *Critical Approaches to Ageing and Later Life*. Buckingham, UK: Open University Press.

Jamieson, L. (1999). Intimacy Transformed? A Critical Look at the "Pure Relationship." *Sociology* 33: 477-94.

Jaques, E. (1970). Death and the Mid-Life Crisis. In *Work, Creativity, and Social Justice* (pp. 38-63). London: Heinemann.

Jirovec, R.L., and Erich, J.A. (1995). Gray Power or Power Outage? Political Participation Among Very Old Women. *Journal of Women and Aging* 7: 85-99.

Joannides, P. (1992). "Primitivism" in the Late Drawings of Michelangelo: The Master's Construction of an Old-Age Style. In C.H. Smyth (Ed.), *Michelangelo Drawings, Studies in the History of Art* 33: 245-61.

Johnson, C.L., and Barer, B.M. (1992). Patterns of Engagement and Disengagement among the Oldest Old. *Journal of Aging Studies* 6: 351-64.

Kaiser, F.E. (1999). Erectile Dysfunction in the Aging Man. *The Aging Male Patient* 83: 1267-78.

Kalisch, D., and Aman, T. (2001). Maintaining Prosperity in an Ageing Society. *Organization for Economic Co-operation and Development Aging Working Papers*. Paris: OECD.

Kalish, R. (1972). Of Social Values and the Dying: A Defense of Disengagement. *The Family Coordinator* 21: 81-94.

Kalish, R. (1979). The New Ageism and the Failure Models: A Polemic. *The Gerontologist* 19: 398-402.

Kaminsky, M. (1993). Definitional Ceremonies: Depoliticizing and Reenchanting the Culture of Aging. In T.R. Cole, W.A. Achenbaum, P.L. Jakobi, and R. Kastenbaum (Eds.), *Voices and Visions of Aging: Toward a Critical Gerontology* (pp. 257-74). New York, NY: Springer.

Kastenbaum, R. (1991). Racism and the Older Voter? Arizona's Rejection of a Paid Holiday to Honor Martin Luther King. *International Journal of Aging and Human Development* 32: 199-209.

Kastenbaum, R. (1993). Encrusted Elders: Arizona and the Political Spirit of Postmodern Aging. In T.R. Cole, W.A. Achenbaum, P.L. Jakobi, and R. Kastenbaum, (Eds.), *Voices and Visions of Aging: Toward a Critical Gerontology* (pp. 160-83). New York, NY: Springer.

Kastenbaum, R. (2000). Creativity and the Arts. In T.R. Cole, R. Kastenbaum, and R.E. Ray (Eds.), *Handbook of the Humanities and Aging* 2nd Ed. (pp. 381-401). New York, NY: Springer.

Katz, S. (1992). Alarmist Demography: Power, Knowledge and The Elderly Population. *Journal of Aging Studies* 6: 203-25.

Katz, S. (1995). Imagining the Life Span: From Premodern Miracles to Postmodern Fantasies. In M. Featherstone, and A. Wernick (Eds.), *Images of Aging: Cultural Representations of Later Life* (pp. 61-73). London, UK: Routledge.

Katz, S. (1996). *Disciplining Old Age: The Formation of Gerontological Knowledge.* Charlottesville, VA: University Press of Virginia.

Katz, S. (1997). Foucault and Gerontological Knowledge: The Making of the Aged Body. In Clare O'Farrell (Ed.), *Foucault: The Legacy* (pp. 728-35). Brisbane, AU: Queensland University of Technology.

Katz, S. (1999a). Charcot's Older Women: Bodies of Knowledge at the Interface of Aging Studies and Women's Studies. In Kathleen Woodward (Ed.), *Figuring Age: Women, Bodies, Generations* (pp. 112-27). Bloomington and Indianapolis, IN: Indiana University Press.

Katz, S. (1999b). Fashioning Agehood: Lifestyle Imagery and the Commercial Spirit of Seniors Culture. In J. Povlsen, S. Mellemgaard, and N. de Coninck-Smith (Eds.), *Childhood and Old Age: Equals or Opposites?* (pp. 75-92). Odense, Denmark: Odense University.

Katz, S. (2000a). Busy Bodies: Activity, Aging and the Management of Everyday Life. *Journal of Aging Studies* 14: 135-52.

Katz, S. (2000b). Reflections on the Gerontological Handbook. In T.R. Cole, R. Kastenbaum, and R.E. Ray (Eds.), *Handbook of the Humanities and Aging* (pp. 405-18). New York, NY: Springer.

Katz, S. (2001). Growing Older Without Aging? Positive Aging, Anti-Ageism, and Anti-Aging. *Generations* 25: 27-32.

Katz, S. (2003). Critical Gerontological Theory: Intellectual Fieldwork and the Nomadic Life of Ideas. In S. Biggs, J. Hendricks, and A. Lowenstein (Eds.), *The Need for Theory: Critical Approaches to Social Gerontology for the 21st Century* (pp. 15-31). Amityville, NY: Baywood Publishing.

Katz, S., and Marshall, B.L. (2003). New Sex For Old: Lifestyle, Consumerism and the Ethics of Aging Well. *Journal of Aging Studies* 17: 3-16.

Katzenstein, L. (1998). *Viagra: The Potency Promise.* New York, NY: St. Martin's Press.

Kaufert, P., and Lock, M. (1997). *Pragmatic Women and Body Politics.* Cambridge, UK: Cambridge University Press.

Kaufman, S. R. (1986). *The Ageless Self: Sources of Meaning in Later Life.* Madison, WI: University of Wisconsin.

Kaufman, S.R. (1993). Reflections on "The Ageless Self." *Generations* (Spring/Summer): 13 16.

Keith, A. (2000). The Economics of Viagra. *Health Affairs* 19: 147-57.

Kelly, J.L. (1957). *So You THINK You're Impotent!* New York, NY: Doubleday.

Kelly, J.R. (Ed.). (1993). *Activity and Aging: Staying Involved in Later Life.* Newbury Park, CA: Sage.

Kemp, C.L., and Denton, M. (2003). The Allocation of Responsibility for Later Life: Canadian Reflections on the Roles of Individuals, Government, Employers, and Families. *Ageing and Society* 23: 737-60.

Kemp, M. (1976). "Ogni dipintore dipinge se": A Neo-Platonic Echo in Leonardo's Art Theory? In C. Clough (Ed.), *Cultural Aspects of the Italian Renaissance: Essays in Honour of Paul Oskar Kristeller* (pp. 311-23). Manchester: Manchester University Press.

Kemp, M. (1977). From "Mimesis" to "Fantasia": The Quattrocento Vocabulary of Creation, Inspiration and Genius in the Visual Arts. *Viator* 8: 347-98.

Kenyon, G.M., Birren, J.E., and Schroots, J.F. (Eds.). (1991). *Metaphors of Aging in Science and The Humanities.* New York, NY: Springer.

Kenyon, G., Ruth, J-E., and Mader, W. (1999). Elements of a Narrative Gerontology. In V.L. Bengston and K.W. Schaie (Eds.), *Handbook of Theories of Aging* (pp. 40-58). New York, NY: Springer.

Kenyon, G., Clark, P. and de Vries, B. (Eds.). (2001). *Narrative Gerontology: Theory, Research and Practice.* New York, NY: Springer.

Killingsworth, J. M., and Palmer, J.S. (1992). *Ecospeak: Rhetoric and Environmental Politics in America.* Carbondale, IL: Southern Illinois University Press.

Kinsey, A., Pomeroy, W.B., and Martin, I. (1948). *Sexual Behavior in the Human Male.* Philadelphia, PA: Saunders.

Kinsey, A., Pomeroy, W.B., and Gebhard, P.H. (1953). *Sexual Behavior in the Human Female.* Philadelphia, PA: Saunders.

Kirk, H. (1992). Geriatric Medicine and the Categorisation of Old Age—The Historical Linkage. *Ageing and Society* 12: 483-97.

Kitzinger, C. (1987). *The Social Construction of Lesbianism.* Newbury Park, CA: Sage.

Klassen, T.R., and Gillin, C.T. (1999). Heavy Hand of the Law: The Canadian Supreme Court and Mandatory Retirement. *Canadian Journal on Aging* 18: 259-76.

Klein, R. (1979). Judgment and Taste in Cinquecento Art Theory. In M. Jay and L. Wieseltier (Trans.), *Form and Meaning: Essays on Renaissance and Modern Art* (pp. 161-69). New York, NY: Viking Press.

Kohli, M (1986a). Social Organization and Subjective Construction of the Life Course. In A.B. Sorensen, F.E. Weinert, and L.R. Sherrod (Eds.), *Human Development and the Life Course: Multidisciplinary Perspectives* (pp. 271-92). Hillsdale, NJ: Lawrence Erlbaum Associates, Publishers.

Kohli, M. (1986b). The World We Forgot: A Historical Review of the Life Course. In V.W. Marshall (Ed.), *Later Life: The Social Psychology of Aging* (pp. 271-303). Beverly Hills, CA: Sage Publications.

Kohli, M. (1987). Retirement and The Moral Economy: An Historical Interpretation of the German Case. *Journal of Aging Studies* 1: 125-44.

Kondratowitz, H-J. von. (1991). The Medicalization of Old Age: Continuity and Change in Germany from the Late Eighteenth to the Early Twentieth century. In M. Pelling and R.M. Smith (Eds.), *Life, Death and the Elderly: Historical Perspectives* (pp. 134-64). London, UK: Routledge.

Kontos, P.C. (1998). Resisting Institutionalization: Constructing Old Age and Negotiating Home. *Journal of Aging Studies* 12: 167-84.

Kontos, P. (2003). "The Painterly Hand": Embodied Consciousness and Alzheimer's Disease. *Journal of Aging Studies* 17: 151-70.

Kris, E., and Kurz, O. (1979 [1934]). *Legend, Myth and Magic in the Image of the Artist.* New Haven, CT and London: Yale University Press.

Kutza, E.A. (1996). The Maturation of an Interdisciplinary Discipline. *The Gerontologist* 36: 827-28.

LaCapra, D. (1985). *History and Criticism.* Ithaca, NY: Cornell University Press.

Lambert, J., Laslett, P., and Clay, H. (1984). *The Image of the Elderly on TV.* Cambridge, UK: Cambridge University of the Third Age.

Lamm, S., and Couzens, G.S. (1998). *The Virility Solution: Everything You Need to Know About Viagra, the Potency Pill that Can Restore and Enhance Male Sexuality.* New York, NY: Fireside Books (Simon and Schuster).

Lancaster, G., and Williams, I. (2002). Consumer Segmentation in the Grey Market Relative to Rehabilitation Products. *Management Decision* 40: 393-410.

Lanspery, S.C. and Hyde, J. (Eds.). (1997). *Staying Put: Adapting the Places Instead of the People.* Amityville, NY: Baywood Publishing.

Laslett, P. (1989). *A Fresh Map of Life: The Emergence of the Third Age.* London, UK: Weidenfeld and Nicolson.

Laslett, P. (1995). The Third Age and the Disappearance of Old Age. In E. Heikkinen, J. Kuuisinen, and I. Ruoppila (Eds.), *Preparation for Aging.* New York, NY: Plenum.

Latour, B. (1986). Visualization and Cognition: Thinking With Eyes and Hands. *Knowledge and Society* 6: 1-40.

Latour, B. (1987). *Science in Action.* Milton Keynes, UK: Open University Press.

Laumann, E.O., Paik, R. and Rosen, R. (1999). Sexual Dysfunction in the United States: Prevalence and Predictors. *Journal of the American Medical Association* 281: 537-44.

Lauretis, T. de. (1987). Gramsci Notwithstanding, or, The Left Hand of History. In T. de Lauretis (Ed.), *Technologies of Gender* (pp. 84-94). Bloomington and Indianapolis, IN: Indiana University Press.

Laws, G. (1995a). Understanding Ageism: Lessons from Feminism and Postmodernism. *The Gerontologist* 35: 112-18.

Laws, G. (1995b). Embodiment and Emplacement: Identities, Representation, and Landscape in Sun City Retirement Communities. *International Journal of Aging and Human Development* 40: 253-80.

Laws, G. (1996). "A Shot of Economic Adrenalin": Reconstructing "The Elderly" in the Retiree-Based Economic Development Literature. *Journal of Aging Studies* 10: 171-88.

Laws, G. (1997). Spatiality and Age Relations. In A. Jamieson, S. Harper, and C. Victor (Eds.), *Critical Approaches to Ageing and Later Life* (pp. 90-101) Buckingham, UK: Open University Press.

Lawton, M.P. (1993). Meanings of Activities. In J.R. Kelly (Ed.), *Activity and Aging: Staying Involved in Later Life* (pp. 25-41). Newbury Park, CA: Sage.

Lawton, M.P., Windley, P., and Byerts, T. (1982). *Aging and The Environment: Theoretical Approaches.* New York, NY: Springer.

Lawton, M.P., Moss, M., and Duhamel, L.M. (1995). The Quality of Daily Life Among Elderly Care Receivers. *The Journal of Applied Gerontology* 14: 150-71.

Layder, D. (1994). *Understanding Social Theory.* Thousand Oaks, CA: Sage.

Lee, R.L.M. (1990). The Micro-Macro Problem in Collective Behaviour: Reconciling Agency and Structure. *Journal for the Theory of Social Behaviour* 20: 213-33.

Lehman, H. (1953). *Age and Achievement.* Princeton, NJ: Princeton University Press.

Lemieux, A. (1995). The University of the Third Age: Role of Senior Citizens. *Educational Gerontology* 21: 337-44.

Leonard, P., and Nichols, B. (Eds.). (1994). *Gender, Aging and the State.* Montreal, QC: Black Rose.

Leonardo da Vinci .(1965). *Leonardo da Vinci on Painting: A Lost Book (Libro A) Reassembled from the Codex Vaticanus Urbinas 1270 and from the Codex Leicester by Carlo Pedretti.* London, UK: P. Owen.

Lewis, M.I., and Butler, R.N. (1972). Why Is Women's Lib Ignoring Old Women? *International Journal of Aging and Human Development* 3: 223-31.

Lind, L.R. (1988). Introduction. In Gabriele Zerbi, *Gerontocomia: On the Case of the Aged and Maximianus, Elegies on Old Age and Love* (pp. 1-22). Philadelphia, PA: American Philosophical Society.

Livesley, B. (1975). *The Osler Lecture of 1975: Galen, George III and Geriatrics.* London, UK: Society of Apothecaries.

Lock, M. (1993). *Encounters with Aging: Mythologies of Menopause in Japan and North America.* Berkeley, CA: University of California Press.

Lock, M. (1998). Anomalous Aging: Managing the Post-Menopausal Body. *Body and Society* 4: 35-61.

Longino, C.F. Jr. (1984). Migration Winners and Losers. *American Demographics* 6: 27-29, 45.

Longino, C.F. Jr. (1989). Migration Demography and Aging. *Gerontology Review* 2: 65-76.

Longino, C.F. Jr. (1995). *Retirement Migration in America.* Houston, TX: Vacation Publications.

Longino, C.F. Jr. (1998). Geographic Mobility and the Baby Boom. *Generations* 22: 60-64.

Longino, C.F. Jr. (2001). Geographic distribution and migration. In R.H Binstock, and L.K. George (Eds.), *Handbook of Aging and The Social Sciences,* 5th ed. (pp. 103-24). San Diego, CA: Academic Press.

Longino, C.F. Jr., and Marshall, V.W. (1990). North American Research on Season Migration. *Ageing and Society* 10: 229-335.

Longino, C.F. Jr., Marshall, V.W., Mullins, L.C., and Tucker, R.D. (1991). On the Nesting of Snowbirds: A Question About Seasonal and Permanent Migrants. *The Journal of Applied Gerontology* 10: 157-68.

Longino, C.F. Jr., Perzynski, A.T., and Stoller, E.P. (2002). Pandora's Briefcase: Unpacking the Retirement Migration Decision. *Research on Aging* 24: 29-49.

Lorand, A. (1912). *Old Age Deferred.* Philadelphia, PA: F.A. Davis Company.

Lunsford, D.A., and Burnett, M.S. (1992). Marketing Product Innovations to the Elderly: Understanding the Barriers to Adoption. *Journal of Consumer Marketing* 9: 53-63.

Lynott, R.J., and Lynott, P.P. (1996). Tracing the Course of Theoretical Development in the Sociology of Aging. *The Gerontologist* 36: 749-760.

Lyotard, J-F. (1984). *The Postmodern Condition: A Report on Knowledge.* Trans. G. Bennington and B. Massumi. Minneapolis, MN: University of Minnesota Press.

Macdonald, B., and Rich, C. (Eds.). (1984). *Look Me in the Eye: Old Women, Aging and Ageism.* San Francisco, CA: Spinsters Ink.

MacLachlan, D. (1863). *Practical Treatise on the Diseases and Infirmities of Advanced Life.* London, UK: John Churchill and Sons.

MacLean, M. J., Houlahan, N., and Barskey, F.B. (1994). Health Realities and Independence: The Voice of Elderly Women. In B. Nichols, and P. Leonard (Eds.), *Gender, Aging and the State* (pp. 133-63). Montreal, QC: Black Rose.

Major, R. (1974). The Revolution of Hysteria. *International Journal of Psycho-Analysis* 55: 385-92.

Mancini, G. (1956-57). *Considerazioni sulla pittura.* Rome: Accademia nazionale dei Lincei.

Manheimer, R.J. (1992). In Search of the Gerontological Self. *Journal of Aging Studies* 6: 319-32.

Mannell, R.C. (1993). High-Investment Activity and Life Satisfaction Among Older Adults: Committed, Serious Leisure, and Flow Activities. In J.R. Kelly (Ed.), *Activity and Aging: Staying Involved in Later Life* (pp. 123-45). Newbury Park, CA: Sage.

Markets. (1996). *American Demographics* (June): 22, 24.

Marneffe, D. de. (1991). Looking and Listening: The Construction of Clinical Knowledge in Charcot and Freud. *Signs: Journal of Women and Culture* 17: 71-111.

Marshall, B.L. (2001a). "The Nature of the Body": Heterogendered Bodies and Sexual Medicine. Paper presented to the British Sociological Association Conference, Manchester, UK, April.

Marshall, B.L. (2001b). Much Ado about Gender: A Conceptual Travelogue. *Advances in Gender Research. Special Issue, An International Feminist Challenge to Theory* 5: 97-117.

Marshall, B.L. (2002). Hard Science: Gendered Constructions of Sexual Dysfunction in the Viagra Age. *Sexualities* 5: 131-58.

Marshall, V.W. (1978). Notes for a Radical Gerontology. *International Journal of Aging and Human Development* 9: 163-75.

Marshall, V.W. (1980). *Last Chapters: A Sociology of Aging and Dying.* Monterey, CA: Brooks/Cole.

Marshall, V.W. (1987). Introduction: Social Perspective on Aging. In V.W. Marshall (Ed.), *Aging in Canada: Social Perspectives,* 2nd ed. (pp. 1-7). Markham, ON: Fitzhenry and Whiteside.

Marshall, V.W. (1994). Sociology, Psychology, and the Theoretical Legacy of the Kansas City Studies. *The Gerontologist* 34: 768-74.

Marshall, V.W. (1996). The State of Theory in Aging and the Social Sciences. In RH. Binstock and L.K. George (Eds.), *Handbook of Aging and the Social Sciences,* 4th ed (pp. 12-30). San Diego, CA: Academic Press.

Marshall, V.W. (1999a). Analyzing Social Theories of Aging. In V.L. Bengston and K.W. Schaie (Eds.), *Handbook of Theories of Aging* (pp. 434-55). New York, NY: Springer.

Marshall, V.W. (1999b). Reasoning with Case Studies: Issues of an Aging Workforce. *Journal of Aging Studies* 13: 377-89.

Marshall, V.W., and Tucker, R.D. (1990). Canadian Seasonal Migrants to the Sunbelt: Boon or Burden? *Journal of Applied Gerontology* 9: 420-32.

Masoro, E.J. (1996). What Are We Talking About? *The Gerontologist* 36: 828-30.

Masters, W.H., and Johnson, V. (1966). *Human Sexual Response.* Boston, MA: Little, Brown.

Masters, W.H., and Johnson, V. (1970). *Human Sexual Inadequacy.* Boston, MA: Little, Brown.

Matthews, S.H. (1979). *The Social World of Old Women.* Beverly Hills, CA: Sage.

Mayer, K.U., and Schoepflin, U. (1989). The State and the Life Course. *Annual Review of Sociology* 15: 187-209.

McCarren, F. (1995). The "Symptomatic Act" Circa 1900: Hysteria, Hypnosis, Electricity, Dance. *Critical Inquiry* 21: 748-74.

McDonald, L. (1997). Invisible Poor: Canada's Retired Widows. *Canadian Journal on Aging* 16: 553-83.

McDonald, K. (2000). Who Will Be Impotent First? *Men's Health* (October): 70-72.

McFadden, B. (1923). *Manhood and Marriage.* New York, NY: McFadden Publications.

McHugh, K.E. (2000). The "Ageless Self"? Emplacement of Identities in Sun Belt Retirement Communities. *Journal of Aging Studies* 14: 103-15.

McHugh, K.E., and Mings, R.C. (1994). Seasonal Migration and Health Care. *Journal of Aging and Health* 6: 111-32.

McKinlay, J.B., Longcope, C., and Gray, A. (1989). The Questionable Physiologic and Epidemiologic Basis for a Male Climacteric Syndrome: Preliminary Results from the Massachusetts Male Aging Study. *Maturitas* 11: 103-15.

McKinlay, J.B., and Feldman, H.A. (1994). Age-Related Variation in Sexual Activity and Interest in Normal Men: Results from the Massachusetts Male Aging Study. In A.S. Rossi (Ed.), *Sexuality Across the Life Course* (pp. 261-85). Chicago, IL: University of Chicago Press.

McLaren, A. (1997). *The Trials of Masculinity: Policing Sexual Boundaries, 1870-1930.* Chicago, IL: University of Chicago Press.

McLeish, J. (1976). *The Ulyssean Adult: Creativity in the Middle and Later Years.* Toronto, ON: McGraw-Hill Ryerson Ltd.

McMullin, J. (1995). Theorizing Age and Gender Relations. In S. Arber and J. Ginn (Eds.), *Connecting Gender and Ageing: A Sociological Approach* (pp. 30-41). Buckingham, UK: Open University Press.

McMullin, J., and Marshall, V.W. (1999). Structure and Agency in the Retirement Process: A Case Study of Montreal Garment Workers. In C. Ryff and V.W. Marshall (Eds.), *Self and Society in Aging Processes* (pp. 305-38). New York, NY: Springer.

McNay, L. (1999). Gender, Habitus, and the Field: Pierre Bourdieu and the Limits of Reflexivity. *Theory, Culture and Society* 16: 95-117.

McNay, L. (2000). *Gender and Agency: Reconfiguring the Subject in Feminist Social Theory.* Malden, MA: Polity Press.

Melchiode, G., and Sloan, B. (1999). *Beyond Viagra: A Commonsense Guide to Building a Healthy Sexual Relationship for Both Men and Women*. New York, NY: Owl Books (Henry Holt and Co.).

Metchnikoff, E. (1903). *The Nature of Man: Studies in Optimistic Philosophy*. Trans. P. Chalmers Mitchell. New York, NY: G.P. Putnam's Sons.

Metchnikoff, E. (1907). *The Prolongation of Life: Optimistic Studies*. Trans. P. Chalmers Mitchell. New York, NY: G.P. Putnam's Sons.

Metz, M.E., and Miner, M.H. (1995). Male "Menopause," Aging and Sexual Function. *Sexuality and Disability* 13: 287-307.

Meyrowitz, J. (1984). The Adultlike Child and the Childlike Adult: Socialization in an Electronic Age. *Daedalus* 113: 19-48.

Micale, M.S. (1985). The Salpêtrière in the Age of Charcot: An Institutional Perspective on Medical History in the Late Nineteenth Century. *Journal of Contemporary History* 20: 703-31.

Micale, M.S. (1989). Hysteria and Its Historiography: A Review of Past and Present Writings I, II. *History of Science* 27: 223-61, 319-51.

Micale, M.S. (1991). Hysteria Male/Hysteria Female: Reflections on Comparative Gender Construction in Nineteenth-Century France and Britain. In M. Benjamin (Ed.), *Science and Sensibility: Gender and Scientific Enquiry, 1780-1945* (pp. 200-39). Oxford, UK: Basil Blackwell.

Micale, M.S. (1995). *Approaching Hysteria: Disease and Its Interpretation*. Princeton, NJ: Princeton University Press.

Midwinter, E. (Ed.). (1984). *Mutual Aid Universities*. London, UK: Croom Helm.

Midwinter, E. (1996). *Thriving People*. London, UK: The Third Age Trust.

Miller, P., and Rose, N. (1990). Governing Economic Life. *Economy and Society* 19: 1-31.

Minkler, M. (1984). Introduction. In M. Minkler, and C.L. Estes (Eds.), *Readings in the Political Economy of Aging* (pp. 10-22). Farmingdale, NY: Baywood Publishing.

Minkler, M. (1990). Aging and Disability: Behind and Beyond the Stereotypes. *Journal of Aging Studies* 4: 245-60.

Minkler, M. (1991). Gold in Gray: Reflections on Business' Discovery of the Elderly Market. In M. Minkler, and C.L. Estes (Eds.), *Critical Perspectives on Aging: The Political and Moral Economy of Growing Old* (pp. 81-93). Amityville, NY: Baywood Publishing.

Minkler, M. (1996). Critical Perspectives on Ageing: New Challenges for Gerontology. *Ageing and Society* 16: 467-87.

Minkler, M. (1999). Introduction. In M. Minkler, and C.L. Estes (Eds.), *Critical Gerontology: Perspectives from Political and Moral Economy* (pp. 1-13). Amityville, NY: Baywood Publishing.

Minkler, M., and Estes, C.L. (Eds.). (1984). *Readings in the Political Economy of Aging*. Farmingdale, NY: Baywood Publishing.

Minkler, M., and Estes, C.L. (Eds.). (1991). *Critical Perspectives on Aging: The Political and Moral Economy of Growing Old*. Amityville, NY: Baywood Publishing.

Minkler, M., and C.L. Estes (Eds.). (1999). *Critical Gerontology: Perspectives from Political and Moral Economy*. Amityville, NY: Baywood Publishers.

Minois, G. (1989). *History of Old Age*. Trans. S.H. Tenison. Cambridge, UK: Polity Press.

Misra, R., Alexy, B., and Panigrahi, B. (1996). The Relationships Among Self-Esteem, Exercise, and Self-Related Health in Older Women. *Journal of Women and Aging* 8: 81-94.

Modell, J. (1989). *Into One's Own: From Youth to Adulthood in The United States, 1920-1975*. Berkeley, CA: University of California Press.

Moody, H.R. (1988a). *Abundance of Life: Human Development Policies for an Aging Society*. New York, NY: Columbia University Press.

Moody, H.R. (1988b). Toward a Critical Gerontology: The Contribution of the Humanities to Theories of Aging. In J.E. Birren and V.L. Bengtson (Eds.), *Emergent Theories of Aging* (pp. 19-40). New York, NY: Springer.

Moody, H.R. (1993). Overview: What is Critical Gerontology and Why is It Important? In T.R. Cole, W.A. Achenbaum, P.L. Jakobi, and R. Kastenbaum (Eds.), *Voices and Visions of Aging: Toward a Critical Gerontology* (pp.xv-xli). New York, NY: Springer.

Moody, H.R. (1998). *Aging: Concepts and Controversies.* 2nd ed. Thousand Oaks, CA: Pine Forge Press.

Morales, A. (1998). Preface. In A. Morales (Ed.), *Erectile Dysfunction: Issues in Current Pharmacotherapy* (pp. xv-xvi). London, UK: Martin Dunitz Ltd.

Morgan, C.M., and Levy, D.J. (1996). Capturing the Mature Marketplace: Boomers Turning 50. *Credit World* (March/April): 19-22.

Morganstern, S., and Abrahams, A. (1988). *Love Again, Live Again.* Englewood Cliffs, NJ: Prentice Hall.

Morgentaler, A. (1999). Male Impotence. *Lancet* 354: 1713-18.

Mumford, K.J. (1992). "Lost Manhood Found": Male Sexual Impotence and Victorian Culture in the United States. *Journal of the History of Sexuality* 3: 33-57.

Munsterberg, H. (1983). *The Crown of Life: Artistic Creativity in Old Age.* San Diego, CA: Harcourt Brace Jovanovich.

Moschis, G.P. (1996). *Gerontographics: Life-Stage Segmentation for Marketing Strategy Development.* Westport, CT: Quorum Books.

Mullins, L.C., and Tucker, R. D. (1988). *Snowbirds in the Sun Belt: Older Canadians in Florida.* Tampa, FL: International Exchange Center on Gerontology, University of South Florida.

Murphy, J.W., and Longino, Jr., C.F. (1998). What Can be Learned from the Arts About Aging? *Journal of Aging & Identity* 3: 77-85.

Myerhoff, B. (1978). *Number Our Days.* New York, NY: E. P. Dutton.

Myerhoff, B. (1986). "Life Not Death In Venice": Its Second life. In V.Turner and E.M. Bruner (Eds.), *The Anthropology of Experience* (pp. 261-86). Urbana and Chicago, IL: University of Illinois Press.

Myles, J. (1984). *Old Age in the Welfare State.* Boston, MA: Little, Brown.

NADBank Survey. (2000). *Toronto: Newspaper Audience Databank Inc.* <www.nadbank.com>.

Napier, A.D.L. (1897). *The Menopause and Its Disorders.* London, UK: The Scientific Press.

Nascher, I.L. (1919). *Geriatrics: The Diseases of Old Age and Their Treatment.* London, UK: Kegan Paul, French, Trubner.

Neugarten, B.L. (Ed.). (1982). *Age or Need? Public Policies for Older People.* Beverly Hills, CA: Sage.

Neugarten, B.L. (1988). The Aging Society and My Academic Life. In M.W. Riley (Ed.), *Sociological Lives* (pp. 91-106). Newbury Park, CA: Sage.

Neugarten, B.L., Havighurst, R.J., and Tobin, S.S. (1961). The Measurement of Life Satisfaction. *Journal of Gerontology* 16: 134-43.

Neugebauer-Visano, R. (1995) Seniors and Sexuality? Confronting Cultural Contradictions. In R. Neugebauer-Visano (Ed.), *Seniors and Sexuality: Experiencing Intimacy in Later Life* (pp. 17-34). Toronto, ON: Canadian Scholars Press.

Newcomer, R., Lawton, J.M., and Byerts, T.O. (Eds.). (1986). *Housing an Aging Society: Issues, Alternatives, and Policy.* New York, NY: Van Nostrand Reinhold.

Neysmith, S.M. (1995). Feminist Methodologies: A Consideration of Principles and Practice for Research in Gerontology. *Canadian Journal on Aging* 14: 100-18.

NIH Consensus Development Panel on Impotence. (1993). Impotence. *Journal of the American Medical Association* 270: 83-90.

Nye, R. (1989). Honor, Impotence, and Male Sexuality in Nineteenth-Century French Medicine. *French Historical Studies* 16: 48-71.

Öberg, P. (1996). The Absent Body—A Social Gerontological Paradox. *Ageing and Society* 16: 701-19.

Ogburn, W.F. (1957). Cultural Lag as Theory. *Sociology and Social Research* 41: 167-74.

Olson, L.K. (1982). *The Political Economy of Aging: The State, Private Power, and Social Welfare.*

New York, NY: Columbia University Press.

O'Malley, P., Shearing, C., and Weir, L. (1997). Governmentality, Criticism, Politics. *Economy and Society* 26: 501-17.

Orloff, A.S. (1993). *The Politics of Pensions: A Comparative Analysis of Britain, Canada, and the United States, 1880-1940.* Madison, WI: University of Wisconsin Press.

Osler, W. (1926). The Fixed Period. In *Aequanimitas* (pp. 389-411). Philadelphia, PA: P. Blakiston.

Ostroff, J. (1989). *Successful Marketing to the 50+ Consumer: How to Capture One of the Biggest and Fastest-Growing Markets in America.* Englewood Cliffs, NJ: Prentice Hall.

Oudshoorn, N. (1994). *Beyond the Natural Body: An Archaeology of Sex Hormones.* London, UK: Routledge.

Owen, A.R.G. (1971). *Hysteria, Hypnosis and Healing: The Work of J.-M. Charcot.* London, UK: Garrett.

Padma-Nathan, H. (1998). The Pharmacologic Management of Erectile Dysfunction: Sildenafil Citrate (Viagra). *Journal of Sex Education and Therapy* 23: 207-16.

Palmlund, I. (1997). The Marketing of Estrogens for Menopausal and Postmenopausal Women. *Journal of Psychosomatic Obstetrics and Gynaecology* 18: 158-64.

Parsons, T. (1968 [1937]). *The Structure of Social Action.* New York, NY: Free Press.

Patterson, I., and Carpenter, G. (1994). Participation in Leisure Activities After the Death of a Spouse. *Leisure Sciences* 16: 105-17.

Patton, P. (2000). *Deleuze and The Political.* London and New York: Routledge.

Pearlman, S.F. (1993). Late Mid-Life Astonishment: Disruptions to Identity and Self-Esteem. In N.D. Davis, E. Cole, and E.D. Rothblum (Eds.), *Faces of Women and Aging* (pp. 1-12). New York, NY: Harrington Park.

Pearsall, M. (Ed.). (1997). *The Other Within Us: Feminist Explorations of Women and Aging.* Boulder, CO: Westview.

Pelling, M., and Smith, R.M. (Eds.). (1991). *Life, Death, and The Elderly: Historical Perspectives.* London, UK: Routledge.

Penning, M.J., and Keating, N.C. (2000). Self-, Informal and Formal Care: Partnerships in Community-Based and Residential Long-Term Care Settings. *Canadian Journal on Aging* 19: 75-100.

Petersen, A., and Bunton, R. (Eds.). (1997). *Foucault, Health and Medicine.* London and New York: Routledge.

Peterson, J.A. (1968) *Married Love in the Middle Years.* New York, NY: Association Press.

Petty, Sir William. (1690). *Political Arithmetick.* London, UK: Robert Clavel.

Phillipson, C. (1982). *Capitalism and The Construction of Old Age.* London, UK: MacMillan.

Phillipson, C. (1998). *Reconstructing Old Age: New Agendas in Social Theory and Practice.* London, UK: Sage.

Phillipson, C. (1999). Population Ageing and The Sociological Tradition. *Education and Ageing* 14: 159-70.

Phillipson, C., and Walker, A. (1987). The Case for a Critical Gerontology. In S. Di Gregorio (Ed.), *Social Gerontology: New Directions* (pp. 1-15). London, UK: Croom Helm.

Pick, D. (1989). *Faces of Degeneration: A European Disorder, 1848-1918.* Cambridge, UK: Cambridge University Press.

Pine, P.P., and Pine, V.R. (2002). Naturally Occurring Retirement Community-Supportive Service Program: An Example of Devolution. *Journal of Aging and Social Policy* 14: 181-92.

Pink, S. (2001). *Doing Visual Ethnography: Images, Media and Representation in Research.* London, UK: Sage Publications.

Pitskhelauri, G.Z. (1982). *The Prolongevity of Soviet Georgia.* New York, NY: Human Sciences Press.

Polivka-West, L.M., Tuch, H., and Goldsmith, K. (2001). A Perfect Storm of Unlimited Risks for Florida Nursing Home Providers. In M.B. Kapp (Ed.), *Liability Issues and Risk Management in Caring for Older Persons. Ethics, Law and Aging Review* 7 (pp. 81-99). New York, NY: Springer.

Pollak, O. (1948). *Social Adjustment in Old Age: A Research Planning Report.* Bulletin 59. New York, NY: Social Science Research Council.

Pratt, H.J. (1993). *Gray Agendas: Interest Groups and Public Pensions in Canada, Britain, and the United States.* Ann Arbor, MI: University of Michigan Press.

Premo, T.L. (1990). *Winter Friends: Women Growing Old in the New Republic, 1785-1835.* Urbana, IL: University of Illinois Press.

Prince, M.J. (2000). Apocalyptic, Opportunistic, and Realistic Demographic Discourse: Retirement Income and Social Policy *or* Chicken Littles, Nest-Eggies, and Humpty Dumpties. In E.M. Gee, G.M Gutman (Eds.), *The Overselling of Population Aging* (pp. 101-13). Don Mills, ON: Oxford University Press.

Pulkingham, J., and Ternowetsky, G. (1999). Neo-Liberalism and Retrenchment: Employment, Universality, Safety-Net Provisions and a Collapsing Canadian Welfare State. In D. Broad and W. Antony (Eds.), *Citizens or Consumers? Social Policy in a Market Society* (pp. 84-94). Halifax, NS: Fernwood Publishing.

Quadagno, J. (1982). *Aging in Early Industrial Society: Work, Family and Social Policy in Nineteenth-Century England.* New York, NY: Academic Press.

Quételet, A. (1968 [1842]). *A Treatise on Man and The Development of His Faculties.* New York, NY: B. Franklin.

Rabinow, P. (1989). *French Modern: Norms of Forms of the Social Environment.* Cambridge, MA: The MIT Press.

Rabinow, P. (1994). The Third Culture. *History of the Human Sciences* 7: 53-64.

Rabinow, P. (1996). *Making PCR: A Story of Biotechnology.* Chicago, IL: University of Chicago Press.

Ray, R.E. (1996). A Postmodern Perspective on Feminist Gerontology. *The Gerontologist* 36: 674-80.

Ray, R.E. (1999). Researching To Transgress: The Need for Critical Feminism in Gerontology. *Journal of Women and Aging* 11: 171-84.

Redvay-Mulvey, G. (2000). Gradual Retirement in Europe. *Journal of Aging and Social Policy* 11: 49-60.

Reinharz, S. (1986). Friends or Foes: Gerontological and Feminist Theory. *Women's Studies International Forum* 9: 503-14.

Reynell, R. (1931) Sexual Neuroses. *Proceedings of the Royal Society of Medicine, Section of Urology* 24 (27 February): 27-36.

Riley, M.W. (1994). *Work, Family and Leisure.* New York, NY: John Wiley.

Ripa, Y. (1990). *Women and Madness: The Incarceration of Women in Nineteenth-Century France.* Trans. C. du P. Menagé. Oxford, UK: Polity.

Robertson, J. (1996). *At the Cultural Center.* Charlotte Harbor, FL: Tabby House.

Robinson, W.J. (1930). *A Practical Treatise on the Causes, Symptoms, and Treatment of Sexual Impotence and Other Sexual Disorders in Men and Women.* 15th ed. New York, NY: Critic and Guide Co.

Rodgers, W., and Miller, B. (1997). A Comparative Analysis of ADL Questions in Surveys of Older People. *Journals of Gerontology: Psychological and Social Sciences* 52B: 21-36.

Rosand, D. (1987). Editor's Statement: Style and the Aging Artist. *Art Journal* (Summer): 91-3.

Rose, N. (1989). *Governing the Soul: The Shaping of the Private Self.* London, UK: Routledge.

Rose, N. (1992). Governing the Enterprising Self. In P. Heelas and P. Morris (Eds.), *The Value of the Enterprise Culture, The Moral Debate* (pp. 141-64). London, UK: Routledge.

Rose, N. (1993). Government, Authority, and Expertise in Advanced Neoliberalism. *Economy and Society* 22: 283-99.

Rose, N. (1996). *Inventing Ourselves: Psychology, Power, and Personhood.* Cambridge, UK: Cambridge University Press.

Rose, N. (1999). *Powers of Freedom: Reframing Political Thought.* Cambridge, UK: University of Cambridge Press.

Rosen, G. (1974). *From Medical Police to Social Medicine: Essays on the History of Health Care.*

New York, NY: Science History Publications.

Rosenthal, E.R. (Ed.) (1990). *Women, Aging and Ageism*. New York, NY: Harrington Park.

Ross, A., and Liebig, P.S. (2002). City of Laguna Woods: A Case of Senior Power in Local Politics. *Research on Aging* 24: 87-105.

Rowles, G.D. (1978). *Prisoners of Space?: Exploring the Geographical Experience of Older People*. Boulder, CO: Westview Press.

Rowles, G.D. (1994). Evolving Images of Place in Aging and "Aging in Place." In D. Shenk and W. A. Achenbaum (Eds.), *Changing Perceptions of Aging and the Aged* (pp. 115-25). New York, NY: Springer.

Rowles, G.D., and Ravdal, H. (2002). Aging, Place and Meaning in the Face of Changing Circumstances. In R. Weiss, and S. Bass (Eds.), *Challenges of the Third Age: Meaning and Purpose in Later Life* (pp. 81-114). New York, NY: Oxford University Press.

Rule, G.B., Milke, D.L., and Dobbs, A.R. (1994). Design of Institutions: Cognitive Functioning and Social Interactions of the Aged Resident. In V.W. Marshall, and B.D. McPherson (Eds.), *Aging: Canadian Perspectives* (pp. 70-82). Peterborough, ON: Broadview Press.

Rush, B. (1947 [1789]). On Old Age. In D.D. Runes (Ed.), *The Selected Writings of Benjamin Rush* (pp. 342-57). New York, NY: Philosophical Library.

Russell, C., Hill, B., and Basser, M. (1996). Identifying Needs Among "At Risk" Older People: Does Anyone Here Speak Health Promotion? In V. Minichiello, N. Chappell, H. Kendig, and A. Walker (Eds.), *Sociology of Aging: International Perspectives* (pp. 378-93). Melbourne, AU: Thoth.

Sawchuk, K.A. (1995). From Gloom to Boom: Age, Identity, and Target Marketing. In M. Featherstone and A.Wernick (Eds.), *Images of Aging: Cultural Representations of Later Life* (pp.173-87). London, UK: Routledge.

Saxe, L.P., and Gerson, N.B. (1964). *Sex and the Mature Man*. New York, NY: Gilbert Press.

Scaff, L. (1998). The "Cool Objectivity of Sociation": Max Weber and Marianne Weber in America. *History of the Human Sciences* 11: 61-82.

Scambler, G. (Ed.). (2001). *Habermas, Critical Theory, and Health*. London and New York: Routledge.

Schaie, K.W., and Willis, S.L. (1999). Theories of Everyday Competence and Aging. In V.L. Bengston and K.W. Schaie (Eds.), *Handbook of Theories of Aging* (pp. 174-95). New York, NY: Springer.

Schlesinger, B. (1996). The Sexless Years or Sex Rediscovered. *Journal of Gerontological Social Work* 26: 117-31.

Schofield, B. (2002). Partners in Power: Governing the Self-Sustaining Community. *Sociology* 36: 663-83.

Schutze, Y. (1987). The Good Mother: The History of the Normative Model "Mother-Love." *Sociological Studies of Child Development* 2: 39-78.

Scientific American (13 May 2002). The Truth About Human Aging. www.sciam.com.

Scott, G.R. (1953). *The Quest for Youth: A Study of All Available Methods of Rejuvenation and of Retaining Physical and Mental Vigour in Old Age*. London, UK: Torchstream.

Sears, E. (1986). *The Ages of Man: Medieval Interpretations of the Life Cycle*. Princeton, NJ: Princeton University Press.

Seiden, O.J. (1998). *Viagra: The Virility Breakthrough*. Rocklin, CA: Prima Publishing.

Settersten, Jr., R.A. (Ed.). (2002). *Invitation to the Life Course: Toward New Understandings of Later Life*. Amityville, NY: Baywood Publishing.

Shabsigh, R. (1999). Efficacy of Sildenafil Citrate (Viagra) Is not Affected by Aetiology of Erectile Dysfunction. *International Journal of Clinical Practice* S102: 19-20.

Shahar, S. (1993). Who were Old in the Middle Ages? *The Social History of Medicine* 6: 313-42.

Shahar, S. (1997). *Growing Old in the Middle Ages*. London and New York, NY: Routledge.

Shahar, S. (1998). Old Age in the High and Late Middle Ages: Image, Expectation and Status. In P. Johnson, and P. Thane (Eds.), *Old Age from Antiquity to Post-Modernity* (pp. 43-63). London and New York, NY: Routledge.

Shaw, S. (1995). Spontaneous Combustion and the Sectioning of Female Bodies. *Literature and Medicine* 14: 1-22.

Sheehan, M.M. (Ed.). (1990). *Aging and the Aged in Medieval Europe.* Toronto, ON: Pontifical Institute of Medieval Studies.

Shenk, D., and Schmid, R.M. (2002). A Picture is Worth ... : The Use of Photography in Gerontological Research. In G.D. Rowles and N.E. Schoenberg (Eds.), *Qualitative Gerontology: A Contemporary Perspective* (pp. 241-62). New York, NY: Springer.

Shenk, D., and Achenbaum, W.A. (Eds.) (1994). *Changing Perceptions of Aging and the Aged.* New York, NY: Springer.

Shilling, C. (1993). *The Body in Social Theory.* London, UK: Sage.

Showalter, E. (1985). *The Female Malady: Women, Madness, and English Culture, 1830-1980.* New York, NY: Pantheon.

Shweder, R.A. (Ed.). (1998). *Welcome to Middle Age! (And Other Cultural Fictions).* Chicago, IL: University of Chicago Press.

Silber, I.F. (1995). Space, Fields, Boundaries: The Rise of Spatial Metaphors in Contemporary Sociological Theory. *Social Research* 62: 323-55.

Simonton, D.K. (1991). Creative Productivity Through the Years. *Generations* (Spring): 13-16.

Simonton, D.K. (1994). *Greatness: Who Makes History and Why.* New York, NY: The Guilford Press.

Simonton, D.K. (1997). *Genius and Creativity: Selected Papers.* Greenwich, CT: Ablex Publishing Corporation

Simonton, D.K. (2002). *Great Psychologists and Their Times: Scientific Insights into Psychology's History.* Washington, DC: American Psychological Association.

Sinclair, Sir John (1807). *The Code of Health and Longevity, Vol. I.* Edinburgh, UK: Archibald Constable.

Singer, L. (1993). *Erotic Welfare: Sexual Theory and Politics in the Age of Epidemic.* London, UK: Routledge.

Sinoff, G., and Ore, L. (1997). The Barthel Activities of Daily Living Index: Self Reporting versus Actual Performance in the Old-Old. *Journal of the American Geriatrics Society* 45: 832-36.

Skae, F. (1865). Climacteric Insanity in the Male. *Edinburgh Medical Journal* 11: 232-44.

Slater, D. (1997). *Consumer Culture and Modernity.* Cambridge, UK: Polity.

Smith, E.D. (1972). *Handbook of Aging For Those Growing Old and Those Concerned with Them.* New York, NY: Barnes and Noble.

Smith, J. (1752 [1666]). *The Portrait of Old Age.* London, UK: E. Whithers.

Smith-Rosenberg, C. (1985). *Disorderly Conduct: Visions of Gender in Victorian America.* New York, NY: Oxford University Press.

Soussloff, C.M. (1987). Old Age and Old-Age Style in the "Lives" of Artists: Gianlorenzo Bernini. *Art Journal* (Summer): 115-21.

Soussloff, C.M. (1997). *The Absolute Artist: The Historiography of a Concept.* Minneapolis, MN: University of Minnesota Press.

Squier, S.M. (1995). Reproducing the Posthuman Body: Ectogenic Fetus, Surrogate Mother, Pregnant Man. In J. Halberstam and I. Livingston (Eds.), *Posthuman Bodies* (pp. 113-32). Bloomington and Indianapolis, IN: Indiana University Press.

Special Committee on Aging, United States Senate. (1987). *Developments in Aging: 1987.* Washington, DC: US Government Printing Office.

Squier, S.M. (1999). Incubabies and Rejuvenates: The Traffic Between Technologies of Reproduction and Age-Extension. In K. Woodward (Ed.), *Figuring Age: Women, Bodies Generations* (pp. 88-111). Bloomington and Indianapolis, IN: Indiana University Press.

Stall, S. (1901). *What a Man of Forty-Five Ought to Know.* Philadelphia, PA: VIR Publishing Company.

Statistics Canada. (2000). Income Levels, Income Inequality, and Low Income among the Elderly: 1980 to 1995. *The Daily* (6 March).

Stearns, P.N. (1977). *Old Age in European Society: The Case of France*. London, UK: Croom Helm.

Stearns P.N. (1980). Old Women: Some Historical Observations. *Journal of Family History* 5: 44-57.

Stearns, P.N. (Ed.). (1982). *Old Age in Preindustrial Society*. New York, NY: Holmes and Meier Publications.

Steers, W.D. (1999). Viagra—after One Year. *Urology* 54: 12-17.

Steinberg, L. (1968). Michelangelo's Florentine *Pietà*: the Missing Leg. *Art Bulletin* 50: 343-53.

Steinberg, L. (1989). Animadversions. *Art Bulletin* 71: 480-505.

Steinberg, S.R., and Kincheloe, J.L. (1997). *Kinderculture: The Corporate Construction of Childhood*. Boulder, CO: Westview.

Stekel, W. (1927). *Impotence in the Male: The Psychic Disorders of Sexual Function in the Male*. London, UK: Bodley Head.

Stephenson, S. (1996). $elling Seniors. *Marketing Strategies* (15 October): 78, 80, 82.

Sterling, B. (1996). *Holy Fire*. New York, NY: Bantam Books.

Stieglitz, E.J. (1949). *The Second Forty Years*. London, UK: Staples Press.

Stoller, E.P., and Longino, C.F. Jr. (2001). "Going Home" or "Leaving Home"? The Impact of Person and Place Ties on Anticipated Counterstream Migration. *The Gerontologist* 1: 96-102.

Stone, C.T. (1938). *Sexual Power*. New York, NY: D. Appleton Century.

Strain, L. (2001). Senior Centres: Who Participates? *Canadian Journal on Aging* 20: 471-91.

Street, D. (1999). Special Interests or Citizen Rights? "Senior Power," Social Security, and Medicare. In M. Minkler, and C.L. Estes (Eds.), *Critical Gerontology: Perspectives from Political and Moral Economy* (pp. 109-30). Amityville, NY: Baywood Publishing.

Sturgis, F.R. (1931). *Sexual Debility in Man*. Chicago, IL: Login Bros.

Summers, D. (1981). *Michelangelo and the Language of Art*. Princeton, NJ: Princeton University Press.

Summers, D. (1987). *The Judgment of Sense: Renaissance Naturalism and the Rise of Aesthetics*. Cambridge, UK: Cambridge University Press.

Swindell, R., and Thompson, J. (1995). An International Perspective on the University of the Third Age. *Educational Gerontology* 21: 429-47.

Taira, E.D., and J.L. Carlson (Eds.). (1999). *Aging in Place: Designing, Adapting, and Enhancing the Home Environment*. New York, NY: Haworth Press.

Tallmer, M. (1996). *Questions and Answers about Sex in Later Life*. Philadelphia, PA: Charles Press.

Terry, J., and Urla, J. (1995). *Deviant Bodies: Critical Perspectives on Difference in Science and Popular Culture*. Bloomington, IN: Indiana University Press.

The Carnegie Inquiry into The Third Age (9 Reports). (1993). Dunfermline, UK: The Carnegie United Kingdom Trust.

Thoms, W.J. (1873). *Human Longevity: Its Facts and Its Fictions*. London, UK: John Murray.

Tietze, H. (1944). Earliest and Latest Works of Great Artists. *Gazette des Beaux-Arts* 26: 273-84.

Tilt, E. (1882). *The Change of Life in Health and Disease: A Clinical Treatise on the Diseases of the Glanglionic Nervous System Incidental to Women at the Decline of Life*. 4th ed. New York, NY: Birmingham.

Tinsley, H.E.A., Teaff, J.D., Colbs, S.L., and Kaufman, N. (1985). A System of Classifying Leisure Activities In Terms of the Psychological Benefits of Participation Reported by Older Persons. *Journal of Gerontology* 40: 172-78.

Tornstam, L. (1989). Gerotranscendence: A Meta-theoretical Reformulation of the Disengagement Theory. *Aging: Clinical and Experimental Research* 1: 55-63.

Troyansky, D. (1989). *Old Age in the Old Regime: Image and Experience in Eighteenth-Century France*. Ithaca, NY: Cornell University Press.

Tucker, R.D., Marshall, V.W., Longino, C.F. Jr., and Mullins, L.C. (1988). Older Anglophone

Canadians in Florida: A Descriptive Profile. *Canadian Journal on Aging* 7: 218-32.

Tucker, R.D., Mullins, L.C., Beland, F., Longino C.F. Jr., and Marshall, V.W. (1992). Older Canadians in Florida: A Comparison of Anglophone and Francophone Seasonal Migrants. *Canadian Journal on Aging* 11: 281-97.

Tulle-Winton, E. (1999). Growing Old and Resistance: Towards a New Cultural Economy of Old Age? *Ageing and Society* 19: 281-99.

Tulle-Winton, E. (2000). Old Bodies. In P. Hancock, B. Hughes, E. Jagger, K. Patterson, R. Russell, E. Tulle-Winton, and M. Tyler, *The Body, Culture, and Society: An Introduction* (pp. 64-83). Buckingham, UK: Open University Press.

Turner, B.S. (1991). The Discourse of Diet. In M. Featherstone, M. Hepworth, and B.S. Turner (Eds.), *The Body: Social Process and Cultural Theory* (pp. 157-69). London, UK: Sage.

Turner, B.S. (1994). The Postmodernisation of the Life Course: Towards a New Social Gerontology. *Australian Journal on Ageing* 13: 109-11.

Turner, B.S. (1995). Aging and Identity: Some Reflections on the Somatization of the Self. In M. Featherstone and A. Wernick (Eds.), *Images of Aging: Cultural Representations of Later Life* (pp. 245-60). London, UK: Routledge.

Twigg, J. (2000). *Bathing—The Body and Community Care*. London and New York: Routledge.

Unruh, D.R. (1983). *Invisible Lives: Social Worlds of the Aged*. Beverly Hills, CA: Sage Publications.

Urla, J., and Terry, J. (1995). Introduction: Mapping Embodied Difference. In J. Urla and J. Terry (Eds.), *Deviant Bodies: Critical Perspectives on Difference in Science and Popular Culture* (pp. 1-18). Bloomington, IN: Indiana University Press.

Urry, J. (2000). *Sociology Beyond Societies: Mobilities for the Twenty-First Century*. London and New York: Routledge.

Van Tassel, D.D., and Stearns, P.N. (Eds.). (1986). *Old Age in Bureaucratic Society: The Elderly, The Experts, and the State in American History*. Westport, CT: Greenwood Press.

Vasari, G. (1962). *La vita di Michelangelo nelle redazioni del 1550 e del 1568*. Ed. Paola Barocchi. 5 vols. Milan: R. Ricciardi.

Vasari, G. (1966). *Le vite de' più eccellenti pittori scultori e architettori nelle redazioni di 1550 e di 1568*. Ed. R. Bettarini and P. Barocchi. Florence: Sansoni.

Veal, A.J. (1993). The Concept of Lifestyle: A Review. *Leisure Studies* 12: 233-52.

Vincent, J. (1999). *Politics, Power, and Old Age: Struggles Over Old Age and Ageing*. Buckingham, UK: Open University Press.

Walker, A. (1981). Towards a Political Economy of Old Age. *Ageing and Society* 1: 73-94.

Walker, A. (1987). Ageing and the Social Sciences: The North American Way. *Ageing and Society* 7: 235-41.

Walker, A. (2000). Public Policy and the Construction of Old Age in Europe. *The Gerontologist* 40: 304-08.

Walters, W. (1997). The "Active Society": New Designs for Social Policy. *Policy and Politics* 25: 221-34.

Walton, C.K. (1993). *The Gulf Coast of Florida Book: A Complete Guide*. Stockbridge, MA: Berkshire House Publishers.

Warthin, A.S. (1929). *Old Age: The Major Involution*. New York, NY: Paul B. Hoeber.

Weiland, S. (2000). Social Science Toward the Humanities: Speaking of Lives in the Study of Aging. In T.R. Cole and R.E. Ray (Eds.), *Handbook of the Humanities and Aging*, 2nd ed. (pp. 235-57). New York, NY: Springer.

Welsch, W. (1999). Transculturality: The Puzzling Forms of Cultures Today. In M. Featherstone and S. Lash (Eds.), *Spaces of Culture* (pp. 194-213). London, UK: Sage.

Wernick, A. (1995). The Dying of the American Way of Death. In C. Hummel and C.J.L. d'Epinay (Eds.), *Images of Aging in Western Societies* (pp. 69-90). Geneva: Centre for Interdisciplinary Gerontology, University of Geneva.

Whitbourne, S.K. (1995). Sexuality in the Aging Male. In R. Neugebauer-Visano (Ed.), *Seniors and Sexuality: Experiencing Intimacy in Later Life* (pp. 73-80). Toronto, ON: Canadian Scholars Press.

Whitehead, E.D., and Malloy, T. (1999). *Viagra: The Wonder Drug for Peak Performance.* New York, NY: Dell Books.

Williams, S.J., and Bendelow, G. (Eds.). (1998). *The Lived Body: Sociological Themes, Embodied Issues.* London, UK: Routledge.

Wolfe, D.B. (1992). Business's Mid-Life Crisis. *American Demographics* (September): 40-44.

Wolfe. D.B. (1994). Targeting the Mature Mind. *American Demographics* (March): 32-36.

Woodward, K. (1991). *Aging and Its Discontents: Freud and Other Fictions.* Bloomington and Indianapolis, IN: Indiana University Press.

Wölfflin, H. (1923). *Kunstgeschichtliche Grundbegriffe.* 6th ed. Munich: Hugo Bruckmann Verlag.

Woodward, K. (Ed.) (1999). *Figuring Age: Women, Bodies, Generations.* Bloomington and Indianapolis, IN: Indiana University Press.

Ylanne-McEven, V. (1999). "Young at Heart": Discourses of Age Identity in Travel Agency Interaction. *Ageing and Society* 19: 417-40.

Young, M., and Schuller, T. (1991). *Life After Work: The Arrival of the Ageless Society.* London, UK: Harper/Collins.

Archival and Primary Resources.

Arts and Humanities Council of Charlotte County

Canadian Snowbird Association News Magazine (Medipac International Communications, North York, Ontario)

Charlotte County Chamber of Commerce: 1999 Visitor's Guide (Charlotte County Chamber of Commerce)

Charlotte County Economic Development Council Profile

Englewood Chamber of Commerce Tour Guide and Directory 1998-99 (Englewood Area Chamber of Commerce)

Englewood Sun Herald

Port Charlotte Sun Herald

Senior Living Guide of South Florida (Orlando: Senior Living Network).

The Globe and Mail (Toronto)

The Toronto Star

<www.mapleleafgcc.com> (Maple Leaf Estates)

<www.charlotte–florida.com> (Charlotte County, Florida)

<www.snowbirds.org> (Canadian Snowbird Association)

<www.warmmineralsprings.com> (Warm Mineral Springs)

<www.theculturalcenter.com> (Port Charlotte Cultural Center)

Index

AARP (American Association of Retired
Persons) Foundation, 212
Achenbaum, W. Andrew, 13, 24, 47, 75–76,
90, 92, 98
Activities of Daily Living (ADL), 129, 138n4
activity, 16, 18, 141, 150, 162, 171
    anti-activity, 131–32
    as cultural ideal, 122
    as empirical and professional instru-
        ment, 126–30
    as a gerontological theory, 123–26
    idealized old age, 127
    in institutional settings, 129–30
    regulatory and instrumental connota-
        tions, 133
    and successful aging, 122
activity checklists, 130–31
activity theory, 124
    criticism of, 125
    in health promotion, 126
    in recreational counselling, 126
adjustment, 123, 125
    problematization, 124, 126–27, 132
ADL. *See* Activities of Daily Living
Adorno, Theodor, 54
adult education, 152–53
    lifelong learning, 19, 99, 146, 154
    Port Charlotte Cultural Center, 220
    U3As, 152–54, 156–58
Age and Achievement (Lehman), 102–3
"age-defying" practices, 17
age-segregated communities, 226
age-stratification theories, 87
Age Studies, 90
ageism, 13, 19, 32, 92, 104
    positive ageism, 163
ageism/sexism link, 39
agelessness, 144, 162
    "ageless" seniors market, 190
agency, 18, 140, 142–43, 149, 157–58

collective, 20, 141, 151, 153
agency and structure dualism, 144, 151, 157
aging
    ageless aging, 180, 182–83
    biological processes of, 193
    commercialization, 198
    contradictory culture of, 140
    as disease, 145
    future of, 229
    global, 14
    hostility to, 167
    negative images, 16, 171, 203
    political economy of, 88–89
    positive aging, 19, 106–7, 178, 183, 193–95,
        199, 229
    post-traditional, 142, 144
    productive, 194
    psychology of, 79–80
    and sexual decline, 164 (*See also*
        menopause; sexual fitness)
    sociology of, 19
    successful, 106, 122, 129, 145, 148–51, 170,
        173, 180, 208
"aging-in-place" debates, 204–6
aging population, 190. *See also* old age;
    senior citizens
    blaming of, 13, 99
aging studies, 38–39
    Americanization, 75–76
    art history and, 16
    connection with women's studies,
        39–40, 49
    gender issues, 37
Alzheimer's, 117n3, 193, 214
American gerontology, 76
American Journal of Sociology, 221
American National Institute on Aging, 92
American policies on aging. *See* social
    policy on aging
American progressive era, 104

American Social Science Research
    Council, 123
animal gland grafts, 168
anti-activity activities, 131–32
anti-ageism, 16–17, 19, 39, 102, 106, 199
anti-aging, 17, 19, 106, 199, 226
    anti-wrinkle industry, 18
    and enhancement technologies, 192
    leading to marginalization, 194
anti-aging culture, 189, 208
art history, 16
artistic creativity, 32, 101–16
    across life-span, 105–7
    old-age style (OAS), 16, 105, 107–9
    peak and decline narrative, 101–5
Assisted Living Facilities (ALFs), 213–14
assisted living services, 206
Australia, 59
    "activity tests" for income support, 137
autonomy, 171

Bacon, Francis, 25, 34n2, 121
    Historie of Life and Death, The, 26, 164
    life-prolonging medicines, 27
bacteriology, 169
Beard, George Miller, Legal Responsibility in
    Old Age, 103
Biggs, Simon, 98
bigotry in older adults, 152
Birren, James, 73–74, 87, 198
Birth of the Clinic, The (Foucault), 124
Blaikie, Andrew, 151, 203, 229
bodies, 42, 53
    hierarchy of, 53
    human body/body politic linkage, 80
    human body/social body connections,
        53
    hysteria, 50
    of older women, 39, 46–47
    problematization of, 136
    sociology of, 40
Bourdieu, Pierre, 12, 15, 86, 94, 98, 142
    "field of artistic production," 116
    habitus, 92–93
    philosophical fieldwork, 93
British Universities of the Third Age. See
    U₃As
Brown-Séquard, Charles E., 168, 170
Burgess, Ernest, 74
"busy ethic" in retirement, 125
Butler, Robert N., 13, 38, 92, 173

Cambridge U₃A, 153
Campbell, Erin, 15, 116
Canadian Club of Charlotte County, 223
Canadian Snowbird Association (CSA),
    222–23
    travel and health insurance packages,
        223
Canadian "snowbird" migrational culture.
    See Snowbird culture
capitalism, 33, 143
    mercantile, 54
    post-modern capitalism, 226
care institutions
    activity work, 130
    Continuing Care Retirement
        Communities (CCRCs), 213–14
    nursing homes, 213–14
Carlisle, Anthony, 35n7
    Essay on the Disorders of Old Age, 28
Cavan, Ruth, 37
Chappell, Neena, 37
Charcot, Jean-Martin, 41–45, 48, 50
    Clinical Lectures On the Diseases of Old Age,
        15, 40, 44, 49
    scientific and sexist biases, 43, 46–47
Charcot's Older Women, 15, 37–50
Charlotte County, Florida, 19, 202, 211
child studies, 78
climacteric, 165–67, 170–71, 174
    in women, 166
cloning and embryonic stem cell technolo-
    gy, 193
Cohen, Lawrence, 90
Cohen-Shalev, Amir, 107
Cole, Thomas R., 13, 24, 32, 83, 92
Commission on Global Aging, 14
community networks, 204, 206–8
constructivism, 19
consumer culture
    "fashioning" aspect of senior worlds, 199
    and gerontological research, 199
    idealization of long life, 24
consumer society, 145–46
consumerism, 16, 189–90, 195, 197
Continuing Care Retirement Communities
    (CCRCs), 213
Cornaro, Luigi, 26–27, 33, 34n2
    How to Live One Hundred Years and Avoid
        Disease, 25
cosmetic and body technologies, 33, 90, 192
Cowdry, Edmund V., 76
    Problems of Ageing, 73, 77–80

creativity. *See* artistic creativity
"Creativity Across the Life Course?", 15
critical aging research, 13
critical curiosity, 16
critical gero-anthropology, 90
"Critical Gerontological Theory," 15
critical gerontology, 13, 85–99, 140, 143–44
cultural gerontology, 144
"cultural lag," 90

Darwin, Charles, 25
Daston, Lorraine, 25
Day, George, 166
De Beauvoir, Simone, 47–44
Dean, Mitchell, 55, 58, 137
death "due to old age," 29
deconstruction, 81
Deleuze, Gilles, 15, 86, 95–96, 98, 190
demasculinization, 168
dementia, 16, 117n3. *See also* Alzheimer's
demography, 98, 229. *See also* population
    alarmist, 13, 99
    in developed *vs.* developing countries,
        14
Dennis, Wayne, 103
dependency, 122, 140, 145, 150, 171, 195
    restructuring, 136
    risk of, 132, 137, 146
    state-supported, 18
    structured dependence theories, 143
developmental psychology
    peak-and decline model, 105
developmental psychology handbooks, 72
Dewey, John, 79
Dickens, Charles, *Pickwick Papers,* 155
dietary, exercise, and behavioural regimes,
    17, 28, 33, 192
disciplinary power, 53–54
Discipline and Punish (Foucault), 53–54, 124,
    137
Disciplining Old Age (Katz), 12, 39–40, 50
disengagement, 87, 124–25, 138n3, 195
Donahue, Wilma, 73
Dubois, W.E.B., 92

early retirement, 150
Ekerdt, David
    on activity theory, 125
elder abuse, 39, 206
elderhood. *See* old age; senior citizens
elderscapes, 19, 202–3, 220

employment, 212. *See also* post-retirement
    work; retired worker
empowerment, 32, 39, 137, 141, 146
    as a governmental strategy, 136, 138n2
    and risks of dependency, 122
Enlightenment, 25–26, 53, 70
erectile dysfunction, 163, 174–75, 181–82. *See
    also* impotence
    as epidemic, 176–77
    equated with loss of life, 179
    fear of, 178
    as "moral disorder," 179
Essay on the Disorders of Old Age, An
    (Carlisle), 28
Estes, Carrol, 37, 88–89, 97, 99, 198
    on activity theory, 125
    "aging enterprise," 88
ethnicity, 33, 124
ethnocentrism, 75, 116n2
ethnomethodological sociology, 88
excessive longevity, 25, 31
"exemplars of retirement," 18, 146–51

Featherstone, Mike, 13, 24, 32–34, 90, 143, 145,
    166, 184n2, 192
female sexuality. *See* sexuality
femininity, 43
feminist gerontology, 90
feminist scholarship, 38–39, 48, 142
    research on Charcot, 15
Foucault, Michel, 12, 39, 41, 53–54, 146, 183
    Anglo-Foucaultian school, 59
    Birth of the Clinic, The, 124
    critical *curiosity,* 16
    Discipline and Punish, 53–54, 124, 137
    genealogical method, 72
    "Governmentality," 14, 54–56, 58
    History of Sexuality, 53–54, 56, 124
    Madness and Civilization, 124
    on power/knowledge, 93
    problematization, 123, 137
    on sexuality, 161–62
Frank, Lawrence K., 78
Freud, Sigmund, 43, 50
Friedan, Betty, 37, 105–7
functionalism, 123, 141

Galton, Francis, *Hereditary Genius,* 103
gender, 33, 37–38, 46–47, 125, 142
    inequalities, 88
    sociological notions of, 124

"the travels of gender," 93
"gender aging theory," 38
genealogical method, 72–73
generation, 124
generational boundaries
    blurring of, 19, 24, 32, 190–91, 209
genetic therapy, 192
geriatrics, 40, 126, 169
    and bodies of women, 46–47
Geriatrics (Nascher), 126
German medical handbooks, 72
Gerontographics (Moschis), 194, 197–98
gerontological criticality. See critical geron-
    tology
gerontological handbooks, 70–82
    as authorities on aging, 71
    criticisms of, 74–76
    as disciplinary practice, 77–81
gerontological knowledge, 39, 50, 76
    multidisciplinarity and professionalism,
        80
    rhetorical aspects, 77
Gerontological Society, 123
Gerontologist, The, 74
gerontology, 16, 29, 40, 81, 104
    activity as gerontological theory, 122
    Canadian, 37
    cultural, 144
    gender issues and, 37–38
    knowledge-production and scientific
        disciplinarity, 71
    mainstream, 38
    metaphorical development and termi-
        nology in, 90
    misrepresenting women, 49
    models of "productivity," 125
    multidisciplinarity, 76
    optimism, 169
    scientific, 79–80
    social, 80
    women scholars, 37–38
gerontology of creativity, 102
gerontology of mobility, 19, 204, 211, 228
Giddens, Anthony, 142, 144
Gilleard, Chris, 143, 199
Gilman, Sander, 43
Ginn, Jay, 38
Girl Scout Handbooks, 72
glands, 30
Global Aging Initiative (GAI), 14
global societies, 229

global transcultural citizens, 210–11
Goffman, Erving, Asylums, 204
Gothic architecture, 95
"Government of Detail, The" (Katz and
    Green), 15, 69
government of knowledge, 56
government of life, 56
governmental policy discourse. See social
    policy
governmentality, 15, 54, 60–61, 65–67, 69, 146
    Marxist criticism of, 58–59
    in relation to social policy discourse
        and practice, 55
"Governmentality" (Foucault), 55–58
Gramsci, Antonio, Prison Notebooks, 91
Greer, Germaine, 37
"grey lobby," 152
"Grey Marketing," 198
grey political movements, 17, 171
Guattari, Félix, 15, 86, 95–96, 98
Gubrium, Jaber F., 132, 204

Haber, Carole, 24, 165
Habermas, Jurgen, 90
    life-world, 89
habitus, 92–93
Halford, Henry, "On the Climacteric
    Disease," 165
Hall, G. Stanley, 40, 92, 104, 106
    Senescence, 98, 104–5, 126
handbook genre, 70–71, 76, 80–82
    contextual nature of, 75
    as genealogical document, 72–73
    as gerontology standard, 72–76
    multidisciplinarity, 78
Harvey, William, 28
    discovery of circulation of the blood, 27
Hazan, Haim, 33, 76
    From First Principles, 153
    Old Age, 74
health, 45, 122, 127, 150, 162, 180
    healthy aging, 226 (See also successful
        aging)
    healthy lifestyles, 146
    traditional health-management tech-
        niques, 216
Health Canada
    impotence warnings (on cigarette pack-
        ages), 180
health care, 137
    consumer-based, 208

out-of-province, 223
privatization, 99
health promotion discourses, 99
    activity theory, 126
    emphasis on sexual function, 179
    on "positive aging," 178
Hendricks, Jon, 39
Hepworth, Mike, 24, 32–33, 90, 143, 145, 166, 184n2, 192, 194
Hess, Beth, 38
(hetero)sexual functionality, 192
Hindess, Barry, 59
history of medicine, 40
History of Sexuality (Foucault), 53–54, 56, 124
Hite, Shere, 173
HMOs (Health Management Organizations), 99
Hochschild, Arlie, 16–17
Holstein, Martha, 125
hormonal enhancements, 192
human agency. *See* agency
humours, 26
hybrid cultures, 210
hygienic reform, 168
hypnosis, 41
hypochondria, 34n2
hysteria, 15, 43, 46, 50
    Charcot's recreation of, 42
    critical hysteria studies, 49
    feminist and cultural histories of, 40
    as performance, 44

identity, 18, 140–42, 144–46, 149, 157–58
    age-identities, 205
    continuity throughout life course, 144
    production-based, 148
    through collective struggle, 158
impotence, 161, 177, 185n5, 186n13. *See also* erectile dysfunction
    early writing on, 164–65
    Health Canada warnings, 180
    as part of aging, 170
    physically derived, 172, 174
    psychology of, 172–73
independence, 16, 127, 140, 150. *See also* dependency
individual body. *See* bodies
individual responsibility, 19, 146, 148, 150
    for sexual fitness, 180
individual rights and freedoms, 54
inequality. *See* social inequality

institutional settings, 129–30
instrumentalism, 85
insurance
    acquiring, 146
    industry, 24
    life, 31
    out-of-province health care, 223
International Association of Universities of the Third Age (AIUTA), 152
Internet, 155
interpretive theories, 144

James, William, 92
Josiah Macy Jr. Foundation, 78
Jung, Carl, 198

Kansas City Study of Adult Life, 124
Kastenbaum, Robert, 152, 192–93
Katz, Stephen, 192
    Disciplining Old Age, 12, 39–40, 50
Kaufman, Sharon
    theory of the "ageless self," 144
Kinsey, Alfred C., 173
    on impotence, 176
knowledge, 56, 93
    Foucaultian subversion of, 94
    gerontological, 39, 50, 76–77, 8077
    medical, 41–42
    popular, 145
    professionalized, 70, 137
    social relations of, 75
    statistical, 57–58
    technical, 56, 58
Kohli, Martin, 189

labour, 32, 124
Laslett, Peter, 153, 155–56
"last-chance syndrome," 105
late-life artistic style. *See* old-age style (OAS)
later life. *See* old age; senior citizens
Latour, Bruno
    "action at a distance," 55
Lawton, George, 79–80, 131
Lawton, M. Powell, 206
Left, decline of, 59
Lehman, Harvey, *Age and Achievement*, 102–3
leisure, 33, 127–28, 190
Leonardo, da Vinci
    on artistic judgement, 114
liberal humanism, 54

liberal power, 54
life course, 24, 142
    connections to consumer society, 190
    marketing segments, 195
    politics, 189
    in postmodern time, 189–93
    studies, 87
life expectancy. *See* life span
life-extension therapies, 192
life insurance. *See* insurance
life span, 23, 144, 164. *See also* longevity
    Bacon on, 27
    discursive or imagined production, 23
    excessive longevity, 25, 31
    John Smith on, 27
    late Renaissance reformulations of, 25
    limits, 23
    as male construction, 35n7
    modern scientific inquiry, 29, 31
    premodern historical literature on,
        24–25
    projections, 193
life-world, 89
lifelong learning, 19, 99, 146, 154
lifestages, 165
    blurring of, 19, 24, 32, 190–91, 209
lifestyle, 17, 142, 158, 162, 189
    and activity regimes, 99
    hierarchies, 33
    industries and practices, 137
local communities, 207
    idealized sense of, 208
    subsidizing government fiscal policies,
        208
Locke, John, 55
loneliness, 136
longevity, 145
    idealization of, 24
    images of in popular medical treatises,
        14
    literature on, 27
    modern scientific inquiry, 29–31
    popular reports of, 28
    revolution, 13
    technology, 144
Longino, Charles Jr., 221–22
Loomis, Alfred, 40, 44
Lorand, Arnold, 30
    Old Age Deferred, 29, 168
Lyotard, François, 94

Madness and Civilization (Foucault), 124
Making PCR (Rabinow), 93
male climacteric. *See* climacteric
"male menopause," 90
male midlife crisis or "viropause," 167
male sexual fitness. *See* sexual fitness
male sexual potency
    nineteenth century views on, 166
male sexuality
    ageing and, 177
    technologization of, 18, 183
mandatory retirement, 150
Manheimer, Ronald, 74
Maple Leaf Estates, 211, 224–28
market-driven programs, 122. *See also* con-
    sumer society
market-driven retirement planning, 208
market segmentation, 197
marketing language, 19, 195, 197
Marshall, Barbara L., 18, 184, 192
    "the travels of gender," 93
Marshall, Victor W., 13, 87–88, 98, 221–22
Martin-Matthews, Anne, 37
Marx, Karl, 90
Marxism, 85–86, 88, 93
Marxist and humanist traditions, 54
Marxist and psychoanalytical meta-theory,
    95
Marxist political economy, 94, 97
masculinity, 180, 184
masking of age, 32, 196
Maslow, Abraham, 198
Massachusetts Male Aging Survey
    (MMAS), 176
maturity, 189
    and consumerism, 197
Mayo, Elton, 92
McDaniel, Susan, 37
McHugh, Kevin, 145, 209
McMullin, Julie, 37–38
media, 146
medical intervention, 28
medical knowledge, 41–42
medical rejuvenation therapies. *See* rejuve-
    nation
medical theatrics, 42
medicalization of old age, 29, 40
medicalization of sexuality, 163, 179
medicalization of truth claims, 175
menopause, 48, 163, 166
Men's Health, 178

Metchnikoff, Elie, 30, 40, 92, 106, 170–71
    Nature of Man, 169
    Prolongation of Life, 29, 104, 169
"Metropolis and Mental Life, The"
    (Simmel), 92
Michelangelo Buonarroti, 101–2, 109, 112
    Early Modern perception, 109–10, 115–16
    Giorgio Vasari on, 114
    Giulio Mancini on, 113
    late style, 113
middle age, 33
    midlife ageism, 18
    midlife crisis, 90, 116n1, 167
    midlife decline, 183
    sexual loss, 170
Midwinter, Eric, 154–55, 158
migrational and mobile retirement cul-
    tures, 203, 209, 211, 229
    Canadian Snowbirds, 19, 204, 211, 214,
        221–26, 228–29
    studies of, 221
Minkler, Meredith, 37, 39, 88–90, 198
    on activity theory, 125
miracles, 25, 27, 216
mobility, 16, 150, 171, 209–11. *See also* migra-
    tional and mobile retirement cultures
mobilization, 141
modernity, 89, 93
Monet, Claude, 109
Moody, Harry, 32–33, 87, 89
    on activity theory, 125
moral economy, 89
moral regulation, 125
Moschis, George, 199
    Gerontographics, 195, 197–98
multidisciplinarity, 73, 76–78, 81, 86–87
    and professionalism, 80
multidisciplinary technique, 72. *See also*
    genealogical method
Myerhollf, Barbara
    "definitional ceremonies," 227

narratives, 144
    of active living, 132–36
    of the self, 122, 142
Nascher, Ignatius
    Geriatrics, 126
Nascher, Ignatz, 40
National Institute of Health
    on aging and male sexuality, 175
National Research Council, 78

naturally occurring retirement communi-
    ties (NORCs), 207
neo-Galenic medical regimes, 27, 32
neoliberal "active society," 18
neoliberal positive-aging parables, 147
neoliberal programs
    to *responsibilize* senior citizenry, 99
neoliberal technologies, 150, 158
neoliberalism, 19, 59, 146, 198
    antiwelfarist agendas, 136
    policies to "empower" older individu-
        als, 122
    social security cutbacks, 194
Neugarten, Bernice, 37, 92, 127, 200n2
new aging, 14, 18, 140–41, 143, 145–46, 148
    new age elderly consumers, 196, 226
    styles defined as deviant and, 195
nomad sciences, 95–96
nursing homes, 213–14

objectivity, 43
old age. *See also* aging; senior citizens
    as clinical problem, 28
    as distinct, developmental stage, 32
    hardships of, 193–95 (*See also* social
        inequality)
    medicalization, 29, 40
    normalization of, 122
    older women, 15, 37–50
    postponing, 145
    special part of life course, 29
Old Age Security "clawbacks," 150–51
old-age style (OAS), 16, 105, 107–9
older populations. *See* aging population
older women, 45
    Charcot's Older Women, 15, 37–50
    negative cultural attitudes toward, 48
optimism. *See also* Enlightenment optimism
    of Metchnikoff and Hall, 106
Osler, William
    "The Fixed Period" speech, 104

Parr, Thomas, 27–31, 33
Parsons, Talcott
    Structure of Social Action, 92
peak and decline narrative, 101–5, 116n2
penile erectility, 163, 180, 182. *See also* erectile
    dysfunction
pensions, 31
person-environment relations, 206–7
Petty, William, 56

phenomenology, 93
Phillipson, Chris, 82, 88
philosophical fieldwork, 92
Pinel, Philippe, 41
police and state bureaucracies, 54, 93
police science (or model), 57–59
political authority, 19, 55
political economy of aging, 88–89
political rationality, 122
Pollak, Otto, *Social Adjustment in Old Age*, 123
popular hygiene literature, 31
population, 16, 56–57. *See also* demography
    disciplinary ruling of, 54
    Foucault on, 53–54
    population *flows*, 209–10
Port Charlotte Cultural Center, 211
    counter space to surrounding commer-
        cial space, 221
    mutual aid society, 220
    volunteer pool, 218, 220
"Port Charlotte University," 220
Portrait of Old Age, The (Smith), 27
positive ageism, 163
positive aging, 19, 106–7, 178, 183, 199, 229. *See
    also* successful aging
    overlooking hardships, 193–95
positivism, 43–44
positivist/interpretive dualism, 141
post-retirement work, 147. *See also* employ-
    ment; retired worker
    advantages of, 149
post-traditional aging, 142, 144
postindustrial society, 188, 209
postmodern life course, 189–93, 209
postmodern timelessness, 18, 24, 191–92
postmodernism, 32–33, 94, 203, 226
postmortem evidence, 28
poverty, 45, 57, 191, 209
power, 53, 93, 141, 146
    disciplinary, 53–54
    liberal, 54
    procreative, 163, 166
    professional, 54
    senior, 220
practices of government, 58
practices of the self, 58, 146
privatization, 13, 99
problematization, 124, 137
    of adjustment, 124, 126–27, 132
    Foucault's use of, 123
    of older bodies, 136

Protestantism, 16–17
psychoanalytic theory, 50
psychology of aging, 79–80
psychology of impotence, 172–73

qualitative/quantitative dualism, 141
quality of life, 129
Quételet, Adolphe, 105
    *Treatise On Man and the Development of
        His Faculties*, 31, 103

Rabinow, Paul
    French Modern, 93
    Making PCR, 93
race, 43, 88, 125
radical theoretical traditions, 85
Ray, Ruth, 82–83
reflexivity, 141
rejuvenation, 168, 179, 192
    culture of, 167–68, 170
    pseudo-scientific experimentation, 168
    surgical, 168
Rembrandt Harmenszoon van Rijn, 108
Renaissance, 25–26
retired worker, 18, 140, 147–50
retirement, 16, 18, 31–32, 144. *See also* Third
    Age
    age, 150
    "exemplars of retirement," 18, 146–51
    market-driven planning for, 208
    new aging images of, 18
    post-retirement work, 147, 149
    "retirement ready," 137
retirement cultures, 85, 124
retirement lifestyles, 90
rhetoric, 39, 61, 77, 80
Riley, Matilda White, 37
risky populations. *See* problem groups
Rose, Nikolas, 55, 146
Rosen, George, 57
Rowles, Graham, 205
Rural Older Women's Project in Minnesota, 203

Saltpêtrière Hospital, 15, 40, 44, 47, 50
    medical knowledge, 41–42
    population, 44–45
    sexual politics of old age and hysteria,
        49
Scientific American, 192
scientific community, 25–26, 39, 192
scientific gerontology, 79–80

Scott, George Ridley, 179
"second chance," 148
self-care, 19, 140
self-help, 146, 152
self-improvement, 99, 137
Senescence (Hall), 98, 104–5, 126
senior centres, 207
senior citizenry, 127
    symbolic and cultural meaning, 191
senior citizens, 124, 194
sex, 27, 131
Sexual Debility in Man (Sturgis), 161
sexual decline, 171
    aging process, 164
    premature, 172
sexual dysfunction, 174. *See also* erectile dys-
    function
sexuality, 18, 177, 183
    female, 48
    Foucault on, 161–62
    male, 18, 83, 177
    medicalization, 163, 179
    repressed, 50
sexualization, 93
Shanas, Ethel, 37
Shenk, Dena, 203–4
Shock, Nathan, 92
Simmel, Georg, 142
    "Metropolis and Mental Life, The," 92
Simonton, Dean Keith, 105
Sinclair, John, *Code of Health and Longevity,
    The,* 28
Singer, Linda, 177
Smith, Adam, 55
Smith, John, *Portrait of Old Age, The,* 27
Snowbird culture, 19, 204, 211, 214, 221,
    224–26, 228–29
    bi-national identities, 223
    Canadian TV and newspapers, 222
    as "flow," 211
    medical resources, 222
    middle class, 222
social gerontology, 80, 96, 204, 229
social mobility, 140
social policy on aging, 53–68
social reproduction, 141
spatial gerontology, 19, 204–5, 229. *See also*
    elderscapes
Squier, Susan, 168
Stall, Sylvanus, *What a Man of Forty-Five
    Ought to Know,* 170

statistical knowledge, 57
Stearns, Peter, 48
Steinach, Eugen, 168, 170
"Steinach operation," 168
Steinem, Gloria, 37
Stekel, William, *Impotence in the Male,* 172
stereotyping, 32, 155, 171, 203. *See also* ageism
    in new market literature, 198
    sociological notions of, 124
Sturgis, F. R., *Sexual Debility in Man,* 161
subjectivity, 141
successful aging, 106, 129, 145, 149–51, 180. *See
    also* positive aging
    activity, 122
Sun Cities, 192, 208–9
    cultural critiques, 229
    developers, 18
Sunbelt culture, 211
surgical rejuvenation, 168

technologies of government, 146
technologization of male sexuality, 18. *See
    also* Viagra
television
    ageist stereotyping, 155
    watching, 131
telomere cellular shortening, 192
Third Age, 145, 151–52, 154–56, 158. *See also*
    retirement
    differentiation, 152–53
Third Agers, 18, 141
    as homogenous, prosperous market, 157
Thom, William J., 31
    Human Longevity, 30
Thompson, E. P.
    moral economy, 89
Tibbitts, Clark, 73, 81
timelessness, 24, 32–33, 189
Titian, 101–2, 109
    Early Modern perception of, 109–10,
        115–16
    late style, 112
Trollope, Anthony, 104
Troyansky, David, 24–25
Turner, Bryan, 191
Twigg, Julia, 98, 206

U₃As, 18, 141, 151, 153–55, 157
    central *vs.* local politics, 154
    commercial *vs. educational interests,* 156
    criticism, 158

denial of objective realities of aging, 156
United Kingdom, 59, 90, 151, 154
    aging society, 157
    cultural constructions of retirement, 203
    health promotion, 99
United States, 14, 47, 71, 90
    gerontology, 37
    HMOs (Health Management
        Organizations), 99
United States Senate Special Committee
    on Aging
    Developments in Aging, 61–63, 66, 68
Universities of The Third Age. See U₃As
urban sociology, 92
Urry, John, 210–11, 222

Vasari, Giorgio, 113, 115
    Lives of the Most Famous Painters, Sculptors
        and Architects, 109
    on Michelangelo, 114
Veronoff, Serge, 168
Viagra, 18, 163, 180, 183
    ever younger market, 182
    iconic status, 181
    reconceptualization of sexuality, 192
Viagra revolution, 18, 163, 174
visual gerontology, 41–42, 203
vitality, 32, 171

Walker, Alan, 74–75, 88
Warthin, Alfred Scott, Old Age, 167
Weber, Marianne, 91
Weber, Max, 54, 91–92, 142
    "spirit of capitalism," 16
welfare, 124. See also social services
welfare state, 88, 140
Wernick, Andrew, 34
wisdom, 195
women
    abuse, 39
    advice literature, 16
    bodies of, 49–50
    Charcot's Older Women, 15, 37–50
    misrepresented by gerontology and
        geriatrics, 49
    post-menopausal, 48
women's studies, 38
    connections with aging studies, 39–40,
        49
Woods Hole Conference, 78
Woodward, Kathleen, 13, 17, 32, 39, 50–51, 90

Young, Michael, 153, 156
youth, 17, 24, 46